Medicine in Society

Medicine in Society

BEHAVIOURAL SCIENCES FOR MEDICAL STUDENTS

Edited by

Christopher Dowrick

*Professor of Primary Medical Care,
The University of Liverpool, Liverpool, UK*

A member of the Hodder Headline Group
LONDON • NEW YORK • NEW DELHI

First published in Great Britain in 2001 by
Arnold, a member of the Hodder Headline Group,
338 Euston Road, London NW1 3BH

http://www.arnoldpublishers.com

Distributed in the USA by
Oxford University Press Inc.,
198 Madison Avenue, New York, NY10016
Oxford is a registered trademark of Oxford University Press

Whilst the advice and information in this book are believed to be true and
accurate at the date of going to press, neither the authors nor the publisher
can accept any legal responsibility or liability for any errors or omissions
that may be made. In particular (but without limiting the generality of the
preceding disclaimer) every effort has been made to check drug dosages;
however, it is still possible that errors have been missed. Furthermore,
dosage schedules are constantly being revised and new side-effects
recognized. For these reasons the reader is strongly urged to consult the
drug companies' printed instructions before administering any of the drugs
recommended in this book.

British Library Cataloguing in Publication Data
A catalogue record for this book is available from the British Library

Library of Congress Cataloging-in-Publication Data
A catalog record for this book is available from the Library of Congress

ISBN 0 340 76027 3

1 2 3 4 5 6 7 8 9 10

Commissioning Editor: Georgina Bentliff
Development Editor: Tim Wale
Production Editor: Wendy Rooke
Production Controller: Martin Kerans

Typeset in 10 on 12 pt Palatino by Cambrian Typesetters, Frimley, Surrey
Printed and bound in Great Britain by MPG Books, Bodmin, Cornwall

What do you think about this book? Or any other Arnold title?
Please send your comments to feedback.arnold@hodder.co.uk

Contents

Preface

Christopher Dowrick

Medical education is experiencing a process of rapid evolution. It remains essential for doctors to understand human structure and function through the study of subjects such as anatomy, biochemistry and physiology. However, we now realize that it is also important for tomorrow's doctors to acquire knowledge about how individuals operate within groups and societies, and to develop ethical perspectives on their patients and on clinical practice. This textbook is designed to meet these new educational needs.

Our intention is to provide a clear and comprehensive introduction to the group of subjects that are collectively known as the *behavioural sciences*.

Behavioural sciences concentrate on the context within which illness and disease occur, and the interactions that take place between patients and health professionals. In general terms, they are concerned with the relationships between individuals and the groups and societies within which they function. They include perspectives drawn from ethics, sociology, psychology, epidemiology, health economics and public administration.

We offer medical students, for the first time, a framework for understanding all of these behavioural sciences within one readable volume. We describe the theoretical bases of these subjects, explain the key concepts which we think it is important for you to know about, and link these concepts to clinical situations and experiences that you are likely to encounter during your training.

We begin by introducing you to the key issues in health care ethics. We then consider sociological perspectives – first a broad approach to the social determinants of health and disease, and then a more specific focus on the interactions between patients and their carers (including both family and professionals). We describe the principles and application of epidemiology (the study of disease in populations), and follow with two linked chapters on psychology, first setting out the theoretical bases of the subjects, and then demonstrating the relevance of psychology to our understanding of health and illness. The latter part of the book is concerned with recent perspectives on behavioural sciences, including health economics and health promotion. Finally, we explore the complex interactions between health and social care, and we consider how and why health systems are likely to change in the future.

Although it is written primarily with the needs of medical students in mind, this textbook should be of considerable relevance to students of dentistry, nursing and the allied health professions.

List of Contributors

Christopher Dowrick Professor of Primary Medical Care, Department of Primary Care, The University of Liverpool, Liverpool, UK

Stephen Abbott Senior Research Fellow, Health and Community Care Research Unit, The University of Liverpool, Liverpool, UK

Alan Beattie Professor of Health Promotion, The University College of St Martin, Lancaster, UK

Peter Bundred Reader in Primary Care, Department of Primary Care, The University of Liverpool, Liverpool, UK

Christine Bundy Lecturer in Health Psychology, Medical School, University of Manchester, Manchester, UK

Simon Capewell Professor of Clinical Epidemiology, Department of Public Health, The University of Liverpool, Liverpool, UK

Lucy Frith Lecturer in Health Care Ethics, Department of Primary Care, The University of Liverpool, Liverpool, UK

Tony Hak Senior Lecturer in Methodology, Department of Methodology, Rotterdam School of Management, Erasmus University, Rotterdam, The Netherlands

Cynthia Iglesias Research Fellow, Department of Health Studies and Centre for Health Economics, The University of York, York, UK

Ann Jacoby Professor of Medical Sociology, Department of Primary Care, The University of Liverpool, Liverpool, UK

Elizabeth Perkins Director of the Health and Community Care Research Unit, The University of Liverpool, Liverpool, UK

Mary Jane Platt Senior Lecturer (Clinical), Department of Public Health, The University of Liverpool, Liverpool, UK

David Torgerson Reader, Department of Health Studies and Centre for Health Economics, University of York, York, UK

Introduction

1

Christopher Dowrick

Behavioural sciences and medicine
Becoming a doctor
The structure of this book

Behavioural sciences and medicine

The study of human beings can be considered from a vast range of perspectives. From the perspective of the subjects that are collectively known as the natural sciences, for example, humans are composed of elementary subatomic particles which unite in various complicated ways to form molecules and cells, and which grow, mutate and die as a result of chemical processes and reactions. Cells may be combined to form organs and whole organisms, which have discrete and describable structures and function in specific ways.

From the perspective of the humanities, we are people situated within a particular culture and history, and past events and experiences have shaped our understanding of the present. We engage in particular methods of allocating power and resources and settling disputes. We have the ability both to destroy and to create, and we have a need or desire to find meaning, understanding and coherence in the world in which we find ourselves.

All of these perspectives are legitimate, and they provide us with essential insight into and understanding of ourselves. No one viewpoint is more accurate than any other. Each is simply considering and describing different aspects of the human self.

Modern medicine takes a wider view of health and illness than it has done in the past, now including both behavioural and physical perspectives. In terms of Table 1.1, it includes all of the perspectives from Level 2 (cells and chemical reactions) to Level 5 (members of groups).

The behavioural sciences, and hence this textbook, are mainly concerned with Levels 4 and 5. The behavioural sciences refer to those aspects of undergraduate medical education which are distinct from the natural sciences, such as anatomy, physiology and biochemistry, and which are best understood within a psychosocial rather than a biomedical paradigm. Behavioural sciences concentrate on the context within which illness and disease occur, and the interactions that take place between patients and health professionals. In general terms, they are concerned with *the interface between the individual and society*. They involve an appreciation of the following:

Table 1.1 Some methods of studying human beings

Perspective	Objects	Disciplines
Natural sciences	1. Subatomic particles	Nuclear physics
	2. Cells and chemical reactions	Molecular biology
		Biochemistry
	3. Organism: structure and function	Anatomy
		Physiology
Behavioural sciences	4. Individuals	Ethics
		Psychology
		Sociology (interpersonal)
		Health care use
	5. Members of groups	Sociology (community)
		Epidemiology
		Health care delivery
Humanities	6. Broader contexts	History
		Politics
		Art and literature
		Theology

- the role and significance of systems of morality and ethics;
- social processes, at the levels of both individuals and populations;
- psychological theories of behaviour, and of health and illness;
- patterns of health and disease (epidemiology);
- how health care is used and organized;
- the relevance of economic considerations for health and health care.

The behavioural sciences do not concern themselves directly with a detailed understanding of physical structure and function, in terms of how human bodies are arranged at an anatomical or cellular level, or with a biochemical or physiological understanding of normal and pathological physical functions. Those areas are the territory of subjects such as anatomy and physiology, biochemistry and pharmacology. They fall within Levels 2 and 3 of Table 1.1, and until recently comprised the overwhelming majority of medical undergraduate studies.

This does not mean that students of medicine and the other health professions can safely ignore the perspectives of subatomic physics, or of the humanities. It is rather a question of emphasis and focus.

It is not usually necessary for medical students to have or to acquire a detailed knowledge of subatomic particles or nuclear physics. However, these subjects are important in that they enable greater understanding of certain aspects of medicine, such as investigation by chest X-ray or nuclear magnetic resonance scan, and treatments such as radioactive iodine for thyrotoxicosis. They also enable one to appreciate the devastating medical consequences of nuclear accidents and the destructive potential of modern warfare.

At the other end of the spectrum, medical students are not usually expected to become proficient in history, politics, art, literature or theology. However, you would probably wish to become aware that each of these can have a major impact on our understanding of diseases and how we manage them.

For example, politics in the UK has a major impact on the level of spending on health care. Through the tax and benefit systems, and through the ways in which the economy and investments are managed, it can have a significant effect on the way in which wealth is distributed within society. As you will see in Chapter 3, this in turn has a marked effect on patterns of health and illness. Political violence, whether local, national or global, is a major cause of death and illness worldwide. Warfare often also leads to a breakdown of civil order, and a consequent increase in infectious diseases and forced migrations.

History has greatly affected our perceptions of illness and health. For example, homosexuality has in various times and places been considered a sin, a normal human experience, or an illness requiring medical attention. In sixteenth-century England, sneezing was considered to be an indication of demon possession, although today we are more likely to regard it as a sign of hay fever or an upper respiratory tract infection. The history of medicine is an important topic in its own right, and one which is now part of the syllabus in certain undergraduate medical courses.

Art and literature are crucial to many people's enjoyment of life, and are often the means whereby we can express ourselves creatively. Studying art and literature enhances our understanding and interpretation of human beings, and may also enable us to find out more about ourselves. The study of languages and linguistics is relevant to our understanding of communication skills. Several medical schools do now run literature courses as part of their undergraduate training programme.

Religious beliefs can have a major effect on attitudes to communication and on relationships between doctors and patients, and there is increasing evidence of their impact on the outcome of serious diseases, including cancer. From a religious perspective, hearing voices and speaking in tongues may be signs of spiritual ecstasy, whereas a psychiatrist would be more inclined to regard them as signs of a severe mental illness. Belief in life after death, in its various forms, can have a profound effect on our patients' attitudes to death and dying.

It should by now be clear that it is no longer possible for medical students to content themselves with learning only about the structure and function of the human body, how it should work, what goes wrong when people get ill, and what are the best ways of preventing, curing or managing the diseases that do occur. Although these remain central to good medical practice, they are not sufficient in themselves to provide the range of experience that is necessary for tomorrow's doctors. This view is now fully supported by the General Medical Council, the governing body of medicine in the UK. In a document on medical training, entitled *Tomorrow's Doctors* (General Medical Council, 1993), the General Medical Council affirms the continued importance of acquiring knowledge of human structure and function. In addition, it places new emphasis on the acquisition of knowledge, skills and attitudes in the following three broad areas:

- individuals, groups and societies;
- communications and consultation skills;
- ethical perspectives both on patients and on clinical practice.

This textbook will provide you with a thorough coverage of the first and third of these areas. It will also give you the basis for understanding the relevance and importance of good communication and consultation techniques, although these are skills which can really only be acquired through direct training and regular clinical practice.

Becoming a doctor

As a first approach to exploring the relevance of the behavioural sciences to medical students, and to students in the allied health professions, let us look at what these perspectives can tell us about a subject which is of direct relevance to the primary readership of this book – that is, to you personally. What can the behavioural sciences tell you about the process in which you are currently engaged, namely that of becoming a doctor?

One of the most obvious points about becoming a doctor is that you are entering a *profession* which is generally held in high regard by society and which, despite the need for rigorous training and continued hard work, is likely to reward you well in terms of both finance and prestige.

What can *sociologists* tell you about what it means to be entering a profession? If you consider groups such as doctors, lawyers or teachers, one way of understanding this concept is to view a profession as having a definable set of knowledge and skills which are used on an altruistic basis, with a commitment to provide services for the welfare of society in general, or for the common good. This may be contrasted with someone who sets up in business as, say, a street trader or a computer analyst, whose primary concern may be personal gain in terms of finance, promotion or prestige. In this sense the professions may be regarded as close to the more old-fashioned concepts of vocation or calling, although nowadays the religious connotations of these terms would not be universally acceptable.

Greenwood (1957) developed a list of five qualities considered to be necessary if an occupation is to be regarded as a profession:

- systematic theory;
- authority recognized by its clientele;
- broader community sanction;
- a code of ethics;
- professional culture sustained by formal professional sanctions.

Medicine has all of these qualities. It has a theoretical basis (although one which, as this book will show you, is not as simple or one-dimensional as we used to believe). Its authority is recognized both by the patients who choose to consult doctors, and by the governments who seek and accept the collective advice of the British Medical Association (BMA) or the Royal Colleges. It can only be practised by suitably qualified people. It is governed by codes of ethics, of which the Hippocratic Oath and the World Medical Association Declaration of Geneva are the most well known, and it has formal internal sanctions for dealing with those of its members who do not behave according to the standards which it lays down for itself (see Chapter 11).

There are also other more critical ways of understanding the professions. These emphasize the concept of *autonomy*, and view membership of a profession as primarily a means of exercising power and control over others. From this perspective, the British Medical Association can be regarded as one of the most successful trade unions in recent British history. Winston Churchill, when he was Prime Minister in the early 1950s, recommended to his ministers that there were three powerful institutions which they should avoid confronting whenever possible. These were the Brigade of Guards, the National Union of Mineworkers and the British Medical Association. However, today, if we take this less altruistic view of medicine, then it would appear that the dominance of the medical profession may be under threat from several quarters. Other health professionals, especially nurses, are rapidly developing a corpus of skills, knowledge and attitudes which are independent of, and often of equal status to, that of doctors. The National Health Service is increasingly influenced by government guidelines and by health managers, both of which tend to influence and limit the extent to which doctors can act independently. The increasing emphasis on patient autonomy and on consumer involvement in decision-making, at both individual and collective levels, means that doctors have to view themselves as partners in decision-making, rather than as the dispensers of wisdom as in the past.

Doctors in the UK continue to receive high incomes compared with society as a whole. This can be explained to a large extent by *health economics*, in terms of the strict rationing and restrictions which stand in the way of successful entry to medical school. It stands in contrast to the situation in southern Europe, for example, where there are many more places available on undergraduate medical courses, and it is much easier to undertake medical training. However, as a result of that situation there are more young doctors qualifying than there are jobs available. In this situation of supply exceeding demand, medical unemployment is much higher, and salaries and incomes are much lower, than is the case in the UK or the USA.

The term *professionalization* refers to the methods by which new recruits are assimilated within an existing professional culture. For previous generations of medical students – the 'boys in white coats' – this involved a gradual process of indoctrination into the closed world of hospitals, which were mainly inhabited by Caucasian men from affluent backgrounds. Knowledge was acquired by exposure to large tracts of factual information, which was presented didactically in lecture theatres, to be uncritically absorbed for later repetition in formal written and oral examinations. The acquisition of skills involved gradual acclimatization to the rudiments of human anatomy and pathology, with the initiation ceremonies of the pre-clinical dissecting rooms at its heart. Attitudes of superiority to patients and nurses were created by the practice of talking from a standing position (vertical) to patients lying in bed (horizontal), and by the habits of deference inculcated among nurses. Among doctors, awareness of the power structures and hierarchy within medicine was enhanced through the ritual testing and humiliation of students and junior doctors by their superiors during teaching ward rounds (Allen, 1994).

Over the past 20 years or so there has been something akin to a revolution in all of these processes of professionalization. The knowledge base of medicine has expanded enormously (hence the need for this textbook!), and the ways in which such knowledge may be acquired have changed, if anything even more dramatically. The emphasis of medical education is now on learning rather than on teaching, with the autonomous, self-directed student at the heart of the process. The emphasis is now on students' own ability – whether individually or, more commonly, as members of small working groups – to generate their own awareness of clinical problems and find their own solutions. Instead of a fully organized and structured curriculum, there may now be a core curriculum, which every student is expected to master, and then a substantial proportion of optional activities which allow the individual to develop his or her own particular interests and skills. This should, if successful, produce a new generation of doctors who are both more self-confident and more self-critical than their predecessors.

Clinical experience, which was previously entirely hospital based, is now as likely to be gained in community-based settings, usually primary care, since an increasing proportion of health care is experienced and delivered in the community rather than in hospital settings. Instead of a doctor-centred universe, medical students now find that health care is multidisciplinary in focus. They are expected to become aware of the necessity of effective teamwork, and the vital and complementary roles played by nurses, physiotherapists, occupational therapists and social workers in providing comprehensive health care for patients.

Medical students themselves have also changed considerably. No longer are the majority of entrants to medical school 18-year-old Caucasian young men from comfortable socio-economic backgrounds, educated at boarding or grammar schools, with A-levels in physics, chemistry and biology. The biggest change is in gender, with most medical schools in the UK now admitting a small majority of women each year. The proportion of medical students from minority ethnic backgrounds is increasing and so too – although more slowly – are the numbers from working-class families. The numbers of mature entrants are increasing. Moreover, a much wider range of previous educational experience is now considered to be acceptable by admissions tutors, including A-levels in humanities subjects such as English or history, which is a reflection of the widening nature of medical curricula.

These changes in the nature, background and experiences of medical students themselves are likely to have an enormous influence on all aspects of medical practice in ways which are as yet largely unpredictable. For example, the high proportion of women entrants is likely to have a beneficial effect on styles and skills in communication and consultations between doctors and patients. Students from a variety of ethnic backgrounds bring with them differing experiences and definitions of health and disease. Working patterns for junior doctors will have to be amended even further, to ensure that the needs of the profession are complementary to rather than in conflict with the needs of young parents who wish to start and raise families.

The *psychological* effects of being a medical student should not be underestimated. Most people find the experience generally enjoyable and fulfilling. However, there are particular stresses associated with being a medical student, in addition to the usual academic pressures of deadlines and examinations. Many students begin medical training with very high expectations of themselves, which have been generated by their families, their schools or themselves. This, allied to the awareness of entering a 'high-status' profession, can lead to the generation of significant internal pressure. Many students have concerns about the likelihood and consequences of failure, and the stigma that this might cause themselves and their families. One recent study found that over half of a new intake of medical students were very stressed at the beginning of their first term, although by the end of the summer term this proportion had decreased to one-third (Miller, 1994). Later in the course, when more time is spent in direct contact with patients and doctors, the sources of stress may be different. Many students find that talking with terminally ill patients, and relationships with consultant colleagues, are aspects of their work which are often particularly difficult to manage (Firth-Cozens, 1986).

The new curricula, with their emphasis on self-directed learning and early exposure to clinical material, should produce more reflective and creative doctors. However, they may also generate new and different stresses among medical students. Direct contact with patients who are in pain or suffering, many of whom may die, may be more difficult to handle at the age of 18 than at the age of 20 or 21 years. The new methods of learning may be experienced as threatening and confusing, as a result of the considerable increase in both uncertainty and responsibility compared to teaching methods on more traditional medical curricula.

Although most students cope well most of the time with the stresses that they encounter, sometimes they resort to stress-relieving methods which are less than beneficial in the long term. A study by Ashton and Kamali (1995) found that one-quarter of medical students were drinking alcohol at levels higher than the recommended low-risk levels, and that there was a 10% increase in self-reported alcohol and illicit drug use among medical students over the previous 10 years. Such patterns, once established, tend to carry on into medical careers, and doctors are at a higher risk than most other occupational groups of developing alcohol problems.

There are better ways of dealing with stress, and a number of suggestions are listed here.

- Perhaps the most important method is to ensure that you have good *support networks*, and that you are happy to use them whenever there is something about which you are worried or concerned. Family and friends are the first port of call for most people, but if this seems difficult, or the problems appear to be more complex, then all medical schools have facilities whereby students have access to personal tutors who are there to provide help on a confidential basis. There should also be easy access to counselling services, either directly or through your general practitioner.

- With regard to your work itself, it is very useful to learn to *prioritise* – to decide what is the most important or urgent task in front of you, and then to delay, delegate or even drop other tasks that are not so vital.
- It is also essential to remember that there is much more to life than studying medicine. Build *enjoyable activities* into your regular routines. These will be personal to you, but might for example include socializing, sport or music. Good mental health requires a balance of achievement and pleasure. Medical students and doctors are generally very good at achieving things, but we are often much less effective at enjoying ourselves. *Carpe diem. . . .*

The structure of this book

This book has 10 main chapters. The next six chapters concentrate on the more theoretical aspects of the behavioural sciences. We begin with the study of medical ethics, since we believe that ethical and moral principles are fundamental to all of our thinking about medicine and health care. The next two chapters consider sociological issues, first in terms of the broad social determinants of health and illness, and then in terms of the ways in which relationships between carers (including doctors) and patients are constructed. We describe the principles and application of epidemiology, and then move on to two linked chapters on psychology. The first of these describes and explains the major theoretical issues in psychology, while the second looks specifically at the ways in which psychology can help us to understand health.

The second part of the book focuses on more recent developments within the behavioural sciences. We first consider the increasingly important field of health economics, and explain some of the different concepts and models which enable us to appreciate how health care may best be delivered. Health promotion is an essential but often neglected part of high-quality medical practice, and we describe the current major approaches in this field. There is growing awareness of the crucial relationship between health and social care, and we place this in its historical and political context. Finally, we consider how health systems are currently operating, where the stresses and strains occur, and how health systems might best be developed in the future.

Each chapter has the same basic structure, which can be summarized as follows.

- It defines the topic.
- It introduces and explains the most important concepts within the topic.
- It provides examples of how these concepts relate to clinical practice.
- It provides discussion points, to encourage reflection and critical thinking.
- It provides a brief list of texts for further reading.

Several chapters also have a *key text* section in which we describe a seminal article, book or report, and explain why it is so important and relevant to modern health care.

All of the chapters are self-sufficient. They can be read in any order you wish. Some topics, such as the aetiology and management of coronary artery disease, and the concept of 'quality of life', are sufficiently important to merit discussion in more than one chapter. You can see where we have done this, either through our cross-referencing in the text, or else via the index. For ease of access, the references cited within each chapter have been collected together at the end of the book.

Medical ethics

Lucy Frith

Introduction

This chapter is an introduction to the subject of medical ethics and will cover the main areas that are essential to a basic understanding of the subject. The chapter will begin by considering why medical students and health care practitioners should study ethics. It will then give a broad definition of ethics and examine the main ethical principles and theories associated with medical ethics for practitioners, namely the four principles, utilitarianism and Kantianism. The more practical issues of consent and confidentiality will subsequently be examined, and the chapter will conclude with a look at some of the ethical dilemmas that could be encountered during medical training.

Why study ethics?

Both professionals and the general public are increasingly aware of the ethical dilemmas that are raised by medicine. The General Medical Council (GMC) report on undergraduate education, *Tomorrow's Doctors* (General Medical Council, 1993), recommended that ethics and law should be included as part of the core curriculum, and postgraduate courses in ethics have flourished in the last 10 years. There is an increasing awareness that there is an ethical dimension to all clinical decisions and that a good clinician is an ethical one.

In *Duties of a Doctor* (General Medical Council, 1995), the GMC set out the basic principles of good medical practice. Many of these principles, such as respect for the patient's views, respect for human life and the right of the patient to be fully involved in decision-making, are ethical principles. *Duties of a Doctor* considers the observance of ethical principles to be a crucial aspect of good medical practice and not merely something subsidiary to clinical factors.

It is necessary to substantiate the above claim that there is an ethical dimension to all clinical decisions and that a good clinician is an ethical one. The fundamental aim of medicine is to promote health in order to enable people to live fulfilled lives. The choice of this aim is an ethical decision based on notions of helping and caring for others in times of physical and mental distress. Professions can be viewed as inherently ethical practices. Medicine seeks to provide a genuine good to its patients, and what constitutes this good is an ethical decision. A genuine good in this context is something we want for its own sake (e.g. health, justice), as opposed to something that we want as a way of acquiring other things (e.g. wealth). By fulfilling one's professional obligations as a doctor, one is already engaged in the pursuit of an ethical goal. Clinical procedures are the means by which we fulfil certain goals, not the goals themselves (which might include a return to health, increased autonomy, etc.), and these goals are determined by ethical criteria.

The appropriate course of action is often conceived in terms of what is the clinically acceptable thing to do – the clinical demands of the situation. However, since the decision concerns another human being, what is appropriate for that individual is almost always a value judgement.

To illustrate this, consider the following case study.

Case study

A woman decides that she wishes to have a home birth, and the general practitioner (GP) readily agrees to this. However, after a routine antenatal visit at 35 weeks it becomes apparent that the baby is in the breech position. After the ultrasound scan it is determined that the baby is a good size for the number of weeks and is unlikely to move. The GP now advises the woman that the home birth might not be such a good idea. However, the woman is reluctant to accept the doctor's advice, stating that breech births used to be routinely delivered at home, and she insists on a home birth. What should the doctor do?

There are two elements in the doctor's assessment of this situation – the clinical element and the ethical one. The breech presentation indicates risk factors that might be better managed in a hospital. These are clinical reasons. However, these have to be weighed against the woman's autonomous decision to direct her care. This is an ethical consideration. The doctor has to consider both respecting the woman's autonomy and trying to promote beneficence for her and the baby. In this decision the clinical and the ethical aspects are interwoven, and in reaching a solution both of these factors will come into play.

As a doctor you will be involved in people's lives in a fundamental and important way, at times of birth, death and terminal illness, as well as during more mundane health care problems. Patients will often be vulnerable due to sickness, worry, inability to work, etc., and how you approach and treat people at these times can make a profound difference to them. As your work is so vital to individuals' welfare, it is important to recognize that not everyone has the same views, values and priorities. Having the ability to clarify and justify your own values will make it easier to understand and analyse other people's views. This understanding makes us aware that not everyone will share the same belief system, and that we should not impose our own values, however unwittingly, on others.

Summary

* Ethics is a core part of the medical curriculum.
* There is an ethical dimension to all clinical decisions.
* The study of ethics can aid our understanding of our own and others' beliefs and values.

What is ethics?

Very broadly, ethics can be defined as the study of the moral aspects of our lives, and it covers a wide range of theoretical and practical areas. Ethics can be divided into three branches – normative, practical and descriptive ethics.

Normative ethics

This is concerned with establishing norms of conduct and developing ethical theories or principles that can govern decision-making and practice. 'Which general norms for the guidance and evaluation of conduct are worthy of moral acceptance and for what reasons?' (Beauchamp and Childress, 1994: 4). For example, this area of ethics would be concerned with examining moral theories to see whether they provide a satisfactory theoretical framework, and considering how acceptable they are as a guide to our actions. In this respect it is not possible to draw a sharp distinction between normative and practical ethics.

Practical ethics

This is the attempt to apply moral theories to practical problems and to reach some conclusions about the morality of a particular situation. For example, if you were faced with the choice of telling a lie to protect one of your friends or telling the truth and them getting into trouble, you could consider how different moral theories might approach such a dilemma and what answer would be produced by applying that theory to this specific situation.

Descriptive ethics

This is a factual investigation of people's moral behaviour and beliefs. For example, a research project was conducted on public attitudes to the ethical acceptability of the reproductive technology *in-vitro* fertilization (IVF). The respondents were asked questions such as whether IVF should be funded from the public purse and how important they considered the problem of infertility to be. This type of research surveys how people feel about moral issues, and it can be useful as a basis for shaping public policy and the medical professions' responses to moral problems.

The main task of studying ethics in a medical context is to be able to understand various normative approaches to medical ethics and to be able to apply these to practical situations and reach a considered and justifiable solution to a particular problem.

Summary

- Ethics can be divided into three branches.
- Normative ethics (ethical theories) can be applied to practical ethical dilemmas in order to reach a considered and justifiable solution to a particular problem.

The four principles of health care ethics

These are as follows:

- autonomy;
- beneficence;
- non-maleficence;
- justice.

In the area of medicine the four principles of health care have become very popular as one particular normative approach to solving ethical dilemmas. The four principles approach, as it has been called, is defended by such authors as Gillon (1986) and Beauchamp and Childress (1994). This approach sets out four principles, namely respect for autonomy, beneficence, minimizing harm and ensuring justice, which can be applied to ethical dilemmas in an attempt to determine what is the right course of action.

Autonomy

The word is derived from the Greek *autos* (self) and *nomos* (rule, governance or law), meaning essentially 'rule of the self'. Autonomy is the doctrine that the individual human will is or ought to be governed by its own principles and laws, and it is closely related to concepts of self-determination and personal freedom. For someone to act autonomously they should be free from limitations that prevent meaningful choice, such as lack of information, and also free from the controlling influences of others. The most concrete way in which patient autonomy is respected in medical practice is by obtaining consent for medical procedures. This encapsulates the belief that it is the patient who should ultimately make the choice as to what procedures to undergo, without undue coercion or influence by the medical practitioner.

Most theories of autonomy incorporate two elements:

1. liberty – freedom from external control or influence;
2. agency – the assumption of a capacity for independent action and the intention to act in a certain way (Beauchamp and Childress, 1994).

It is often not possible in the real world of medicine for people to act in a fully autonomous way. There will always be certain controlling influences on us (e.g. family and finance), and patients may not always have a full and complete understanding of their treatment. What we should be aiming for is substantial autonomy – that is, a degree of understanding and freedom from overt controlling influences, enabling patients to make meaningful decisions about their care (Harris, 1985). For example, a patient, due to lack of medical training, may not be able to understand every aspect and nuance of the treatment they are going to receive, but they can understand the overall risks, side-effects and prognosis of the treatment and thus make a substantially autonomous decision as to whether to go ahead with it.

Beneficence

Beneficence is the act of doing good. It is a stronger word than benevolence (wishing good), since it assumes action. It includes preventing harm, removing harm and actively promoting good. 'The *principle of beneficence* refers to a moral obligation to act for the benefit of others' (Beauchamp and Childress, 1994: 260). Thus it covers all possible aspects of medical activity, from disease prevention, through cancer surgery to advanced pharmacotherapeutics. Health care professionals have an actual duty to do good for their patients, which is often expressed as a duty of care and describes the special relationship that doctors have with their patients. In our personal lives we are under no obligation to act as good Samaritans to others, but simply to refrain from harming them, whereas to those with whom we are in some form of special relationship (e.g. parent and child) we have similar obligations of beneficence.

Non-maleficence

The duty to minimize harm, or non-maleficence, is historically rendered in the Latin phrase *primum non nocere*, or 'first do no harm'. The principle of non-maleficence is often seen as the other side of the beneficence coin and, as Gillon points out, the two principles are closely related, as doing good often implies not harming. When considering non-maleficence it is important to have some notion of what we mean by harm, and this is a difficult concept to pin down. Many health care interventions involve pain and discomfort but, as Gillon says, 'The traditional Hippocratic moral obligation of medicine is to provide net medical benefit to patients with minimal harm – that is, benefi- cence with non-maleficence.' (Gillon, 1986: 185).

One doctrine that is associated with the principles of beneficence and non- maleficence is *paternalism*. It is often stated that traditionally medical practice was paternalistic in nature, operating under the adage that the doctor knew best. The *Oxford English Dictionary* defines paternalism as 'the principle and practice of paternal administration; government as by a father; the claim or attempt to supply the needs or to regulate the life of a community in the way a father does of his children.' Medical paternalism essentially involves the doctor adopting the role of father. With superior knowledge and training the doctor is in a better position to decide what is in the best interests of the patient. As Beauchamp and Childress state, 'Paternalism, then, is the inten- tional overriding of one person's known preferences or actions by another person, where the person who overrides justifies the action by the goal of benefiting or avoiding harm to the person whose will is overridden.' (Beauchamp and Childress, 1994: 274). The key elements of paternalism are that the person's decision and or/action is overridden, and that this is done on the grounds that it is for their own good. For example, a very nervous and unstable patient comes to see their doctor for the results of a biopsy. The results indicate a carcinoma, but the doctor decides – on the grounds of doing no harm to the patient – to act paternalistically and not tell the truth about the results. The patient is being protected from the truth as, in the doctor's view, this is in their best interests.

Justice

Justice is broadly fair, equitable and appropriate treatment. It implies free- dom from discrimination or dishonesty and impartiality. It is often restated as 'distributive justice' or the determination of rights, and it stipulates that the benefits and burdens of society should be distributed fairly in accor- dance with a particular conception of what are considered to be similarly deserving cases. This is the formal principle of justice – that equals should be treated equally. The difficult question here is how equality should be defined. Should it mean equal wealth, equal intelligence, equal need or equal deservingness? In health care, equal intelligence does not seem to be a just way of distributing health care resources, but an argument can be made that it is a just way of distributing places at universities. Equal need appears to be a better definition of equality on which to base the just distri- bution of health care resources, but this approach is not without problems, as a person may greatly need health care but it would not prolong their life, or they might not 'deserve it' due to having contributed to their own ill health. In modern health care, principles of justice are particularly relevant. For example, when considering how limited resources should be deployed, should money be spent on coronary artery bypass grafting or on the management of incontinence?

Here is a simple example of the application of the four principles of health care approach to ethics.

Case study

A patient comes into the surgery, violent and angry, shouting at the staff and those in the waiting-room and threatening to harm himself. This patient has a history of self-harm and at times this abuse has nearly proved fatal. The doctor attempts to calm the patient, but he says that he wants to be allowed to leave and that he will try to kill himself when he gets home. What should the general practitioner do?

If the GP thinks that respecting the patient's autonomy is the most important principle, then she will decide that the best course of action is to let him leave, as he wishes to do. However, allowing the patient to leave conflicts with the doctor's duty to act beneficently towards the patient – that is, to take the course of action that would do the greatest good for him. It could be argued that the patient should be restrained and protected from harming himself. The GP might also want to consider the principle of justice and determine which course of action would involve the most efficient use of resources. She might reason that it would be unjust to allow the patient to go home, as a subsequent episode of self-harm would require the emergency services and the casualty department. By giving the patient medication in the surgery, despite his wishes, she would be taking into account the needs of future patients who might need the emergency services.

This illustrates the fact that the main difficulty with applying the four principles in practice is deciding what course of action we should take if two or more of the principles conflict. What should we do if doing good for a patient involves restricting his autonomy? Which principle should take precedence? In this situation, using the four principles approach, the GP would have to weigh respect for the patient's autonomy (by allowing him to go home) against trying to promote beneficence for the patient (by instigating some form of restraint).

This is often seen as the main criticism of the four principles approach, namely that it gives no guidance on how to act when two or more of the principles conflict. The four principles are only prima facie obligations – that is, the obligations must be followed unless they conflict with another obligation that is equal or stronger – giving us no clear guidance as to which principle should take precedence. This requires us to think about the relative weight of the principles, and there is no easy way of establishing which is the most important principle to follow in a particular case. It is often argued that patient autonomy should take precedence, as freedom of action is regarded as an unqualified good in our society, and any measures that limit people's freedom are viewed as unwarranted. Consequently, there has been a move away from paternalism in medicine, which limits the patient's autonomy for their own good. This is reflected in the increasing concern to ensure that patients give their informed consent to treatments, and patient-centred care is becoming a key principle in modern medical practice. However, some argue that we have swung too far the other way in allowing such unfettered patient autonomy, and that this threatens doctors' ability to do the best for their patients. Despite the questions that the four principles approach leaves unanswered, the approach can indicate elements that should be brought to bear on a situation and hence can provide broad guidance, if not definitive answers, with regard to ethical dilemmas.

Summary

- There are four principles of health care ethics.
- These principles are prima facie obligations, to be followed unless they conflict with another principle.
- This approach does not give us guidance on which principle should take precedence, but it does indicate which elements should be brought to bear on a particular situation

Moral theory

Moral theories are frequently used in medical ethics to provide a framework within which practitioners can evaluate the acceptability of moral actions and judgements. Moral theories are again part of the normative approach to ethics – they attempt to tell us what we should do and give us guidance with regard to what actions are acceptable. There are various components to moral situations, including the agent, the action, the means, the ends (the consequences, the intentions and motives of the person acting, and the side-effects) and so on. The two most frequently used moral theories in medical ethics are utilitarianism and Kantian ethics. Utilitarianism concentrates on the consequences of action, whereas Kantian ethics concentrates on the intentions and actions of the agent.

In utilitarianism:

- the consequences of an action are the only morally important aspect;
- utilitarians determine what is right by examining the particular situation;
- the aim is the greatest happiness for the greatest number;
- the ends justify the means.

In Kantian ethics:

- the intention of the agent and the action itself are the most important aspects;
- Kantianism is a rule-based morality;
- one should act according to the categorical imperatives:
  (i) only act on those maxims which you can will to become universal laws;
  (ii) act so that you always treat humanity, whether in your own person or that of any other, as an end, never as a means.

Utilitarianism

Utilitarianism is concerned with the consequences of an action, which is judged to be right or wrong depending on the good or bad consequences it produces. When thinking about a particular action (e.g. whether you should lie to your friend and tell her she looks good in her new dress), you should consider what action produces the best consequences. Thus in this example you might decide that lying to your friend produces the best consequences, as she will go out feeling happy and your friendship will not be harmed.

Jeremy Bentham (1748–1832) and John Stuart Mill (1806–1873) developed the theory of utilitarianism. Bentham argued that morality should not be about pleasing God, but about producing the greatest happiness for the greatest number. For a utilitarian an action is good or bad depending on the amount of happiness or unhappiness it creates. For Bentham there was only one moral principle, the Principle of Utility, which means that when faced with a choice of actions we should choose the one that produces the best consequences for everyone concerned. The Principle of Utility has two elements. First, we should be concerned about producing happiness, and secondly, this happiness should be for the greatest number. Utilitarianism is often summed up as 'the greatest happiness for the greatest number'.

For the utilitarian there is nothing intrinsically good or bad about any action. For instance, in the above example of lying to a friend, in another set of circumstances it might be wrong to lie, if it produced bad consequences. Thus a utilitarian would not say that lying is wrong. They would examine the particular circumstances and then decide whether a lie would produce the greatest happiness for the greatest number. In the same way, a utilitarian would not think that all killing was wrong. They would examine the particular case and decide whether killing in that instance produced good or bad consequences. For a utilitarian the end justifies the means, and the end is what matters morally about an action, not the means used to achieve it. Consider the following example.

Case study

A patient suffering from end-stage cancer asks the doctor to 'put him out of his misery'. The patient wants a lethal injection that will kill him quickly and painlessly. Leaving aside the legal issues, the doctor, who is a utilitarian, decides to weigh up the consequences of this request. The doctor decides that giving the patient what he wants will produce the best consequences, and he gives him the injection.

Here the means (giving the lethal injection) are justified on the grounds of the good consequences that will be produced (the patient will no longer be suffering, the patient's request is honoured and hospital resources will be saved by not having to care for this patient). However, another doctor considering the same case may come to a different decision about what action would produce the best consequences. This second doctor could argue that giving a patient a lethal injection could have detrimental consequences for the medical profession as a whole. If patients think that doctors could justify killing them, then the doctor–patient relationship could be harmed, as patients would no longer trust their doctors and might fear for their own lives. Thus although in the above case such an action (giving the lethal injection) might produce the best consequences for the patient, that action might also harm the general community of patients.

STRENGTHS OF UTILITARIANISM

1. Consequences are an important factor when we are thinking about whether to perform a particular action. A doctor has to think how their actions will affect others, and whether they will produce the best consequences for their patient. People are judged morally on the basis of the consequences that they produce, and thus they form part of everyday moral reasoning.
2. By recognizing that what is important is the greatest happiness for the greatest number, utilitarianism can be said to be impartial, as no one person's interests are regarded as more important than those of anyone else – we all count as one unit and our interests are considered equally.
3. Matters of morality can be decided by empirical calculation of the consequences. Thus in health care this could be regarded as a useful advantage – we do not have to debate complex philosophical problems in order to determine what is the right action, but rather we can calculate it empirically.

WEAKNESSES OF UTILITARIANISM

1. Counter-intuitive results are obtained – it is often argued that utilitarianism is incompatible with important moral principles. For example, producing the greatest happiness for the greatest number might involve the persecution of a minority. This does not seem to be morally acceptable, as it would be unjust to persecute a group simply because that pleased the majority and, furthermore, this would not respect the rights and autonomous wishes of the minority.
2. There are problems with regard to how one defines happiness. This question is crucial to utilitarianism because, in order for the theory to have the empirical foundation that is claimed for it, we need to have an adequate definition of happiness. Bentham simply stated that happiness is what everyone aims for, and Mill attempted to refine this definition by dividing pleasures into two categories – higher pleasures (those of the intellect and produced through endeavour and hard work) and lower pleasures (those of the body, such as eating, drinking, and so on). However, in a practical health care context the definition of what constitutes the production of happiness will depend on one's values, and there is no universal agreement on such values.

3. There are problems with the calculation. Even if we assume that it would be possible to establish a universally agreed definition of happiness or good consequences, utilitarianism might still be difficult to apply in practice.

   - How does one distribute utility? A health authority might have a certain amount of money left over from the budget, say £50 000, and might decide to distribute it on utilitarian grounds. They narrow the possibilities down to a choice between two options – either fund 10 infertility treatments or fund the health promotion team to distribute leaflets about child nutrition. They work out that both choices will produce 100 units of happiness, but the infertility treatment option will produce this for 10 couples and the health promotion option will produce this for 1000 children. Thus, although both options produce the same amount of happiness, it does not tell us how to distribute this happiness, as it would raise the questions of whether it is better to make one person very happy or several people moderately happy.

   - Another problem is the complexity of the calculation. In practice it might be impossible to determine accurately what the consequences of one's actions might be. Are we only responsible for the consequences we have intended? Or for the likely or rationally expected consequences? Or for the consequences that we have not intended or could not foresee? As often happens, the best laid plans go astray and we may perform an action believing that it will produce the best consequence, but later find out that it in fact produces bad consequences that we had not foreseen. In circumstances like this we often refer to the *intention* of the person doing the action, even if we are harmed by them. If we believe that they did not intend to cause harm and that they performed the action with our best interests in mind, we are inclined to forgive them.

I shall now turn to a moral theory that is concerned with the intentions of the agent and not the consequences of an action.

Kantian ethics

For Immanuel Kant (1724–1804) it is not the consequences of an action that are important – it is the intention of the agent that determines whether an action is morally acceptable. We can never be certain what will happen as a result of our actions, so it is important to concentrate on what we actually *do*. For Kant, morality is linked to rationality. As humans we are rational beings – that is, we have the capacity to think and to deliberate and choose what actions we will perform. Kant argued that animals act out of instinct. For example, a dog will bark not because it chooses to, but because it is compelled to do so out of instinct. The freedom to choose one's actions is central to Kant's ethics. Humans can be held responsible for their choices, whereas animals cannot be held responsible in the same way.

Kant stated that all actions are performed on the basis of some maxim, some kind of 'ought' (e.g. I ought to go to the bank, I ought not to tell a lie), and he called these imperatives. He divided these imperatives into two types – moral and non-moral imperatives. The non-moral type of imperative Kant called *hypothetical imperatives*. Thus the imperative 'I ought to go to the bank' would be a non-moral imperative, as it would depend on your having a particular desire to go to the bank, and this would be a purely personal imperative, not something that would apply to everyone. Kant called moral imperatives such as 'I ought not to tell a lie' *categorical imperatives*. We must all follow these imperatives, and they are not dependent on our individual circumstances or desires.

One formulation of the categorical imperative is: 'I ought only to act on those maxims that I can at the same time will to be universal laws.'

What distinguishes hypothetical from categorical imperatives is that the latter can and should be universalized – that is, everyone is bound by them. If you want to distinguish between a moral and a non-moral imperative, you could determine whether it could be universalized – that is, see whether everyone could follow it all the time. For example, the maxim 'I ought not to tell a lie' can be universalized, as everyone could and should follow it. However, the maxim 'I ought to tell a lie' could not be universalized because, as Kant says, it would be self-defeating. If everyone lied there would be no point in lying, as the purpose of a lie is to deceive while people believe it to be the truth. If everyone lied, no one would believe it to be the truth.

Another formulation of the categorical imperative is: 'Act so that you treat humanity, whether in your own person or that of any other, always as an end and never as a means.'

Kant argued that because we are rational beings we are valuable and deserve respect, and that to treat someone as a means to an end is morally wrong. However, it would appear that we treat people as means to ends all the time. For example, I treat the bus driver as a means of getting to work. However, for Kant this is acceptable, but what we should not do is treat people *merely* as means. We are treating someone merely as a means to an end when we involve them in an action in which they have no share. By this Kant means that they have not consented to that action or they have been coerced into participating in it. Therefore in the above example the bus company would be using the bus driver as a means to an end if he had been enslaved and had no say over whether he drove the bus. However, in normal circumstances a bus driver would have voluntarily decided to work for the bus company and would be paid for his work.

A person can also be used as a means to an end if he has been deceived or deliberately misled. If a doctor wishes someone to consent to an operation and they lie to the patient when they are asked a question about the possible side-effects, this would be morally wrong according to Kant. It is wrong because it does not respect the patient as a person. By not telling him the truth the doctor is preventing the patient from making a fully autonomous decision. The doctor is coercing the patient by manipulating the information and steering him towards a particular conclusion that he might not have reached if he had known the whole truth. Thus according to Kant we should act out of duty – that is, as rational beings we should consider our actions and what maxim guides them and act according to the categorical imperative. For Kant, some actions (e.g. lying or stealing) are always wrong regardless of the circumstances of the action. For example, suppose that a patient in your care has just experienced a protracted and painful death. When the relatives ask you if he suffered any pain, should you tell them the truth, or should you lie and say he died peacefully in his sleep, knowing that this will give some comfort to his relatives? According to Kant you should tell the truth despite the bad consequences that will follow from it. The relatives will be distressed and have painful memories of the death of their loved one for the rest of their lives.

STRENGTHS OF KANTIAN ETHICS

1. Respect for autonomy – Kant's dictum that one should always treat people as ends and not means – is useful in health care and it forms the basis of the principle of autonomy. As stated above, it is very important to respect a patient's autonomy, and Kantian ethics provide a solid theoretical basis for why we should value people as ends in themselves. The doctrine of informed consent (see below) is based on this notion of respecting autonomy and allowing patients to have all of the available information so that they can make their own choices and decisions.
2. Kantian ethics sets out moral rules that should not be broken, and you could argue that this gives people a firm moral code that they can follow. Unlike utilitarianism, Kantian ethics does not depend on complex deliberations about each circumstance. Whereas utilitarianism sanctions the breaking of rules (e.g. the prohibition of killing) if this would produce good consequences, Kantian ethics does not allow moral principles to be sacrificed to the contingencies of the particular situation.

WEAKNESSES OF KANTIAN ETHICS

1. Kantian ethics is not concerned with the consequences of an action. Thus you may follow the categorical imperative and produce very bad consequences. This would not be a problem for Kant, as he would say that as long as you have acted in the right way you are not responsible for the bad outcome. However, in practice we might think that a small lie (e.g. in the above case about the dying relative) that protects someone or does not cause hurt is justified.
2. Kant provides no guidance if moral rules are in conflict with each other. If you had a choice between lying to save someone or telling the truth and allowing them to be captured and killed, what should you do? This would be a conflict between the moral rule 'it is wrong to lie' and the moral rule 'it is wrong to let innocent people be murdered'. In this case you would have to choose which of the absolute moral rules to break, as there is no mechanism for ranking moral rules in order of priority. Thus although we might think that it is better to lie than to let someone be killed, there would be no formal justification for this within Kant's moral theory.

Both utilitarianism and Kantianism seem to capture something important about actions. When judging people's actions we do tend to think both of the motive and of the consequences of their actions. However, although we might not want to adopt either theory as a complete guide by which to live, they are useful in that they indicate the types of benefits and/or problems that focusing on the action itself or focusing on the consequences of an action produces.

Summary

- There are two main moral theories used in medical ethics, namely utilitarianism and Kantianism.
- Moral theories attempt to tell us what we should do and give us guidance on which actions are acceptable.
- Utilitarianism focuses on the consequences of actions.
- Kantianism focuses on the intentions and the actions of the agent.

Informed consent

Consent is one of the most important topics in medical ethics, and is often seen as the bedrock of ethical medical practice. Consent is essentially the agreement of the patient to the treatment or intervention. Consent can be given explicitly either orally and/or by the signing of a form, or tacitly (e.g. by extending an arm for an injection). The ethical foundation of consent is respect for autonomy, and consent is the foremost way in which patient autonomy is respected in health care. The patient is recognized as a competent individual who should be allowed to make decisions with the doctor about their own health care. In the British Medical Association's view this respect for autonomy is at the heart of the consent debate, recognizing that patients are usually the best judges of what is in their best interests (British Medical Association, 1993). Legally, consent must be obtained before any medical intervention, and this rests on the common law assumption that everyone has the right to have their bodily integrity protected against invasion by others. A common law duty is an enforcement of morals by law (Mason and McCall-Smith, 1999: 191). If an intervention was to be undertaken without consent the doctor would be committing a battery against that person.

Consent can be divided into three main elements as follows:

1. threshold elements:
    competence;
    voluntariness;
2. information elements:
    disclosure;
    understanding;

3. consent elements:
   decision;
   authorization.

I shall now consider each of these elements in turn.

Threshold elements

COMPETENCE

If a patient is competent, they have the right to consent to or refuse any medical treatment. When a competent patient consents to a treatment offered by a doctor there is generally no source of conflict. It is over refusal of consent to treatments that conflicts can arise. A competent adult has the right to refuse treatment for any reasons which they deem to be appropriate. An ethical dilemma is raised when a patient refuses life-saving treatment. Lord Donaldson has said that doctors should consider the capacity of the patient to make the decision, and the more serious the decision the greater is the capacity required (British Medical Association, 1993). If the patient is determined to have the relevant capacity to understand and appreciate the consequences of their refusal, then that refusal has to be respected. A competent patient has an absolute right to withhold consent to medical treatment. Lord Donaldson recommended that in cases of uncertainty about the competence of the patient the doctor should approach the courts to establish whether it would be lawful to override the wishes of the patient. There have been cases where the courts have supported the giving of life-saving treatment after a refusal by the patient, on the grounds that the patient's competence was in doubt and thus that doubt should be resolved in favour of giving the treatment and preserving life. For example, consider the case of *Re T*. T was involved in a car crash and rushed to hospital. After a conversation with her mother, who was a Jehovah's Witness (although T was not), she indicated that she did not want a blood transfusion. T's condition deteriorated and she needed a blood transfusion to save her life. The Court of Appeal decided that her refusal of the blood transfusion should be disregarded because she was unable to make a genuine decision and her capacity was in doubt (McHale *et al.*, 1997).

VOLUNTARINESS

Consent should be given voluntarily – that is, with no undue coercion or influence. For example, a doctor should not threaten to remove someone from their list if they do not consent to a treatment, or try to bribe patients to accept interventions. The patient should be presented with a range of options, as far as that is possible, and the doctor should not try to influence the patient unduly by only telling one side of the story or dismissing any objections that the patient may have. In most cases the doctor will be attempting to influence the patient for their own good, and advising and recommending a treatment is clearly a central part of the doctor's role.

However, if this slips into coercion then the patient is not being given the opportunity to make an autonomous decision.

Information elements

DISCLOSURE

In order for consent to be a true reflection of the patient's autonomy, the patient must be fully informed about the treatment, and this is known as *fully informed consent*. This notion of fully informed consent is ethically and legally complex. Legally there is no delineated concept of informed consent, and broadly the Bolam test is applied to information giving. The Bolam test states that the doctor should give as much information as would be given and upheld by a reasonable body of medical opinion. This is called the *prudent professional standard*. The main reason for not giving information is usually that such information-giving would result in harm to the patient. For example, telling a patient that there is a slight risk of scarring from an operation might distress them too much, and therefore it might be better not to tell them. The General Medical Council (1999) advises doctors that they should only withhold information on the grounds that the information would cause the patient serious harm, and that in such cases the decision to withhold information should be recorded.

Ethically it can be argued that the prudent professional standard does not constitute an adequate standard of information-giving. This standard can be seen to be rather paternalistic in that doctors are allowed to decide how much the patient should know. A different standard that is often advanced is the *prudent patient standard*. This focuses on what the patient would like to know, and it is often argued that this standard results in greater information-giving, as patients are not being 'protected' from 'harmful' information.

It is difficult to set out strict criteria on how much information should be given to patients. In general, patients want to know about any risks inherent in the treatment, the likely success rate, the side-effects and comparisons with other treatment options. The General Medical Council (1999) states that individual patients will require different amounts of information, and that the doctor should do his or her best to find out what the patient's individual needs and priorities are, and to tailor their information-giving accordingly.

Box 2.1 Informed consent: how much information should be given to the patient?

The prudent professional standard
The doctor gives as much information as a reasonable body of medical opinion would sanction

The prudent patient standard
The doctor gives as much information as the prudent patient would like to know about the procedure

---

UNDERSTANDING

An important part of information-giving is to ensure that the patient has understood what has been imparted. This is a crucial aspect of obtaining consent from patients, in that it is not enough to run through the information and then get a signature. The patient must understand what they have been told. This leads us to the final aspect of consent.

Consent elements

DECISION

It is important to regard consent as a process rather than a one-off authorization. First, the doctor has to build up a relationship with the patient (as far as is possible) and to ascertain the information needs of the patient. The British Medical Association (1993) states that ideally the doctor–patient relationship is one of partnership, with the doctor's clinical expertise and the patient's individual needs and perspectives being shared in order to reach a joint decision. Secondly, once the patient's information needs have been established, the doctor has to decide how best to give the information to the patient. Fact sheets, websites or books can be recommended. All of the information does not have to be given at once, and the understanding of the patient can be fostered over time, particularly if it is a long-term chronic condition where there is time to discuss treatment options.

AUTHORIZATION

Once the patient has made the decision as to what treatment to have, and the consent form has been signed, this does not mean that the information-giving process is over. The patient should be informed throughout their treatment with regard to what is going on and how they are progressing. Giving information about even minor matters such as temperature and blood pressure can be very important to the patient, and it shows respect for their autonomy.

Difficult cases

It is not always possible to obtain consent from patients, either due to the circumstances or due to the patient's competence, and this puts the medical staff in a difficult position both morally and legally.

EMERGENCIES

When patients are brought into the Accident and Emergency department there is often little time to seek consent. The assumption is that the patient should be given the necessary treatment (and no more) to preserve life, and then they can be consulted about the longer-term measures. However, if the patient has left clear instructions that they do not wish to have a particular treatment (e.g. Jehovah's Witnesses refusing a blood transfusion), then this should be respected.

Another difficult area concerns cases of attempted suicide where the person has left a note asking not to be resuscitated. The debate is whether such a document constitutes a valid refusal of treatment, as it could be argued that the person was not competent to make such a refusal at that time. As stated above, the general assumption is that one should treat the patient, give them the minimum treatment necessary to restore life, and then ascertain their competence. If there is any doubt about the patient's competence to refuse consent, then they should be treated and the matter addressed when they are stabilized.

MINORS

Anyone over 16 years of age has a statutory right to consent to treatment. A child under 16 years may be able to consent, without parental approval, if the doctor thinks that they have reached a significant understanding and have the intelligence to enable them to understand fully the information that has been given to them (Gillick competence). Thus a 14-year-old girl requesting contraception could, if the doctor thought that she understood all of the risks, benefits and implications of her request, be prescribed the pill without recourse to her parents. It is seen as good practice that even very young children, while not being able to consent legally, should be involved as much as possible in the decision and the treatment. Although minors may be able to consent, they do not have the corresponding right of refusal of consent, and this holds for parents as well. Thus parents cannot refuse consent for a treatment that the medical team thinks is in the child's best interests. For example, a Jehovah's Witness could not refuse consent for a life-saving blood transfusion for their child. In such a case the child would be made a ward of court and the treatment would be given.

IMPAIRED CAPACITY

As mentioned above, it is generally a requirement that patients must have a higher level of capacity to refuse consent, particularly of life-saving treatment, than they need to consent to treatment. If a patient is deemed to be incapable of making their own decisions, then these can be taken by others so that the patient's best interests can be safeguarded. The British Medical Association produces guidelines on the treatment of such patients.

Summary

- Informed consent is the main practical way in which a patient's autonomy is respected.
- Consent is both a legal and an ethical requirement.
- There is much debate over how much information needs to be given to the patient in order to satisfy both legal and ethical requirements.

Confidentiality

Confidentiality is another concept that has an important place in good medical practice. Like consent, confidentiality is a legal and ethical requirement of doctors, who have a common-law duty to respect the confidences of their patients. A doctor faces professional misconduct charges and can be removed from the medical register if they are responsible for unauthorized breaches of confidentiality. Ethically, respecting patients' confidences respects their autonomy, as it gives them control over information about themselves and protects them from having it divulged in contexts to which they have not consented.

Confidentiality was part of the Hippocratic Oath and has been restated in most codes of medical ethics. For example, the International Code of Medical Ethics states that the doctor must preserve absolute confidentiality on all that they know about their patient, even after the patient's death. The reasons for patient confidentiality can be broadly summarized as follows.

1. Patient confidentiality ensures that patients will come for treatment and not be worried about their information being divulged to other parties. It is essential for good medical practice that patients can speak freely to their doctors. Only in this way can doctors receive the information that they need in order to provide the best possible care.
2. Patients give information to doctors on the basis that it will be kept confidential, and thus it respects their autonomy as it allows them to have control over their personal information.
3. Confidentiality respects patients' rights to privacy. The right to privacy is enshrined in the United Nations and the European Declarations of Human Rights, and with the Human Rights Act 1998 these rights are part of English law.

Breaches of confidentiality

Medical confidentiality is not absolute in the way that confessions to a priest are, as there are occasionally circumstances when it is both legally and ethically necessary to breach confidentiality. It is the decision as to when to breach confidentiality that creates ethical dilemmas for practitioners. The GMC (General Medical Council, 1995) issues guidelines as to when it is acceptable to breach confidentiality, and these will now be considered in turn.

1. *When the patient (or legal adviser) consents.* Patients may consent to the release of information about themselves (e.g. for insurance purposes or for a medical report for an employer). The doctor should, as far as he or she is able, make sure that the patient fully understands what they have consented to and that they can see any report written about them if they so wish.
2. *Information can be shared within the health care team.* It is often not feasible in modern medicine for the doctor to be the only person responsible for the

patient's care, and health care is now usually delivered by teams. For this reason, information-sharing between members of the team is not regarded as an unacceptable breach of confidentiality, and the General Medical Council (1995) recommends that patients be made aware that this is the case. The information should be directly relevant to the care of the patient, and if a patient wishes you to keep certain information from the rest of the team you must respect their request.

3. *Disclosure in the patient's best interests*. In rare circumstances, if it is judged that it would be in the patient's best interests for information to be given to a third party then confidentiality can be breached. For example, if a patient was suffering from a terminal illness and they did not want to know the full prognosis, the doctor might think that this information should be given to a relative. Difficult cases of this kind of breach are cases of abuse. If the abused person is an adult, the doctor should endeavour to persuade this person to report the abuse to the relevant authorities. If the person refuses to do so, then the doctor has to weigh the harm caused by breaching confidentiality against the harm caused by allowing the abuse to continue. Good practice suggests that every effort should be made to persuade the patient, and the patient's view cannot be ignored. Counselling and support should be offered to help the patient to make a decision and consent to the divulging of the information. Ultimately, if it can be shown that the breach was made in the patient's best interests and the efforts to persuade them are recorded, then the doctor would be considered to be acting ethically. In the case of child abuse, the British Medical Association (1993) recommends that any disclosure should be discussed with the child first and made on the grounds that it was in the child's best interests. Disclosure should be made to the appropriate person or statutory authority.

4. *Disclosure in the public interest*. If the doctor considers that maintaining confidentiality will result in harm to the public, they are justified in breaching confidentiality. Common examples of this situation include the following.

   (i) *Fitness to drive*. The General Medical Council (1995) states that if a patient continues to drive against medical advice when they are unfit to do so, then the medical adviser of the Driver and Vehicle Licensing Agency (DVLA) should be informed. Again, good practice suggests that the patient should be told and counselled about their condition and why they should not drive, and given the opportunity to tell the DVLA themselves. The doctor should try to persuade the patient not to drive, and this may include telling their next of kin. If all attempts at persuasion fail, the doctor should then inform the patient that they will tell the DVLA, and once this has been done it should be confirmed in writing to the patient.

   (ii) *HIV infection*. HIV has caused many confidentiality dilemmas for practitioners, and the General Medical Council has produced a separate booklet on HIV in the pack entitled *Duties of a Doctor*. For a patient who is HIV-positive the usual confidentiality provisions apply, except in situations where there is a possibility of harm being caused to another person. For example, if a GP is treating a married man who is found to be HIV-positive, should the GP tell the patient's wife? The GP has two tasks here – first, to ascertain whether the patient's wife is at risk, and secondly, to counsel and persuade the patient to tell her himself. If after persuasion and ample opportunity to tell his wife the patient still refuses to inform her, the doctor would be within his rights to tell the wife himself. 'The GMC believes that most such patients will agree to disclosure in these circumstances, but where such consent is withheld the doctor may consider it a duty to seek to ensure that any sexual partner is informed, in order to safeguard such persons from infection.' (General Medical Council, 1995: 9). It could be argued that this could have long-term detrimental effects on patients with HIV who would feel that they could not visit their doctor in confidence and therefore might not seek treatment. The GMC states that such a breach of confidentiality should only be made after extensive counselling, and hopefully with the right support these types of situations will be rare.

5. *Statutory requirements*. There are various statutory requirements concerning the disclosure of certain information. For example, the Public Health (Control of Disease) Act 1984 requires certain diseases (e.g. cholera, plague and smallpox) to be notifiable. Venereal disease legislation and the Police and Criminal Evidence Act also require specific medical information to be released.

6. *Research*. Information can be released for the purposes of research, and if the data cannot be made anonymous then consent should be sought from the patients concerned.

In summary, two important elements need to be addressed when considering breaches of confidentiality.

1. The burden of proof is on the practitioner to justify any breach. Confidentiality is assumed unless there are good reasons for a breach. Thus the doctor has to weigh the harm against the benefits caused by breaching confidentiality. Here good record-keeping would be essential to show the reasons for the breach and, if appropriate, the attempts to persuade the patient to consent to the breach.

2. Confidentiality should be breached in an appropriate way – that is, in the right circumstances and to the right person. The New Zealand case of Duncan v The Medical Practitioners Disciplinary Committee illustrates this point. After a bus driver had undergone a triple coronary bypass operation, his GP thought that he was not fit to drive, and began to advise passengers not to take the bus when this man was driving. The doctor was subsequently found guilty of professional misconduct. Although the judge recognized that it was an acceptable breach of confidentiality, as the man should not have been driving and was a danger to his passengers, the way in which the doctor had breached confidentiality, by informing the passengers, was unacceptable.

Summary

- Confidentiality is both an ethical and a legal requirement.
- Confidentiality enables patients to speak freely to their doctor and have control over their personal information.
- The main ethical dilemma for doctors is when to breach confidentiality. The doctor should be able to provide a clear justification for the breach.
- Confidentiality should be breached in an appropriate way to the appropriate individuals or bodies.

Ethics and medical students

There are a number of ethical issues that are of particular relevance to doctors when qualifying.

Consent

When patient consent is sought for students to be present during a consultation, it is important that the patient is given a genuine choice. Asking for consent when the student is already seated in the room makes it difficult for the patient to refuse. It is better to ask the patient before the consultation, and to explain fully the role and involvement of the student, so that the patient can make an informed decision.

A further issue is whether a patient's consent is valid when he or she agrees to a doctor carrying out the procedure, but it is performed by a student doctor instead. There was outrage in 1995 when a student on work experience at Bradford Hospital stitched a patient's wound. The Joint Consultants Committee later agreed on a set of safeguards to govern procedures carried out by non-medically qualified people, which stated that the patient had to be told of the training and status of those operating on them and give their fully informed consent.

Confidentiality

Medical students often have access to confidential patient information, and it is important that students recognize that they have a duty of confidentiality to the patient in the same way as the practitioner does. Although the doctor who is responsible for the student may be liable for the breach, the student has an ethical obligation not to carelessly divulge information to which they have access in the course of their training or research.

Students as research subjects

The use of students as healthy volunteers for medical research is common, partly because students are easily recruited by university research teams, and also because they are a low-income group that finds the financial remuneration useful. Students must ensure that they understand the full implications of participating in any research project, including the risks and possible side-effects that they may encounter. The Royal College of Physicians (1985) has published guidelines entitled *Research on Healthy Volunteers*, which recommend that it is undesirable to recruit students who are in close contact with the investigator (e.g. a professor recruiting a member of his class): 'This is because students are, or may feel, vulnerable to pressure from someone in a position to influence their careers.' The guidelines further recommend that any student involved in a clinical trial should notify the Dean of the medical school. This ensures that the student cannot enter several trials simultaneously, and that the medical school is aware of the student's activities.

Conclusions

An understanding of the ethical dilemmas raised in medical practice and a clear impartial mechanism for achieving some practical resolution of these dilemmas is essential for all health care professionals. The study of ethics can also help doctors to understand and appreciate the different values and beliefs that are held by patients, and aid communication between all parties.

Discussion points

Here are some general issues in medical ethics that raise particular problems for practitioners.

- How much information about a procedure should a patient be told in order to ensure that they have given fully informed consent?
- When is it ethically justifiable to breach a patient's confidentiality?
- How should the health care budget be ethically distributed?
- Are there some procedures that should not be given on the NHS? For example, should some types of cosmetic surgery or breast implants not be given?
- How should a doctor respond to the dilemma that in doing the best for a particular patient they are taking resources away from other patients?
- Are there any areas of your medical training that you think raised ethical dilemmas? These might include, for example, consent for inoculations or being asked to do things by a senior colleague that you did not agree with.

Further reading

Beauchamp T and Childress J (2001) *Principles of biomedical ethics*, 5th edn. Oxford: Oxford University Press.

Boyd K, Higgs R and Pinching A (eds) (1997) *The new dictionary of medical ethics*. London: BMJ Publishing.

Downie R and Calman K (1994) *Healthy respect: ethics in health care*. Oxford: Oxford Medical Publications.

Dowrick C and Frith L (eds) (1999) *General practice and ethics: uncertainty and responsibility*. London: Routledge.

Gillon R (1986) *Philosophical medical ethics*. Chichester: John Wiley & Sons.

Harris J (1985) *The value of life*. London: Routledge.

Social determinants of health and illness

Ann Jacoby

Introduction

Levels of health and ill health are not evenly distributed across populations, but vary according to a range of factors, including age, gender, social class, ethnic group, region and country. Such variations exist whatever measure of health or ill health we choose to examine, be it mortality, 'hard' measures of morbidity (e.g. consultation rates) or softer subjective measures (e.g. self-assessed health status). The way in which health and ill health are socially patterned is further complicated by interactions between the various contributing factors. This chapter will address the following areas.

- We shall begin by considering the various ways in which health, or the lack of it, can be measured.

- We shall examine the concept of 'social class', which has been demonstrated to be a major determinant of health and illness, and discuss how social scientists have attempted to measure social class.
- We shall consider the evidence for the link between social class and inequalities of health, and the extent to which this link is simply a reflection of differences in wealth.
- We shall examine opposing perspectives on the causes of inequalities in health and the weight of evidence supporting each of them.
- We shall consider the link between different types of 'social stress' and the predisposition to poor health, and the possible mediating effects of social support.
- We shall explore the influence of factors such as gender and ethnicity on levels of health and ill health, and the extent to which these differences are attributable to biology or social role.
- Finally, we shall consider what remains a key text on this topic, namely the Black Report, which was first published in 1980, but is still highly relevant to the 'social determinants' debate (Townsend and Davidson, 1988).

The idea that ill health and disease are determined by factors other than those which are the focus of biomedicine has been a concern of sociologists since Emile Durkheim published his study of suicide in 1897 (for a translation, see Spaulding and Simpson, 1951). Durkheim was not concerned with the act of suicide at the level of the individual, but with the suicide rate as a social phenomenon. He showed that the rate varied with age, gender, marital status and religion. Although he accepted that some individuals were psychologically predisposed to the act, Durkheim interpreted suicide as an expression of social rather than psychological forces (Aron, 1970). Durkheim's work was important both in developing the sociological concept he termed *anomie* (the weakening or loss of social norms and values), which he regarded as central to explaining the suicide rate, and for 'its methodological emphasis on social facts as a distinct category of analysis' (Siegrist, 2000). It was the foundation-stone for the plethora of subsequent socio-epidemiological studies which have linked health and ill health to sociological constructs such as social class (see below) and demonstrated the importance of social as well as biological factors in explaining patterns of health and illness.

The social patterning of health has been a concern of governments as well as social scientists since the routine collection of population statistics began. The practice of classifying the UK population by occupation and industry began at the time of the first Census in 1851, and the first formal measure of social classification, the Registrar General's Social Classes (RGSC) was developed specifically to examine differences in mortality rates between different occupational groups. The application of the Registrar General's scheme was central to a major intellectual debate of the time – that between eugenicists and environmentalists about differential fertility rates between the different social classes. Stevenson, the initiator of the Registrar General's Social Classes, stood firmly in the environmentalist camp and so intended it as 'an assertion of the importance of social factors in accounting for observed trends in fertility and mortality' (Rose and O'Reilly, 1997).

Consideration of the way in which health and ill health are socially determined raises two related but distinct questions. The first is why levels of health vary across subgroups in the population. The second is why, *within* particular subgroups, some individuals have poorer health than others. Studies which focus on the first question tend to concentrate on external determinants of health (e.g. social class position, income or geographical placement). Studies which focus on the second question tend to be concerned with the role of particular social stressors (e.g. major life events) and, as a corollary, with factors such as social support, which may counteract their effects. Beyond this, the role of internal psychological characteristics such as personality type, coping style and locus of control have also been examined in terms of whether they promote or protect ill health. As this and subsequent chapters will show, no one set of factors of itself provides an adequate explanation for the differences that are observed.

Understanding the way in which a complex set of social and psychological (as well biological) circumstances combine to produce good or poor health is important for a number of reasons. It is vital to the formation of appropriate public health policies aimed at minimizing differences in the level of health across different population groups. It is also the key to providing appropriate health and medical care at the level of the individual patient. In this chapter, we shall examine the evidence for the uneven distribution of health and ill health and some possible explanations for this unevenness. We shall also consider the way in which the different explanations offered differ in their implications at the level of health policy. However, since any discussion of the way in which health and ill health are patterned rests on their sound measurement, we shall begin with a discussion of how this can best be achieved.

Measuring health

The most commonly used measure of health and ill health is mortality. The standardized mortality ratio (SMR) is the measure used to compare death rates in different groups of the population, taking into account differences in the composition of the groups (e.g. differences in the age or sex structure). The SMR of the standard population is 100, and the mortality of any particular group is higher than expected when the SMR is above 100, and lower than expected when it is below that figure. Since the registration of deaths began in the UK in the middle of the nineteenth century, mortality across all age–sex groups has declined (see Figure 3.1). Death rates in England fell from 18 per 1000 in 1896 to 11 per 1000 in 1996. Statistics from the Office of National Statistics show that between the years 1984 and 1994, mortality rates fell by 35% for infants under 1 year of age, by 22% in young adults aged 15–19 years and by 10% in adults aged 75 years or over (Dunnell, 1995). Life expectancy has also increased. For example, between 1970 and 1990, life expectancy at birth rose from 69 to 73 years for men and from 75 to 79 years for women (Dunnell, 1995).

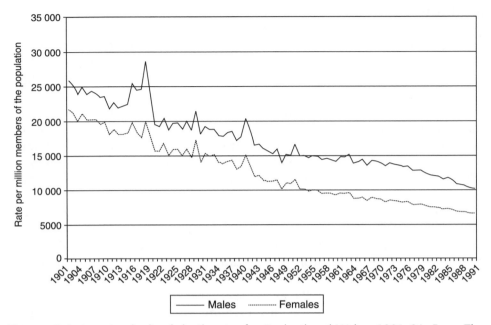

Figure 3.1 Age-standardized death rates for England and Wales, 1901–91. From *The health of adult Britain 1841–94*.

Mortality is the traditional measure for describing the health of populations, because it is regarded as objective and reliable evidence. In Chapter 5 we shall explain more about how it is used to understand patterns of health and disease. However, its objectivity has been questioned by sociologists such as Prior (1985), who examined the way in which mortality statistics are collected and processed, and by Samphier *et al.* (1988), who looked at the way in which causes of death as recorded on death certificates varied according to social class. Morbidity rates offer an alternative method of considering the distribution of health and ill health, possible indicators being GP consultation rates, hospital out-patient attendance, hospital in-patient admissions, prescription rates, rates of work or school absenteeism, sickness certifications, and self-reported illness, symptoms and health status.

Opting for morbidity measures is potentially more problematic than using mortality rates for a number of reasons. First, when based on consultation rates, they may be more representative of illness behaviour than of true morbidity. The term 'illness behaviour' refers to how a person interprets the symptoms of possible ill health and decides whether, when and how to act upon them, including whether or not to consult a health professional. Studies have shown that the frequency and visibility of symptoms are only two of a whole host of factors which determine whether or not a person will seek medical help (Zola, 1973; Mechanic, 1978). Of equal importance are factors such as the significance accorded the symptoms, the degree of disruption that they cause to daily life, and the degree to which seeking medical help is sanctioned by others. In a study by Wadsworth *et al.* (1971) of the illness experience and behaviour of adults over a 2-week period, about 20% reported having symptoms of illness for which they were taking no action, and over 50% reported having symptoms for which they were taking only non-medical action. The message from studies such as this is that there is a 'whole iceberg of ill health' which would not be detected by collecting information about consultation rates.

The second potential difficulty when using morbidity data is that if such data are based on self-reports of health or ill health, they involve subjective judgements on the part of the person from whom information is obtained. Since subjective data have often been criticized as being 'soft' (Fallowfield, 1990), we shall now consider the appropriateness of using them in more detail.

The rationale for the development of self-report measures of health and morbidity derives from studies by social scientists that have examined concepts of health held by lay people, and which have shown that such conceptualizations differ from the traditional biomedical model in which illness is attributed to 'invariant biological structures and processes' (Atkinson, 1988). Blaxter (1990) asked over 9000 adults in the UK to describe what, for them, constituted good health. Some of them proffered ideas which paralleled the biomedical model, in as much as they defined health as the absence of disease or illness. Others viewed it rather differently – for example, in terms of possessing an inborn health reserve, being fit or leading a healthy life, maintaining positive social relationships or having high levels of energy, vitality and well-being. It has also been shown that lay concepts of health and illness vary according to people's cultural and social situation (Herzlich, 1973; Pill and Stott, 1982; Cornwell, 1984; d'Houtard and Field, 1984; Blaxter, 1990; Howlett *et al.*, 1992). For example, Blaxter (1990) reported that concepts of health differed according to gender and through the life course:

> Younger men tend to speak of health in terms of physical strength and fitness . . . Young women, though they also talk of fitness or its appear-ance, favour ideas of energy, vitality and ability to cope. In middle age, concepts of health become more complex, with an emphasis upon total mental and physical well-being. Older people, particularly men, think in terms of function, or the ability to do things, though ideas of health as contentment, happiness, a state of mind – even in the presence of disease or disability – are also prominent.
>
> (Blaxter, 1990: 30)

Howlett and colleagues undertook a secondary analysis of Blaxter's data to compare concepts of health held by people from different ethnic groups (Howlett *et al.*, 1992). They found that, compared to white respondents, Asian people were more likely to define health in terms of their ability to perform everyday tasks, and Afro-Caribbean people defined it in terms of energy and physical strength.

Research has also shown (unsurprisingly, given the differences described above) that people who are ill often have different concerns about their illness and different expectations about the outcome of their care to those of the health professionals who are treating them. The implication of such findings is that what constitutes good or poor health and successful or unsuccessful treatment for illness is necessarily subjective. These insights from research are consistent with the shift within modern health care systems towards self-management of their illness by patients, increased patient participation in treatment decisions and the decline of medical paternalism (Coulter, 1999). They also fit within the wider context of the development of the concept of consumerism in Western societies. Importantly, they have acted as a catalyst to the development of measures of health (or the lack of it), and measures of the outcomes of care, in terms that are meaningful and important to the users of health and medical services, rather than to the providers. Such measures are designed to be completed by users themselves and to document their subjective assessments of their health. A large number of well-validated measures are now available (Bowling, 1991, 1995), and these are commonly used alongside more traditional measures of health and health outcomes, including mortality and objective measures of morbidity. It is worth noting that self-report measures of health, despite their subjective nature, have been shown to be significantly associated with health service use and mortality.

Other possible *objective* measures of health could include standard physiological measures, such as blood pressure or lung function, height at a given age, levels of obesity or dental health. For example, the UK national study of health and growth in schoolchildren showed that the average height of 7-year-old boys was 1.1 cm taller in 1994 than in 1972. The average height for girls of the same age increased by 1.6 cm over the same period. The UK Department of Health has conducted a series of surveys of dental health in both adults and children, which incorporated a standardized dental examination. They showed a dramatic decrease in the proportion of children with decayed permanent teeth, another positive indicator of health, between 1973 and 1993 (Todd, 1975; Todd and Dodd, 1985; O'Brien, 1994). Less encouragingly, the number of overweight adults in the population is increasing rather than decreasing. Figures from Government surveys show that between 1980 and 1993, the proportion of the UK population who were classified as overweight or obese increased from 39% to 56% for men and from 32% to 46% for women.

The Health and Lifestyles Survey (Blaxter, 1990) provides valuable information about morbidity. It documented the experienced health of over 9000 adults in the UK in both objective and subjective terms. Four components of health were measured, namely levels of fitness (based on standard physiological measurements such as blood pressure, lung function and body mass index), disease and disability (based on reported medically defined conditions), experienced illness (based on self-reports of symptoms) and psychosocial health (based on reports of psychosocial symptoms). From these data, Blaxter calculated *standardized health ratios* (SHRs) equivalent to the standardized mortality ratio (SMR) referred to above. For each of the components, values over 100 represented poorer health and values under 100 represented better health. Figure 3.2 shows the way in which the four components varied with age and gender.

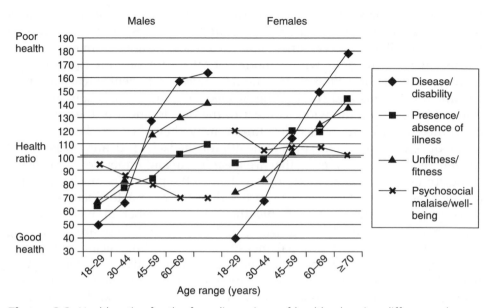

Figure 3.2 Health ratios for the four dimensions of health, showing differences by age and gender (total population mean = 100). From Blaxter N (1990) *Health and lifestyle*. London: Tavistock.

Summary

- Mortality is the most commonly used measure of health and ill health. Since record-keeping began in the mid-nineteenth century, mortality in the UK has fallen across all age–sex groups.
- Morbidity rates are another way of measuring health, but may be as much a reflection of illness behaviour as of true morbidity.
- Self-reported health status measures, although often criticized for lacking objectivity, are significantly associated with 'hard' measures of health such as health services use and mortality.
- Self-report measures emphasize the social nature of health and ill health. Their use has demonstrated that patients' views about health and the outcomes of health care may be very different to those of the health professionals who care for them.

The concept of class

A considerable part of the work examining social determinants of health and illness and seeking to explain their uneven distribution has focused on the concept of social class, 'if only because there is more evidence to go on' (Townsend and Davidson, 1988) than for other possible contributory variables. In this section, we shall consider the way in which sociologists have tried to conceptualize class, and the way in which agencies and researchers have operationalized it in health and social studies.

The term *social stratification* refers to the way in which societies are hierarchically structured. In western industrial societies, the underlying hierarchical principle has been given the name *social class*. Other systems of social stratification include the caste system in the Indian subcontinent and serfdom in feudal societies. Karl Marx was the first sociologist to develop the concept of social class. He maintained that, in order to belong to a social class, people must both share a common attribute and be conscious that they do so (Cuff *et al.*, 1992). Within Marxist theory about capitalism, there were only two social classes – the capitalists who owned the means of production and the workers whom they exploited. In as much as the former had a strong commitment to maintaining the status quo, while the latter had a strong interest in destroying it, class was seen by Marx as vital to the process of social and economic change. The German sociologist, Max Weber, refined Marxist theories by arguing that the concept of class as it relates to ownership of the means of economic production can be overlaid by a second dimension, namely that of status. By 'status', Weber was referring to the positive or negative estimations of honour accorded to a person or persons by the rest of society. In his view, 'stratification by status goes hand in hand with a monopolization of ideal and material goods and opportunities' (Weber, *Essays*, cited in Bendix, 1966).

Present-day social-class theorists are still grappling with the question of whether 'social stratification can be conceptualized as some single, homogeneous ... dimension (e.g. of prestige or status) rather than as some more complex structure grounded in relations within the social divisions of labour' (Goldthorpe, 1988). Goldthorpe identifies three different types of stratification principle, which he describes as *official* (or *quasi-official*), *occupational* and *class*. The Registrar General's Social Classes are an example of the first type. Occupational scales include *reputational scales*, such as the one developed by Goldthorpe himself, which measure the general desirability of occupations, and *associational scales*, which are concerned with differences in lifestyle as reflected in patterns of marriage, friendship, and so on. Class schemata are based on classical sociological theory, such as the theory of Wright (1985), which is derived from Marxist theories of class domination.

The Registrar General's Social Classes are the most commonly used measure of social class in the UK. They were developed by Stevenson, a medical statistician working in the General Register Office,[*] and first used to analyse data on infant mortality from the 1911 Census (Goldblatt, 1988). The original eight-category scheme ranked occupations according to their status and 'general standing' in the community. In recent decades, more emphasis has been placed on level of occupational skill, reflecting the change towards a 'knowledge-based' society. It was revised in 1921 and on several occasions subsequently (most recently in 1990), to take account of

---

[*] Later the Office of Population Census and Surveys (OPCS) and now part of the Office for National Statistics (ONS).

changes in the structure of occupations, the creation of new job titles and the demise of old ones. By the 1930s it had become an explicitly ordinal scale, running from Social Class I (professional occupations) down to Social Class V (unskilled manual occupations). It has retained that format ever since. The RGSC currently consists of six categories (five social classes, but with social class III subdivided into skilled non-manual and skilled manual occupations).

Table 3.1 Occupations within social class groupings

Social class	Classification	Occupation
I	Professional	Accountants, engineers, doctors
II	Managerial and technical Intermediate	Marketing and sales managers, teachers, journalists, nurses
IIIN	Non-manual skilled	Clerks, shop assistants, cashiers
IIIM	Manual skilled	Carpenters, goods-van drivers, joiners, cooks
IV	Partly skilled	Security guards, machine-tool operators, farm workers
V	Unskilled	Building and civil engineering labourers, other labourers, cleaners

Source: Drever F and Whitehead M (1997)

The Registrar General's Social Class Scale has been heavily criticized by sociology theorists for lacking any theoretical base. It has been described as 'arbitrary and crude' (Brewer, 1986), even if commonsensical. One concern that has been raised about it is the question of whether the current assignment of occupations across the six categories discriminates between them adequately. Another concern is that, because of the historical context in which it was developed, it reflects a gendered occupational structure (Hardey, 1998). By tradition, it defines class according to the occupation of the male head of household, so discounting the changing socio-economic position of women. A third major criticism hinges on the fact that because it classifies individuals on the basis of their current employment, it ignores the question of how people who are unemployed or retired, or more critically who have never worked, place themselves in social class terms. Set against these criticisms is the fact that the RGSC is strikingly successful in producing a sharp and consistent upward gradient in standardized mortality rates from Class I to Class V. Its predictive success explains why over time it was adopted as the standard measure of social class, and accounts for its abiding popularity in socio-medical research.

In 1951, a second official classification system, known as Socio-Economic Groups (SEG), was introduced. Since then, SEG has been coded alongside the RGSC in the analysis of data from successive Censuses. It uses the same basic information to classify occupations deemed to be of similar social and economic status into 17 groups. Although it is less widely used than the RGSC, it is generally considered to be a better measure due to the fact that it 'comes closer to being a measure of employment relations and therefore to a sociological measure of class' (Rose and O'Reilly, 1997). It has been shown that SEG, when collapsed into fewer categories, produces variation which is more theoretically supported (e.g. that self-employed people are more likely to vote Conservative).

The scope for refining the Registrar General's Social Classes has been seen as limited by the need for continuity – it has been used in every Census since it was introduced in 1911. However, both RGSC and SEG are set to disappear following a review commissioned by the Office for National Statistics and conducted by the Economic and Social Research Council (ESRC). The remit of the ESRC group was to devise a new socio-economic classification which would unite the most important features and advantages of the RGSC and SEG and be bridgeable to them, while having a clearer conceptual base and wider population coverage. The new classification, which will be known as the National Statistics Socio-Economic Classification (NS-SEC), will replace the RGSC and SEG in the 2001 Census. It is also based on occupation, but is explicitly concerned with employment relations and conditions rather than, as for RGSC, occupational standing. Because what it is measuring is made explicit, it should in principle be easier to suggest reasons for the associations shown between SEC and outcomes of interest such as health, education or income. It is to such associations that we shall turn next.

Summary

* Systems of social stratification include the caste system, serfdom in feudal societies and social class in Western industrial societies.
* Sociologists do not necessarily agree about the dimensions by which social class can be conceptualized. Some adhere to Marxist theories about class dominance and ownership of the means of production. Others have espoused Weberian ideas about the importance of status and prestige in determining a person's class position.
* The Registrar General's Social Classes is the most used measure of social class in the UK, but has been heavily criticized for lacking any real theoretical basis. A new classification is set to replace it in future Government statistics.

Health inequalities

The World Health Organization (WHO) has proposed that, in health terms, 'ideally everyone should have the same opportunity to attain the highest level of health and, more pragmatically, none should be unduly disadvantaged' (World Health Organization, 1985). The concept of health inequalities focuses on differences in the distribution of health which are generated by social or economical forces rather than the result of 'natural physiological constitution or process' (Townsend and Davidson, 1988). In 1985, the European Region of

WHO adopted a common health strategy, with a central theme of health equity and the reduction of health inequality as one of its major targets.

In the UK, health inequalities have been a major political concern since the publication of the Black Report (Townsend and Davidson, 1988) in 1980. The report (which will be discussed in detail later in this chapter) had a major impact on the UK research and political agendas for health inequalities, and was followed by a series of Government and quasi-government sponsored reports and papers addressing the topic. In 1986, the Health Education Council commissioned an update on the original findings of the Black Report, published in 1988 under the title *The Health Divide* (Whitehead, 1988). At the same time, it established an independent multidisciplinary committee to examine the effectiveness of existing public health policy and stimulate the development of new national strategies, including ones to promote equal opportunities for health. In the early 1990s, the Chief Medical Officer set up a subgroup to consider *The Health of the Nation* and what could be done to reduce what it preferred to describe as 'variations in health.' Under the current Labour Government, the health inequalities debate has acquired new impetus. The Government Green Paper, *Our Healthier Nation* (Department of Health, 1998), acknowledged that 'poor people are ill more often and die sooner' than richer people. A structure by which improvements in the health of the worst off and a reduction in the health gap could be achieved was set out in the accompanying White Paper, *The New NHS* (Department of Health, 1997). At the same time, an Independent Inquiry into Inequalities in Health (Acheson, 1999) was charged to summarize 'the evidence for inequalities of health and the expectation of life in England and identify trends [and] priority areas for future policy development . . . likely to offer opportunities for Government to develop beneficial, cost-effective and affordable interventions to reduce health inequalities'.

The Independent Inquiry was guided in its consideration of the available evidence by a socio-economic model of health (see Figure 3.3), in which its main determinants are represented as layers of influence. Individuals are placed at the center, shown as endowed with unalterable characteristics (e.g. age, sex and constitution), and surrounded by layers which can potentially be altered (e.g. personal lifestyle, social and economic conditions and environment). It is these potentially changeable characteristics and the interactions between them that are of greatest interest to social scientists and public health physicians. Although the Black Report concentrated on differences in health associated with social class, it and subsequent research have also examined inequalities associated with other indicators, such as unemployment, income and material or social deprivation, and with factors such as gender and ethnicity. In the following sections, we shall consider the evidence for the relationship between such factors and inequalities in health.

Social class and health

We can examine the relationship between social class and health by considering each of the measures of health discussed above – mortality, objective

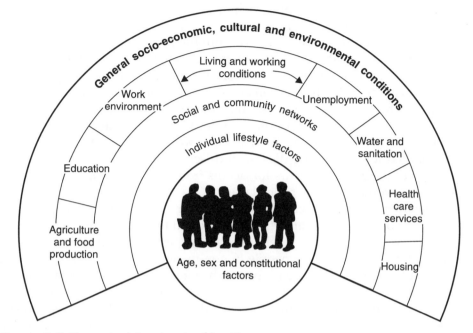

Figure 3.3 The main determinants of health.

indicators of morbidity and subjective health status. Infant mortality (deaths in the first year of life per 1000 live births) has proved to be a particularly useful indicator of health since Stevenson first analysed its relationship to occupational group. Figures collected routinely for perinatal mortality (still-births or deaths in the first week of life), neonatal mortality (deaths from 7 to 28 days) and post-neonatal mortality (deaths from 28 days to 1 year) show that rates for all three have fallen steadily in the UK over the course of the last century. Overall infant mortality rates fell from over 80 per 1000 in 1921 to under 8 per 1000 in 1991. However, The Black Report showed that despite this overall decline, there was a clear social class gradient in risk of death in the first year of life, and that this gradient, although narrowing, persisted into childhood. Whitehead (1988) confirmed these findings, showing that social class differences in deaths at various stages in the first year of life meant that children from social class V were almost twice as likely to die as children from social class I.

Social class differences in mortality are not confined to childhood. Data from the Office of Population Censuses and Surveys Longitudinal Survey, which is following a cohort of 1% of the population drawn from the 1971 Census, show that social class differences in mortality continue into adult-hood and older age (Harding, 1995). During the period 1976–89, mortality rose progressively from social class I to social class V among men of working age (15–64 years), which means that men in social class I had an SMR of only 66, compared to an SMR of 134 for men in social Class V (see Table 3.2). Moreover, although social class differences narrowed with age, the gradient remained even after retirement, which means that in old age men from social class V had a mortality rate more than 50% higher than the rate for men in social class I. There was also evidence from the Longitudinal Survey that the class gradient widened rather than narrowed in the 1980s (see Table 3.2).

This class gradient is seen not only for the mortality rate overall, but also in relation to causes of death. For men of working age, it is most marked for lung cancer and respiratory disease, so that the risk of dying from respiratory disease in the period 1979–83 was six times higher for men in social class V than for men in social class I. For women of working age, the differences are most marked for respiratory disease and ischaemic heart disease. A notable reversing of the gradient occurs for deaths from breast cancer, which is more common in women of higher social class.

This pattern of a clear social class gradient for mortality is also apparent for morbidity. For example, White *et al.* (1993) found that people in manual social classes were nearly twice as likely to report experiencing breathlessness and bringing up phlegm as were people in non-manual social classes. They were also less likely to describe themselves as being in good health. Data from the General Household Survey (GHS) show that the social class gradient for morbidity is steepest for limiting long-standing illness, and less steep but still marked for less serious illness. For both categories, class differences are greatest in middle age, suggesting that there is a cumulative effect of life circumstances on health. Findings from the Health and Lifestyles Survey (Blaxter, 1990) echo those of the GHS. The health of those who took part was classified across four different measures of morbidity. People from lower social classes fared worse on each measure, reporting more common symptoms such as headache or backache, higher rates of disease such as bronchitis and arthritis, higher rates of psychosocial malaise such as sleep problems, and poorer self-assessed health status. At the start of adult life, the differences were small, but they widened by middle age and persisted into older age for the more subjective measures, even though they narrowed for the more objective ones.

The social class gradient is also clear across a whole range of other measures of health. For example, data from the 1995 Health Survey for England show that, overall, for men under 55 years of age the accident rate is higher for manual than non-manual workers. The 1980 Survey of Height and Weight showed that, in almost all age groups, people from manual households were shorter on average than people living in non-manual households. Childhood obesity was also more common in manual households. The 1978 Adult Dental Health Survey (Todd *et al.*, 1982) found that the proportion of people with no natural teeth was much lower in social class I than in social class V. A parallel survey in children (Todd and Dodd, 1985) found that 5-year-olds from manual households had twice as many actively decayed teeth and more teeth missing because of decay as children from non-manual households.

Because they collect data at only one time point, studies such as these can only suggest associations between different variables. However, a few studies have followed people over time in order to investigate the causal effects of factors such as social class on health. Power *et al.* (1996) analysed data from

Table 3.2 Mortality of men aged 15–64 years at death by social class in 1971 and period of death

Social class in 1971	Period of death											
	1976–81		1982–85		1986–89		1976–89	
	Deaths	SMR	Deaths	SMR	Deaths	SMR	Deaths	SMR
I	159	69	87	61	93	67	339	66
II	749	78	424	78	362	80	1535	79
IIIN	524	103	280	98	214	85	1018	97
IIIM	1698	95	1052	101	931	102	3681	99
IV	913	109	507	113	414	112	1834	111
V	425	124	240	136	222	153	887	134
Armed Forces	25	102	18	98	19	88	62	96
Inadequately described	92	173	40	144	37	145	169	159
Unoccupied	272	212	99	165	83	137	454	182
All men aged 15–64 years	4857	100	2827	100	2375	100	9979	100

Source: OPCS longitudinal study on social class differences in mortality in men (Harding, 1995).
SMR, standardized mortality ratio.

the National Child Development Study, in which a cohort of children born in one week in 1958 have been followed into adulthood. At the age of 33 years, there was a clear association between poor health (albeit self-rated) and social class for both men and women, which could be accounted for by prior poor health and social class at birth and at ages 16 and 23 years. The key message is that differential lifetime socio-economic circumstances, of which social class is an important indicator, play a major role in creating health inequality.

Poverty and health

The notion that 'wealth buys health' (*The Observer*, 9 January 2000) is certainly supported by research evidence. It has been shown that not only are poorer people more likely to experience ill health, but they are also less likely to survive it. For example, 5-year survival rates for cancer differ by up to 16% between the most affluent and the poorest people in the UK (Coleman *et al.*, 1999). Kaplan and colleagues (Kaplan *et al.*, 1996) looked at the relationship between income inequality and mortality in the USA. Income inequality was defined as the percentage of total household income received by the less well off 50% of all households in each US state. It was significantly correlated with all-cause and age-specific mortality, as well as with other measures of health, including rates of low birth weight (the single most important predictor of death in the first month of life), work disability and expenditure on medical care. Income inequality was a strong predictor of trends in mortality between 1980 and 1990, states with greater inequality showing smaller declines in mortality through the decade.

Other indicators of wealth, such as housing tenure and car ownership, have also been shown to be associated with mortality rates. Filakti and Fox (1995) used data from the UK Londitudinal Study (see above) to examine the relationship between these two surrogates for wealth and mortality rates. The highest rates were among people living in local authority accommodation and those without access to a car (see Table 3.3). Moreover, although the mortality rates declined for all groups over the period that was studied, the differentials between them widened rather than decreased. Differences have also been found in levels of morbidity. Breeze and colleagues (Breeze *et al.*, 1999) used Longitudinal Study data to examine the rates of limiting long-standing illness in old age, and reported a clear association between ill health and earlier socio-economic status as measured by housing tenure and car ownership. Eachus and colleagues used the Townsend deprivation score (calculated on the basis of housing tenure, car ownership, level of overcrowding and employment status) to examine levels of morbidity among people in one UK health region, and found that material deprivation was strongly linked with many common diseases, especially diabetic eye disease, bronchitis, asthma and depression (Eachus *et al.*, 1996). Consistent with these findings, 'low-income' respondents in the Health and Lifestyles Survey (those whose household income was £100 per week or less) had clearly poorer than average health and were significantly more likely to report more than one health problem (Blaxter, 1990).

Table 3.3 Direct age-standardized all-cause mortality rates by housing tenure and car access: 1971 and 1981 Census cohorts

| | Death rates per 1000 population 1981–89 | |
	Males	**Females**
Owner occupiers	9.5	5.7
Private renters	11.3	6.8
Local authority tenants	12.7	7.5
1+ cars	9.2	5.8
No cars	13.0	7.2

Source: Population Trends 81, Autumn 1995.

Such findings beg a number of questions, the first being whether the differences in mortality and morbidity that have been shown by social class are simply the result of differences in level of wealth. Based on data from the Health and Lifestyles Survey, Blaxter (1990) concluded that they are, since the apparently strong association between social class and health appears to be 'primarily an association of income and health'. Other research indicates that the situation may be more complex. The Whitehall studies (Marmot *et al.*, 1984a, 1991) followed two very large cohorts of civil servants, none of whom were 'poor by any absolute standard' (Marmot, 1995). They were all people in white-collar jobs, in stable employment and living in one part of the country, so that many of the factors that could contribute to socio-economic differences in health were in effect controlled for. Despite this, there was a clear gradient in mortality by employment grade for all major causes, as well as for rates of non-fatal disease and sickness absence. This implies that although the link between poverty and health is important, other factors also play a part in the creation of health inequalities.

The second question is whether the association between poverty and poor health can be influenced by changes in income distribution. Although the answer may seem to be self-evident on the basis of the evidence presented above, it is the subject of a perennial debate in the literature on the causes of health inequalities and how they might best be reduced. We shall consider this debate in more detail in the next section.

Summary

- The concept of health inequality focuses on differences in the distribution of health generated by socio-economic forces rather than biology. The reduction of health inequalities is a major target for the World Health Organization.
- A series of studies have demonstrated that there is a clear association between health inequality and social class. Social class differences in health are apparent across all age groups and for a variety of health indicators.
- Longitudinal studies show that social class exerts a long-term effect on health. Poor health and low social class at birth and in childhood are followed by poor health and low social class in adulthood.

- Poverty is another important determinant of health inequality. There is considerable support for the argument that social class differences in health are largely a reflection of differences in wealth. However, research suggests that other facets of social class may also be important and exert independent effects.

The materialist debate

There is a fundamental divide between people who attribute inequalities in health to structural aspects of society and those who view them as being generated by individual behaviour. Proponents of the *structuralist* or *materialist* perspective emphasize factors which are external to the individual (e.g. poverty, poor housing and work conditions and environmental pollution) as the causes of poor health. The Black Report, while acknowledging the potential role of other non-structuralist factors, aligned itself clearly with the materialist position. While acknowledging overall improvements in living and working conditions during the twentieth century, the authors of the Black Report emphasized their concern with the effects of *relative* material deprivation and accompanying *relative* health disadvantage. Support for their position comes from a recent analysis by Wilkinson (1992), which showed that in a sample of industrialized countries, life expectancy increased as the distribution of wealth became more egalitarian, but was only poorly correlated with average income. The implication of Wilkinson's findings is that the doubling of UK household disposable incomes in the last two decades (Pullinger and Summerfield, 1998) is of considerably less significance than the increase in the proportion of people with a net disposable income below average in explaining the persistent 'health gap' between the well off and the less well off.

It has been estimated by one supporter of the materialist perspective that at least 20% of the NHS clinical budget is spent on trying to cure illness caused by structuralist factors such as unemployment, poverty, bad housing and environmental pollution (Lawson, 1996). The authors of the Acheson Report, although cautious about making a direct link between poverty and ill health, recognized that people living on low incomes have insufficient money to buy items and services such as food and fuel, which are essential to good health. They proposed changes in taxation to shift the tax burden from lower-income groups, along with changes in the welfare benefits system, which would target the most disadvantaged groups in society.

In contrast to the structuralist position, the *cultural/behavioural* perspective proposes that differences in *individual* behaviour and lifestyle (e.g. smoking, diet, alcohol consumption and exercise) are the key to understanding inequalities in health. This concentration on the role of the individual fits within a wider sociological debate about whether the concept of class still has meaning in contemporary society, where the emphasis is on self-identity, consumption and lifestyle (Annandale, 1998). The behavioural perspective was the one adopted by the last Conservative government in its document *The Health of the Nation* (Department of Health, 1992), which focused attention squarely on such factors in its discussion of how to reduce excess morbidity and mortality. It implies that since improvements in health can be achieved through changes in personal activities, what are most needed are educational initiatives to encourage such changes. It also raises the uncomfortable underlying question of whether people with non-health-promoting lifestyles which they are unwilling to change 'deserve' good health and health care. Seen in this light, the concept of health promotion becomes a highly political one in that it effectively ignores structural disadvantage as a cause of health inequality. Indeed, it has been argued that health promotion campaigns are no more than a way of deflecting public attention from the failure of government to address structural issues. Such campaigns may even, it is suggested, accentuate rather than lessen health inequalities by appealing more to higher-income groups (Bunton, 1995) and being more easily taken up by them.

It has been suggested that the argument between the materialist and behaviouralist perspectives is a sterile one, since both views are correct. Certainly, interpreting the evidence is difficult and highlights the complexity of the link between socio-economic position and lifestyle. We know, for example, that poverty, poor housing and smoking behaviour are interconnected (Graham, 1993). Some authors contend that a position which emphasizes 'the social rootedness of lifestyles' while largely discounting 'any influence of the social and material environment' is unhelpful (Davey Smith *et al.*, 1990). Others are of the opinion that the two cannot realistically be separated. For example, it has been suggested that indices such as income may do more than just measure contemporary material circumstances. They may also act as proxy measures for psychosocial stressors which influence health (Der *et al.*, 1999). The argument being made here is that people who are socio-economically disadvantaged are also subject to a greater number of life stresses, which increases their susceptibility to poorer health. In the next section, we shall consider further what is known about the relationship between psychosocial stress and health.

Summary

- The materialist perspective on health inequalities emphasizes the importance of factors such as poverty and unemployment, poor housing and environmental pollution. It is concerned with the effects of *relative* rather than *absolute* material deprivation and health disadvantage.
- The cultural/behavioural perspective views health inequalities as being rooted in individual behaviour and lifestyle. Factors such as diet, smoking habits, alcohol consumption and exercise are regarded as critical to the maintenance of health and avoidance of ill health.
- Some researchers maintain that lifestyle factors are clearly separate from factors relating to the socio-economic environment, while others maintain that the two are inextricably linked.
- The materialist–cultural debate is a politically highly charged one, since proponents of the one position emphasize the role and responsibilities of

society, while proponents of the other emphasize the role and responsibilities of the individual.

Social stress and health

The relationship between psychosocial stressors and ill health can be approached in a number of different ways. Some researchers have focused on the idea that particular periods of life (e.g. adolescence) create stress, while others have been more interested in the way in which a person's life course can configure to produce stress. Some have examined the particular stresses of family life, while others have looked at those of the workplace. Some have studied the impact of specific individual life events (e.g. bereavement, unemployment), while others have focused on the longer-term effects of occupying particular social roles and positions. All of these competing explanations of the relationship between stress and health have to a greater or lesser degree been absorbed into our everyday understanding of the causes of illness, so that we often attribute our own ill health to one or other of them. Another important focus of study has been the way in which a person who is exposed to a particular life stress can utilize personal resources to mitigate its effects. Here again different approaches have been taken, with some researchers focusing on the importance of internal psychological resources (e.g. coping responses) and others concentrating on the importance of external factors (e.g. the level of available social support).

Life change and ill health

One focus of research has been on the way in which significant changes in a person's life and social circumstances create stress and so contribute to ill health. For example, studies have looked at the effects of becoming unemployed, and have shown that people who do so are at increased risk of chronic physical ill health and of dying from conditions such as heart disease and lung cancer. They are also at increased risk of poor mental health, manifested at its most extreme by higher rates of suicide and attempted suicide. One study showed that the likelihood of the latter increased as the duration of unemployment extended (Platt and Kreitman, 1984). Conversely, a recent study has shown that the suicide rate in England and Wales is decreasing in line with rising levels of employment (McClure, 2000). The link between unemployment and ill health was highlighted in a study by Banks and Jackson (1982) which assessed the mental health of adolescents before and after they left school. Those who went on to employment showed improved mental health after leaving school, whereas those who were unable to find work had poorer mental health, yet there were no differences between the two groups while these individuals were at school. The deleterious health effects of being unemployed are also supported by the finding that the mental health of people re-entering the work-force after a period of unemployment is significantly improved (Whitehead, 1988). Another important finding is that the effects of unemployment on ill health are not limited to people who find themselves in this position, but extend to other family members.

Another change in social circumstances that is known to be associated with ill health is bereavement. At every age, people who are widowed have an increased mortality risk compared to those who are married, although the excess risk is greater for men than for women, particularly in the earlier months of their bereavement. People who are widowed have also been shown to consult doctors more often, take more medication, have higher symptom and illness rates and poorer mental health than their married counterparts. The apparently protective effect of marriage on health is supported by findings from a study in the USA, which followed deaths among both widowed and married people over a 12-year period. Mortality rates were found to be higher among the widowed, but the likelihood of dying was reduced by remarriage (Helsing *et al.*, 1981). The seemingly self-evident conclusion is that grief is bad for your health, and that people can indeed die from a 'broken heart'. The reality is, of course, that the process by which the one translates to the other is complex and allows for a number of different possible mechanisms (Bowling,1987), including the following:

- grief precipitates changes in the endocrine and central nervous systems, reducing resistance to illness through the so-called 'desolation effect';
- widowed people become socially isolated and lonely because their social ties are weakened, with knock-on effects for their mental health if not their physical health;
- widowed people, particularly men, are also subject to a 'disorganizational effect' resulting from the loss of the person who provided them with material and task support, and they may adapt less than well to having to acquire a new role.

The relationship between widow(er)hood and mortality may, of course, be a combination of all of these effects. Equally, it may be that none of them is really important and the relationship is artefactual – the product of a process of 'selective mating' whereby people of similarly poor health status marry, or widowed people who are in better health remarry. Whatever the explanation, the important point is that studies such as those of unemployment or bereavement are concerned with examining the loss of a particular social status and the acquisition of a less desirable one, and the health costs that are consequent upon the change. Change that is represented as loss is stressful and thus increases a person's vulnerability to ill health.

Life events and health

Another set of theories about the effects of stress on health concerns the idea that particular life events, as opposed to status changes, are stressful and so precipitate ill health. Holmes and Rahe (1967) drew up a scaled list of events, the Social Readjustment Rating Scale (SRRS), which could reasonably be regarded as disruptive to the normal pattern of a person's life (see Table 3.4).

The life events included in the list ranged from the death of a spouse (considered to be the most traumatic) to a minor violation of the law (considered to be the least traumatic). Values for each event were determined by asking a sample of people how much readjustment they would require, relative to marriage. For any individual completing the scale, their score is the sum of the values for each event that they have experienced in the recent past. Research

Table 3.4 Social Readjustment Rating Scale

Rank	Life event	Mean value
1	Death of spouse	100
2	Divorce	73
3	Marital separation	65
4	Jail term	63
5	Death of close family member	63
6	Personal injury or illness	53
7	Marriage	50
8	Fired at work	47
9	Marital reconciliation	45
10	Retirement	45
11	Change in health of family member	44
12	Pregnancy	40
13	Sex difficulties	39
14	Gain of new family member	39
15	Business readjustment	39
16	Change in financial state	38
17	Death of close friend	37
18	Change to different line of work	36
19	Change in number of arguments with spouse	35
20	Mortgage over $10 000	31
21	Foreclosure of mortgage or loan	30
22	Change in responsibilities at work	29
23	Son or daughter leaving home	29
24	Trouble with in-laws	29
25	Outstanding personal achievement	28
26	Wife beginning or stopping work	26
27	Beginning or ending school	26
28	Change in living conditions	25
29	Revision of personal habits	24
30	Trouble with boss	23
31	Change in work hours or conditions	20
32	Change in residence	20
33	Change in schools	20
34	Change in recreation	20
35	Change in church activities	19
36	Change in social activities	19
37	Mortgage or loan less than $10 000	18
38	Change in sleeping habits	17
39	Change in number of family get-togethers	16
40	Change in eating habits	15
41	Vacation	13
42	Christmas	12
43	Minor violations of the law	11

Source: Holmes and Rahe (1967).

by the scale's authors showed that there was a relationship between high scores on the scale and poor health. For example, 49% of a group of physicians who were classed as 'high risk' by virtue of their recent life events reported ill health over a 9-month period, compared with only 25% of their 'medium-risk' counterparts and 9% of their 'low-risk' counterparts.

Although the ideas behind the SRRS make intuitive sense, it has been heavily criticized. The main arguments against it are as follows.

- The assumption is that the events contained in the SRRS are necessarily negative. However (as discussed above), just as judgements about what constitutes good or poor health have been shown to be subjective, so is the experience of life events. What is traumatic and health-threatening for one person may be benign or even actively health-promoting for another. Any assessment of the impact of life events would therefore need to allow for this possibility. Equally, no allowance is made for the possibility that, even if the events included in the SRRS are all universally viewed as negative, their effects may be mitigated by other unrecorded positive events in a person's life.
- If information about life events is collected retrospectively, it is open to selective recall and bias. A person who is asked about such events may either over- or underestimate their occurrence, and may assess their impact differently depending on whether they are now ill or well. One of the findings of sociological studies of chronically ill people is that they try to make sense of their illness by searching for explanations in their past behaviour and life course (Williams, 1984). As a result, they may place more emphasis on the significance of experienced life events than they would have done if they had remained well.
- Although they are assumed to be discrete, life events may interact with one another, either intensifying or mediating their individual effects. The SRRS makes no allowance for such interactions, and is over-simplistic in its treatment of the impact of different events as cumulative. In addition, it does not make any allowance for events which do *not* occur, as opposed to those that do, so it ignores the possibility of the negative impact of a hoped for event that did not materialize.
- A high score can be obtained in a number of different ways. It could be the result of one major life event or of several minor ones, and there is no evidence to support the implicit assumption that the outcome for health would be the same.

Summary

- Research into the relationship between social stress and health has explored the influence of particular life events, specific life phases, occupying particular social roles and the impact of status changes.
- A considerable body of research which has examined the association between behaviour and ill health suggests that grief is bad for one's health, and a number of possible mechanisms by which the one translates to the other have been suggested.

- People who become unemployed are at increased risk of physical and mental ill health and death. Re-entry to the labour force has a positive effect on health.
- The idea that specific life events can contribute to ill health was first developed by Holmes and Rahe. Using a scale that ranked a range of life events from the most serious to the least serious, they found a relationship between high scores on the scale and poor health.
- It would appear that both longer-term and more immediate stressors can contribute to the loss of health.

Social support and health

If we accept the basic premise that stress predisposes people to ill health, we next need to explore why it is that only some people who experience particular life events or occupy particular unfavourable social positions or social roles become ill. One explanation that has been alluded to above concerns the meaning that individuals attach to their situations. Another which has received considerable research attention and to which we shall now turn is the potentially protective effect of social support. The basic thesis is that social support or the lack of it can influence health either directly or indirectly by acting as a buffer against stress. Just as grief is bad for your health, so social support, it is maintained, is good for it.

Social support is linked to, although conceptually distinct from, the concept of social networks. Network analysis was developed by sociologists and social anthropologists, who argued that the characteristics of social networks were important determinants of the behaviour of individuals involved in them (Bowling, 1991). Social networks are the set of people with whom we maintain contact and have some kind of social bond. Clearly, while such networks can be highly supportive, they may also fail to provide support, depending on their size, geographical dispersion, level of integration, composition, frequency of contact, and level of intimacy and reciprocity. However, when they are good, social networks are known to lengthen life and improve health (Wilkinson *et al.*, 1998). The concept of social support is concerned with the extent to which individuals feel themselves to be held in high regard by the members of their social network (Cobb, 1976). Schaefer and colleagues distinguish three different types of support – *emotional* (intimacy and attachment), *tangible* (provision of direct aid or services such as money or goods) and *informational* (information, advice and feedback on how a person is doing) (Schaefer *et al.*, 1981). It would appear that the first of these is the single most valued feature of social support (Gottlieb, 1978). Their preoccupation with the notion of social support as an explanatory variable in health and social behaviour means that social scientists have developed a large number of scales purporting to measure it – one recent review identified 33 of them (O'Reilly, 1988).

One of the pivotal studies of the relationship between social support and health was the Alameda County study in the USA, which followed nearly

7000 adults over a period of 12 years (Berkman and Syme, 1979). Mortality from all causes was found to be greater in people with low levels of social support, independent of factors such physical health, socio-economic status, lifestyle and life satisfaction. Subsequent studies have confirmed the health-promoting effects of social support. For example, one of the most famous studies of the link between social factors and health showed that women who lacked an intimate friend were at significantly higher risk of depression (Brown and Harris, 1978). The UK Health and Lifestyles Survey (Blaxter, 1990) showed that illness, psychosocial ill health and disease or disability were all reported more often by people with low levels of social support and integration. Health, especially psychosocial health, showed a marked decline for both men and women as social integration declined – those with the weakest ties had the lowest level of well-being. Perceived social support was also clearly related to illness and psychosocial malaise. In people over 40 years of age, having little social support was unimportant with regard to health if income was high, but made more difference if income was low. For younger men, income was unimportant as long as they had good social support, and for younger women, social support was more important than income (see Figure 3.4).

The main hypotheses about the way in which the effects of social support are bestowed include the theory that it affects health directly and the theory that it acts as a buffer to stress. Although both hypotheses can be supported by the available evidence, support is stronger for the former than for the latter (Radley, 1994). It is still unclear whether social support influences health by altering a person's behaviour, physiology, perceptions, or all three (Cohen and Syme, 1985). The Acheson Report on health inequalities recognized the importance of social support in mediating the effects of low socio-economic status, and argued for housing policies that allow people to maintain their social networks and systems of social support. However, it has been argued that the health-promoting effects of social support cannot cancel out the health-damaging effects of poverty, and that the danger of the social support thesis is that it may have political appeal in a way that direct action to improve living conditions does not (Oakley, 1992).

The concepts of social support and social networks are not new to the social sciences. They extend back as far as Durkheim's theory of 'anomie'. A new spin on them has been given by the concept of *social capital*, which is concerned with social connections and 'the features of social organization, such as trust, norms and networks that can improve the efficiency of society by facilitating co-ordinated actions' (Putnam, 1994). The availability or lack of social capital to particular groups in the population will, its theorists maintain, have a major impact on the quality of their lives, including the level of their health.

Summary

* Just as stress appears to predispose people to the loss of health, so social support appears to help to preserve it.

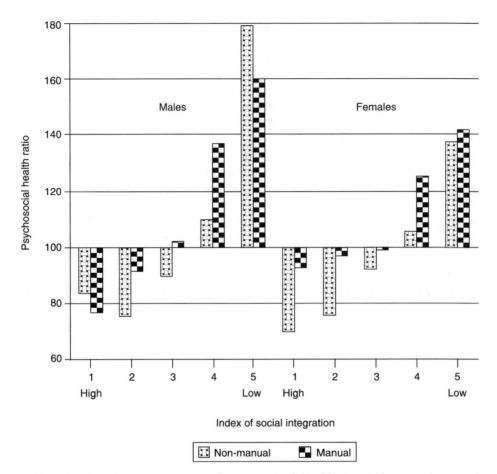

Figure 3.4 Social integration, social support and health. Note that a value on the psychosocial health ratio of 100 represents the mean. A lower value represents less ill health; a higher value represents greater ill health. From Blaxter N (1990) *Health and lifestyle*. London: Tavistock.

* Social support may influence health directly, by altering a person's behaviour.
* It may also influence health indirectly, by acting as a buffer against stress.
* The health-promoting effects of social support are unlikely to cancel out the health-reducing effects of poverty and socio-economic deprivation.

Gender and health

One of the findings that has emerged from research into the relationship between particular life events and ill health is that men and women express concern about different types of events, and react to the same events with different symptoms (Conger *et al.*, 1993). This touches on a much wider debate within the field of sociology of health and illness, about the importance of gender as a determinant of health, and the extent to which the recorded differences in health and ill health between men and women are the product of biology or of social role. As we shall see, proponents of the latter view argue that the stress of the social role that women occupy is key to understanding the observed differences. So what are these differences?

It has been described as an 'established sociological wisdom' (Annandale, 1998) that in modern western societies men are at higher risk of death, while women are at higher risk of ill health. However, we know that women have not always been in a position of mortality advantage (nor are they today in other parts of the world). Historical studies suggest that in the sixteenth and seventeenth centuries men fared better than women, but by the early nineteenth century their position was equal. By the second half of the twentieth century the position was reversed, so that women had a higher life expectancy than men, and the most recent evidence indicates that their relative advantage over men may now be waning (Annandale, 1998). Women's acquired health advantage can be attributed to both medical and social factors. Improvements in reproductive practices and in the management of pregnancy and childbirth reduced women's risk of mortality, while at the same time changes in their social status and economic circumstances played an important role. Speculation about the causes of the suggested reduction in this advantage hangs on the notion that women now behave 'more like a man', as evidenced by their increased levels of cigarette and alcohol consumption.

Despite their advantage (at least for the present) in terms of mortality, research has repeatedly shown that women experience, or at least report, more illness than men. For example, in the Health and Lifestyles Survey, women reported a higher average number of symptoms than men, and twice as many women as men reported experiencing at least six symptoms over a 1-month period. Women are more likely to experience depressive and other mental illness than men and to be admitted to hospital because of such illness. Women also fare less well in terms of their general well-being. Data from the Oxford Healthy Lifestyles Survey (Jenkinson *et al.*, 1996) show that women of all ages have poorer self-assessed health than men. Finally, women seek medical help more often than men (see Table 3.5).

Table 3.5 GP consultations: percentage of individuals who consulted a doctor in the 14 days before interview: UK, 1991

Economic activity status	Men (age in years)				Women (age in years)			
	16–44	45–64	65 and over	Total	16–44	45–64	65 and over	Total
Working	8	9	12	8	14	15	10	14
Unemployed	10	11	0	10	25	13	0	22
Economically inactive	18	22	19	20	20	20	19	20
All persons	9	11	18	11	17	17	19	17

Source: Office of Population Censuses and Surveys 1993.

There are some important caveats to the seemingly self-evident conclusion to be drawn from such data, namely that women have poorer health than men. For example, it has been argued that the finding that they experience higher rates of mental illness may simply reflect the generation of new categories of mental illness and the 'medicalization' of women's problems by a male-dominated medical profession, and so should not necessarily be taken at face value (Hardey, 1998). The differences in self-reported health status between men and women that were reported in the Oxford study were often small and unimportant, and may have been the product of differences in their perceptions of symptoms and in their propensity to report them. It also appears that a large part of the difference in consultation rates can be accounted for by conditions relating to reproduction. Macintyre *et al.* (1996) analysed two large data sets and concluded that in fact morbidity is consistently higher for women only with respect to psychological symptoms, while with regard to some physical symptoms, women actually do better than men.

If we accept that the picture is not quite so simple as it first appears, in the context of the present discussion we need to consider to what extent the greater ill health of women can be attributed to their social role and its associated stresses. To do this, we must first revisit the earlier discussion about the protective effect of marriage. We have already seen that married people have a lower risk of mortality than those who are not married. Married people also fare better on objective measures of morbidity. For example, blood pressure levels have been found to be significantly lower among married people than in those who are single (Macintyre, 1992). The explanation which is commonly offered for such findings is that in modern western societies marriage gives meaning and significance to daily life, and hence promotes a sense of well-being. The decline in the popularity of marriage and the accompanying trend towards cohabitation makes the relationship between marriage and health more difficult to evaluate than when many of the original studies were conducted. However, the limited data available suggest that the health of cohabitees parallels that of married people more closely than it does that of those who are single (Hardey, 1998).

That said, it is also the case that the health gains from marriage are greater for men than for women, even after other social factors that are known to be important have been taken into account. Early proponents of social role theories about the relationship between gender and health generally took the view that the emotional and physical labour that women commit themselves to in marriage explains its contribution to gendered health inequality. Women have poorer health because they occupy multiple social roles and so find themselves in an inherently more stressful position than men. Certainly studies have repeatedly shown that despite the fact that in the majority of present-day families both parents work outside the home, the domestic division of labour remains unequal, with women carrying much greater responsibility for mundane domestic tasks. The same appears to be true in relation to childcare, where women are most often responsible for the routine aspects and men for the more enjoyable ones (Burghes *et al.*, 1997). Marriage would thus appear to impose a greater role strain on women, who are consequently more vulnerable to ill health.

However, subsequent research has shown that to attribute women's health problems to the conflict caused by their adopting multiple roles over-simplifies the issue. In fact, it has been shown that it is those women who stay at home who report the worst health (Kane, 1994), while employment outside the home appears to confer a positive effect (Nathanson, 1980) by promoting a sense of self-esteem and satisfaction and providing valued social relationships. Arber *et al.* (1985) showed that paid work was beneficial to women of all ages without children, and to women over 40 years of age with children (presumably by providing them with a valued role), whereas women under 40 years with children appeared to be more subject to role strain and thus to ill health. In contrast, in one study conducted in four European countries, women who worked were much healthier overall than women who stayed at home, but their levels of anxiety were much higher – perhaps indicative of the role strain that they were experiencing. Annandale (1998) pointed out that what such apparently conflicting pieces of information should remind us is 'that knowing a person occupies a particular role or social position tells us very little about their experience of it.' She highlights the importance of trying to take into account both the quality of the role and the meaning given to it by its occupier. If men and women, or women at different life stages, attach different meanings to their work, marital and family roles, the associated health benefits or disbenefits may also be different.

One further factor to be added to this already complex equation is that gender differences in health are compounded by other social situational differences. Women are economically disadvantaged compared to men. If they are in paid work, they are likely to be in lower-status jobs and earning less. They also more often work part-time and so are less well protected with regard to insurance schemes. At home, the distribution of labour and resources similarly disadvantages them (Pahl, 1990). As a result, they are more likely to be living in poverty than men, and as we showed earlier this is a major determinant of health.

Of course, none of the above should be taken to imply that biological factors are unimportant in accounting for the health differences between men and women. Women do appear to enjoy some advantage both from the positive health effects of the female hormones and from differences in genetic make-up, which may confer on them an increased resistance to infectious disease (Radley, 1994). Nonetheless, studies of large data sets support the view that 'gender differences in health are rooted in social roles, against a backdrop of some male biological disadvantage' (Macintyre *et al.*, 1996).

Summary

- Gender differences in health may be rooted in biology. Alternatively, they may reflect the differing social roles of men and women.
- An 'established sociological wisdom' is that men are at higher risk of death and women are at higher risk of ill health. However, the most recent evidence suggests that women's relative health advantage may be diminishing.

- Women report more ill health than men and seek medical help more often, but there are important caveats to the conclusion that they are less healthy.
- Marriage provides more of a health-promoting effect for men than it does for women, perhaps because for the latter group it imposes a greater role strain.
- Counter to this argument, researchers have shown that women who are employed outside the home have better health than those who stay at home.
- Gender differences in health are complicated by other social situational differences – for example, women are more likely to live in poverty than men.

Ethnicity and health

Another relationship in which both biology and social context appear to be important is that between health and ethnicity. In this section, we shall look briefly at the evidence linking these two variables and highlight some problems in doing so.

The first of these problems, according to Annandale (1998), is that effective research has been hampered by 'a lack of sensitivity to the meaning of categories such as "race", ethnicity and the concept of racism'. For example, the terms 'white' and 'black' fail to take into account the heterogeneity of subgroups contained within these broad categories. A second problem is that much of the research on which we can draw is now rather dated, it relies on information about country of birth rather than ethnic status (and thus ignores the issue of how patterns of health and ill health may change across different generations of people from ethnic minority groups) and it tends to be limited to the analysis of mortality rather than morbidity. A third problem concerns the relationship between 'race' and social class, and the way in which they may interact to produce inequalities in health. The danger here, on the one hand, is that issues of ethnicity are regarded as important only in as much as people from ethnic minorities are socially and economically disadvantaged, rather than as having a significance of their own. On the other hand, the importance of socio-economic disadvantage may be overlooked, and health inequalities by ethnicity may be viewed simply as the product of cultural norms, which therefore need to be changed.

The 1971 Census was the first UK Census in which respondents were asked to provide information about the country of their birth, and which therefore allowed an analysis of mortality rates in people born outside the UK, compared with those born within it. From the data, Marmot *et al.* (1984b) were able to show that the causes of death differed markedly between different migrant groups. For some causes of death, Marmot and colleagues found a clear and persisting effect of the country of origin (the mortality risk of the immigrant populations was similar to that for their place of birth), while for others the pattern was less stable. This suggests a highly complex interplay of genetic, early and later environmental risks and the process of 'acculturation'. This issue has subsequently been explored in studies of, for example, Japanese migrants to the USA (Syme *et al.*, 1975) and Polish migrants to the UK (Adelstein *et al.*, 1979), which have shown that the patterns of mortality between immigrant and native populations tended to converge over time.

In contrast to those investigations, Harding *et al.* (1996), who studied mortality rates in second-generation Irish immigrants living in the UK, found a clear inter-generational effect both for mortality overall and for cause-specific mortality. Socio-economic indicators such as social class and housing tenure could not account for this inter-generational health disadvantage, but the authors suggested a number of alternative explanations, including lifestyle factors, the breakdown of family ties (and hence of social support) and the loss of cultural identity.

In 1991, the Census questions were changed and respondents were asked to identify their ethnic status, as opposed to their country of birth. This allowed researchers to explore the link between ethnic status and self-reported health. Reported rates of limiting long-standing illness were found to be lowest among people who identified themselves as Chinese, and were highest for Pakistani men and women and Bangladeshi men (see Figure 3.5). Other recent studies (Health Education Council, 1994; Fenton *et al.*, 1995) have indicated that people from minority ethnic groups tend to rate their health as poorer than the UK population as a whole. For example, in the study by Fenton *et al.* (1995), the proportion who described their health as

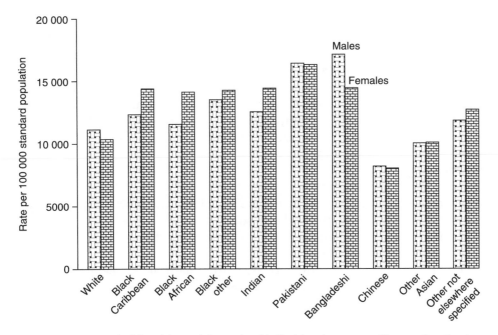

Figure 3.5 Household residents (all ages) with limiting long-term illness: directly standardized rates by ethnic group and sex, 1991, UK. From Charlton J, Wallace M and White I (1994) Long-term illness: results from the 1991 Census. In: *Population trends 75. Spring 1994*. London: HMSO.

only fair or poor was 43% among Black Caribbean people, 41% among Indian people, 44% among Bangladeshis and 61% among Pakistanis, compared to a figure of 29% for respondents in the Health and Lifestyles Survey. Some studies have indicated that people from minority ethnic groups also make greater use of the health services, although others have shown no difference (Smaje, 1995).

A recent review of the literature on ethnicity and health (Ahmad *et al.*, 1996) focuses on differences according to ethnic group in rates of ill health across three major areas, namely cardiovascular disease, mental health and haemoglobinopathies. The review shows that:

- South Asian and Afro-Caribbean populations in the UK experience significantly elevated rates of cardiovascular disease;
- men and women born in the Caribbean are at greater risk of schizophrenia;
- people born in South Asia are at lower risk of psychological morbidity;
- the rates of particular disorders of the haemoglobin (specifically, sickle-cell disorders and thalassaemia) are higher in certain ethnic groups.

The authors of the review point out that such differences should not be viewed as natural and inevitable, or as the result of undesirable cultural practices. They may in part be the result of structural inequalities and associated barriers to the accessibility of high-quality health care. Nazroo (1998) has emphasized that not only socio-economic position, but also the experience of harassment and discrimination, may be important in explaining the variations in health across different ethnic groups.

The message from all of this is that there are important differences in health and ill health in relation to ethnicity, but that the pattern of disadvantage is not uniform, and its existence and relationship to other factors are not yet fully understood. Furthermore, the issue of ethnicity and health is one that is currently relatively under-researched and, in the view of some (Annandale, 1998), limited by an 'intellectual apartheid' in which 'simple, rigid and essentialist notions of culture' are employed and the concept of health is viewed from 'an often undisclosed "white" standard.'

Summary

- Research into ethnicity and health is limited, but suggests a complex interplay of genetic, environmental and social factors.
- Studies have shown that the health of minority ethnic groups is subject to clear inter-generational effects.
- Differences in health by ethnicity are neither natural nor inevitable.
- Such differences may in part be the product of socio-economic disadvantage and societal stigma.
- Effective research into the health of minority ethnic groups has been hampered by a lack of cultural and terminological sensitivity and, perhaps, by a lack of interest.
- This has been described as a form of 'intellectual apartheid'.

Key text: the Black Report

In this section we shall critically review the Black Report, a text which has become fundamental to any discussion of social determinants of health. The Black Report has been described as 'perhaps the first [example] anywhere in the world of an attempt authorized by Government to explain trends in inequalities in health and relate them to policies intended to promote as well as restore health' (Acheson, 1999). It was published in 1980, much to the chagrin of the then Government, which gave it what its authors describe as 'a frosty reception'. The brief given to the working group appointed in 1977 and chaired by Sir Douglas Black, a former Chief Scientist at the Department of Health, was to assess national and international evidence of inequalities in health and the policy implications for reducing them. In the event, the implications were so great that the then Secretary of State found himself 'unable to endorse the Group's recommendations.'

So what did the Black Report say that caused such dissent? As already outlined above, its main message, after reviewing the available research, was that structural factors were major determinants of health or the lack of it. In reaching this conclusion, the authors also considered three other possible explanations of the health inequalities that they documented, which they referred to as follows:

- artefactual explanations;
- theories of natural selection;
- cultural/behavioural explanations.

The last explanation (and their preferred one) has been described earlier in this chapter, but it is also worth giving some attention to the other two.

The *artefactual explanation* suggests that both health and class are artificial variables developed in the course of attempts to measure social phenomena, so that any relationship between them is of no real significance. Artefactualists maintain that the failure to reduce the health gap is the product of changes in the occupational structure and the resultant reduction in the proportion of people in the lowest social classes. However, the pattern of widening differentials persists even when classes are combined, thus diluting the effects of mortality rates in the extreme group.

Another argument by the artefactualists rests on the way in which mortality statistics are derived. Since rates are calculated from two different sources – death registration certificates and Census data – it follows that an individual may be assigned to one social class at the time of Census and another at the time of death, if his or her occupation is described differently at these two events. Researchers on the UK Longitudinal Study aimed to eliminate this problem by categorizing social class at death according to the class of those concerned at the time of the 1971 Census, and they concluded that such discrepancies are relatively infrequent and not of any real significance. Under reclassification, the social class differences remained, although they were slightly smaller. Finally, it has been argued that cause-specific death rates may be biased because clinicians recording the cause of death are influenced in their attributions by their knowledge of the dead person's social class (Bloor *et al.*, 1987). If this is so, the apparent differences in cause of death by social class may not be *real* differences. The validity of artefactual explanations has been relatively poorly researched, but what evidence there is would seem to argue against it. The authors of the report themselves dismissed it by arguing that evidence from successive Census reports failed to support the postulated contraction of the lowest social classes, and that indicators of poor health applied to much wider sections of the population.

Theories of natural selection start from the premise that health determines social class, rather than that social class determines health. This happens through a process of social mobility whereby the healthy move up the social hierarchy, while the unhealthy move down it. The authors of the Black Report have been challenged about the comment in their discussion of natural selection theories that men and women are destined to be consigned to the lower social classes by virtue of their 'innate physical characteristics'. The implication is, it has been argued, that there is a genetic rather than a social basis to individuals' health prospects – a position at odds with the structuralist view which the Black Report concluded was most satisfactory.

The relationship between social mobility and mortality was investigated in the UK Longitudinal Study (Fox *et al.*, 1990), which failed to demonstrate such an association. Some people who moved from one social class to another between the 1971 and 1981 Censuses had higher mortality than the class they had left, while others had lower mortality. Moreover, the mortality of those who changed class did not differ markedly from that of those who did not change. The movement of individuals between social classes had little effect on social class mortality differentials. A mismatch between the (younger) age at which mobility generally occurs and the (older) age at which impaired health is prevalent made it unlikely, in the researchers' view, that ill health had any significant impact on mobility. However, there is some evidence that unhealthy people do experience downward mobility. Wadsworth (1986) showed that men who had been seriously ill in childhood were more likely to experience this phenomenon than others, regardless of their original class position.

It has been suggested by Annandale (1998) that disagreement about the validity of the natural selection explanation has more to do with the way in which it is framed than with its basic premise. Social sorting is likely to be as much a product of negative social discrimination against people who are ill as of any physical properties of their illness *per se*. Downward mobility, or the failure to become upwardly mobile, may also reflect the contribution of factors operating indirectly. For example, it has been shown that people who are ill in childhood tend to underachieve academically, with consequent knock-on effects for their occupational advancement.

To a large extent, support for the various explanations offered in the Black Report during the years since its publication has been a matter of political conviction. However, it has been considered unfortunate that its authors in effect dismissed all explanations but the materialist one. As the above discussion makes abundantly clear, it is likely that materialist, cultural and social selection theories all have something to offer to our understanding of the problem. In opting for one theory in preference to the others, the authors of the report not only generated an antagonistic response from government in the immediate term. In the longer term, they set the scene for a polarized debate which may have deflected attention from exploring the complex pathways by which these three different sets of factors interact to produce and maintain inequalities in health (Macintyre, 1997).

One other possible contributor to inequalities in health was given considerable attention in the Black Report, namely the matter of inequality with regard to the availability and accessibility of health services. Although its authors were quick to point out that this could never be more than a partial explanation, they nonetheless supported the notion of the 'inverse care law' (Tudor-Hart, 1971), according to which those who are in most need receive the least care. For example, they quoted research using GHS data which showed that although it appeared, on the basis of consultation rates alone, that people in lower social classes were higher GP attenders, they in fact consulted less when their health needs were taken into account. We also know that people in lower social classes make less use of preventive health and screening services, such as immunization programmes and ante- and postnatal care.

Summary

* The Black Report on inequalities in health was published in 1980.
* Its authors considered four different explanations for the evidence on health inequalities – artefactual, natural selection, cultural/behavioural and materialist.
* They made clear their support for the materialist position.
* As a result, the report was viewed as highly controversial and became the focus of considerable political dissent.

Determinants of health: the example of low birth weight

In this last section, we shall consider one commonly cited indicator of health, namely birth weight, and the influence of different types of health factors in determining whether a newborn's weight is 'normal' or 'low'. The importance of the problem of low birth weight rests on the wealth of accumulated evidence from research into the fetal origins of adult disease, which indicates that it predisposes to a wide range of developmental and health problems and can have not just short-term but also far-reaching health consequences (Barker, 1997, 1999; Hogan and Park, 2000). For example, studies have shown that small size at birth is associated with an increased risk of coronary heart disease, stroke, hypertension and diabetes in adult life.

The history of medical interest in the subject of low birth weight is summarized by Oakley (1992) in her book, *Motherhood and Social Support*. She points out that birth weight, although now regarded as an objective biological fact, is nevertheless a 'socially constructed' phenomenon. In pre-industrial societies, babies were not weighed at birth. Early interest in the birth weight of newborns stemmed from the concerns of eighteenth and nineteenth century physicians about the greater likelihood of boy babies than girl babies dying, rather than any interest in birth weight *per se*. Indeed, Oakley points out that in many societies the belief was widely held that weighing a baby was unlucky and a weighed baby would fail to thrive. The regular weighing of infants as a means of monitoring their development was first advocated in 1852, but it did not become common practice in the UK until the beginning of the twentieth century. However, from 1945, birth notifications to local authorities routinely included birth weight, and so it became one key element of modern UK national statistics.

In present-day Britain, two slightly different definitions of low birth weight are operational. These are the World Health Organization International Classification of Diseases (ICD) definition, which categorizes as of low birth weight any child weighing less than 2500 g, and the Department of Health definition, which defines a low birth weight as 2500 g or less. The arbitrariness of these definitional cut-off points is highlighted by Oakley's observation that the adoption of the ICD criterion in the UK in 1980 resulted in 1990 babies previously considered to have a 'low' birth weight being reclassified as 'normal'. This might be unimportant were it not for what Oakley refers to as the 'problematization of birth weight' (perhaps as one means by which the medical profession has been able to claim expertise over childbirth) and its application as a 'moral category' against which judgements about the quality of mothering can be made. Around whichever of the two current classifications the information is analysed, the point remains that low birth weight is the strongest identified risk factor for infant mortality. Babies who weigh less than 1500 g at birth have a 90 times higher risk of dying in infancy than babies who weigh 3000 to 3500 g (Botting, 1997).

Early research into the epidemiology of low birth weight focused on the role of clinical factors such as maternal age, height, parity and placental size (Smith, 1970), and there is renewed interest in maternal characteristics such as height and weight, as a result of the work by Barker and his colleagues on reduced fetal growth. The relationship between the quality of antenatal care and birth weight has also been investigated (Greenberg, 1983; Florey and Taylor, 1994), and the conclusion was that the former has an effect which is independent of other possible contributing variables. However, given the discussion earlier in this chapter about the link between social class and health, it should come as no surprise that low birth weight, as well as being what a Department of Health Committee reporting in 1989 described as a 'profoundly difficult biological problem', is also a social one, being considerably more common in children born to women of lower social class (see Table 3.6). Figures for 1994 show that the mean birth weight increased from 3310 g in children born to social class V fathers to 3420 g in children of social class I fathers (Botting, 1997).

Table 3.6 Mean birth weight by father's social class: England and Wales, 1994

Father's social class	Mean birth weight (g)	
	Inside marriage	Outside marriage
I	3420	3360
II	3400	3360
IIIN	3380	3280
IIIM	3350	3280
IV	3320	3280
V	3310	3230
England and Wales	3370	3280

Source: Reproduced with kind permission from Drever and Whitehead (1997).

The following question then arises. Given the list of factors now identified as predisposing to low birth weight, what – if anything – can be done to reduce the risk? From the materialist position, the solution might be thought to be to reduce material disadvantage and improve the living conditions of women in the lower social classes. There is evidence from the USA, for example, that increasing the minimum income of pregnant women increases the birth weight of their offspring (Kehrer and Wolin, 1979). From the cultural/behavioural position the best approach might be to target factors such as maternal diet or smoking patterns, for which there is considerable evidence of a link with poor fetal growth (Simpson and Armand Smith, 1986; Eskenzai and Bergmann, 1995; Perry, 1997). Evidence that major life events (Newton and Hunt, 1984) and role stresses (Pritchard and Teo, 1994) are associated with an increased risk of low birth weight would suggest to proponents of these theoretical concepts that efforts need to be directed towards reducing stresses in pregnancy, or at least providing social support systems for pregnant women who experience those stresses.

One study that set out to investigate the value of social support in reducing stress and so improving pregnancy outcomes was the one referred to above by Oakley (1992). Oakley found that fewer babies of very low birth weight were born to women who received social support that was additional to standard antenatal care (a programme of home visits and telephone calls from a midwife during the course of the pregnancy) than to women who received only standard antenatal care. She also found that both mothers and babies in the supported group were healthier in the early postnatal period. This suggests that social support can have a mediating effect on factors predictive of a poor health outcome of pregnancy, as it also appears to have with regard to other measures of health.

Discussion points

- The use of subjective, user-based measures of health status has been described as a 'new paradigm' in medicine. Governments, health care purchasers and providers and the commercial sector are all interested in using evidence derived from the application of such measures. However, their critics argue that user-based measures of health lack objectivity compared to clinical indicators such as lung function or blood pressure, and so are an unreliable guide to the effectiveness of treatment. How valid is this criticism? How valuable do you think such subjective measures are in assessing the effectiveness and cost-effectiveness of health care? What measures would you choose as indicators of the success or otherwise of a new treatment?

- Tackling health inequalities has been cited as an explicit priority in the Government papers *The New NHS* and *Our Healthier Nation*. Despite this, health inequalities appear to be increasing rather than diminishing. In your opinion, what is the most likely explanation for this? Health inequality has been described as the single most serious problem facing public health (Reid, 1997), and the reduction of poverty its single most important remedy. The recently formed UK Public Health Association has nailed its colours clearly to the materialist mast and is calling for a redistribution of wealth through taxation. Do you agree with the Association's position? Would eradicating poverty solve the problem of health inequalities, or are there other important factors to blame?

- The Inverse Care Law was developed almost 30 years ago and has become a classic reference in the health inequalities literature. This law states that 'the availability of good medical care tends to vary inversely with the need for it in the population served' (Tudor-Hart, 1971). If valid, the law provides another set of explanations for the poorer health of people who are in poorer socio-economic circumstances. Their health is worse quite simply because their care is worse. How convincing an explanation for health inequalities is the Inverse Care Law? Would the improvement of health services at a local level have an impact on the nation's health? Some researchers argue that the health service has only a minor role to play in determining levels of health. Do you agree with them? Even if there are limits to the role of the health care system in reducing health inequalities, it has been argued that universal access to high-quality and effective care should be part of any advanced civilized society (Marmot, 1999). Do you agree with this view?

- 'The primary determinants of disease are economic and social, and therefore its remedies must also be economic and social. Medicine and politics cannot and should not be kept apart' (Rose, 1992). To what extent do you agree with this statement? What should the role of Government be in tackling the determinants of disease? The present Government has created a new post of 'Minister of Public Health'. How can the creation of such a post make a useful contribution? In your view, what other strategies should the Government be adopting?

- It has been shown that targeted interventions can reduce health equalities (Gepkens and Gunning-Schepers, 1996). The types of interventions tested to date include those that are informational only, those that provide information in combination with personal support and those that provide information in combination with structural measures, such as the installation of heating systems in houses that lack them. Which types of interventions do you think would prove most effective, and why?

- Health Action Zones (HAZs) are a new initiative to bring together organizations within and outside the NHS to develop and implement a locally agreed strategy to improve the health of local people. The fundamental principle behind their development is that closer collaboration between the various public agencies can influence levels of health in communities. HAZs will pilot major changes in the organization of primary, secondary and tertiary care, in health promotion and education, and in the relationship between health authorities and local government. Among the facilities that patients in HAZs can expect to find are one-stop primary care centres (including pharmacy, dental, optician and GP services), one-stop clinics to investigate and treat health problems, and healthy living centres to offer advice on diet and fitness. How appropriate a model of health care do you think this is? How would you set out to evaluate the effectiveness of HAZs in improving the health of the population at the local level?

- 'Food poverty' refers to the lack of money, inadequate shopping facilities and poor transport options that deny poorer people healthy food choices (Webster, 1998). Food poverty is one form of health inequality, as it contributes to the reduced life expectancy of poor people and their increased propensity to serious ill health. What steps could be taken to tackle the problem of food poverty? How realistic is the view that healthy eating is possible even on a low income? The Acheson Report focused on the problem of food poverty, suggesting that one vehicle for addressing it might be the Health Action Zone. How effective do you think such an approach might be?

- It has been argued that the search for differences in health that are attributable to gender has led researchers to neglect gender similarities. Annandale and Hunt (1990) suggest that such differences and similarities are better explained by the concept of 'gender-role orientation' – that is, the degree to which men and women adopt 'masculine' or 'feminine' behaviours. How useful do you think their suggestion might be in explaining the observed gender patterning of health?

- It has been suggested that current interest in issues of ethnicity and health is a form of 'covert racism', in which the cultures of minority ethnic groups are often negatively stereotyped and the ways in which they experience ill health are ignored. To what extent do you think such a position might explain the finding that there are higher rates of schizophrenia among Afro-Caribbean men and women? Does such covert racism help to account for the fact that Afro-Caribbean people with schizophrenia are more often dealt with through the criminal justice system than through primary care? Could it help to explain why people born in the Caribbean are treated with more intensive pharmacological regimes, and less often receive psychologically based treatments?

- Blane (1999) has shown that birth weight acts as a marker both of parental social position and of a child's social conditions in later life. Poorer parental social class increases the risk of low birth weight, and low-birth-weight babies are more likely to grow up in less well-off families and poorer quality housing. This suggests what Blane refers to as 'an accumulating chain of disadvantage', in which a number of factors which may be individually unimportant combine to exert a major influence on health. How convincing is this as an explanation of the social gradient in health? The idea of 'critical social transitions' has been proposed by social scientists as being analogous to the concept of critical periods in biological development. What implications does this perspective have for health and social policy?

Acknowledgements

I would like to thank my former colleague, Roger Thomas, for his contribution to the section on the concept of social class in this chapter.

Further reading

Brown G and Harris T (1978) *The social origins of depression*. London: Tavistock.

Dunnell K (1995) *Are we healthier?* Population Trends No. 82. London: Office for National Statistics.

Macintyre S, Hunt K and Sweeting H (1996) Gender differences in health: are things really as simple as they seem? *Social Science and Medicine* **42**, 617–24.

Marmot M (1995) In sickness and in wealth: social causes of illness. *MRC News* **Winter issue**, 8–12.

Townsend P, Davidson N and Whitehead M (1988) *Inequalities in health*. Harmondsworth: Penguin.

Patients and carers

Tony Hak

Introduction

Health care in a broad sense (i.e. including preventative action, cure and care) entails a wide range of activities such as prescribing and taking medicines, providing and consuming healthy food, taking sufficient exercise and rest, etc. The major part of health care is not undertaken by professionals, such as doctors and nurses, but by lay people, by the patients themselves and by their informal carers. Doctors examine, prescribe and perform surgery, but mothers and spouses prepare food and shelter, monitor the health of their dependants and occasionally bring them to doctors. The outcomes of these activities (e.g. better health, a longer life and a better quality of life) depend on how they are performed and how they are co-ordinated. In this chapter we shall explore this type of work which is done by patients and their informal carers. This work will be discussed in terms of the main concepts listed above.

The sociological approach to these issues of lay health work is defined by two questions.

1. What is the *meaning (significance)* of the discussed phenomenon (complaint, disability, illness, treatment, etc.) to the individuals involved (patients, relatives and carers)?
2. How is their behaviour *organized and co-ordinated*?

These two questions point to pertinent aspects of health and illness that cannot be 'seen' from the biomedical perspective. The difference between the biomedical perspective and the sociological approach can be illuminated by the difference between the concepts of the (biomedical) *body* and the (social) *person*. Bodies have diseases but people feel sick and 'fall ill'. There is no direct relationship between these two types of event. A person's body might host a virus or a tumour without the person feeling sick or being a patient. On the other hand, a person might feel sick and seek medical help without having a disease or an observable physical disorder. Biological and medical events, on the one hand, and social and psychological events, on the other, are different *types* of events. Medicine is not just applied biology (or applied biochemistry or applied genetics, for that matter), because the *object* of medical intervention (cure and care) is not only the physical body but also the social person who happens to *inhabit* or rather *be* that body. Although this may seem rather obvious, many problems in health care occur because this apparently obvious difference is neglected.

From a natural science perspective with its focus on physical or biochemical mechanisms, a disorder of the body is just one of the many possible states of an organism. However, the term 'disorder' introduces a normative element into the description. It is a description not only of a physical state of the body but also of a situation that must be changed. The disorder must be brought back to order again. Medicine, as applied natural science, is rooted in this notion that some states of the body need to be changed (but others do not). It is obvious to us why this normative approach to the body exists, because we have all experienced – albeit to different degrees – pain, suffering and fear. In its simplest form medicine can be regarded as a response to a person's request to be helped in becoming free from pain and suffering. In other words, it seems obvious to us that there is an intimate relationship between medicine and healing. Viewed from this perspective, medicine is the institutionalized response to a person's request to be helped. *Note that in this account medicine and healing are intrinsically linked with a notion of society as consisting of mutually supportive relationships between people.* The concept of disorder (and the concept of dis-ease, for that matter) thus invokes a normative 'order' as well as a positive, humanistic vision of society in which individuals are not only able to identify needs in others but are also able and willing to respond to such needs.

It is a matter of historical, anthropological, philosophical and perhaps evolutionary investigation whether the idea (or myth) of society as originating from the need and willingness to provide mutual help can withstand scrutiny. However, irrespective of the historical or other plausibility of this idea, it is a useful device for identifying some basic sociological questions about the social arrangements that exist in our society with regard to illness and the response to it, such as the following.

- What is the relationship between medicine and healing, *cure and care*?
- Who is *entitled* to receive cure and care, and what type and to what extent?
- How is *need* identified?

The main message of this chapter is that all such questions are basically moral in character. Whether someone's cry for help will be heard will depend on a judgement as to whether the request is (morally) justified. An alleged cheater will not, or only reluctantly, be helped. People can be seen as asking too much. Why are some people attended to, while others receive less attention or none at all? Thus it is not only a moral imperative but also a very practical one that patients present themselves as 'good' people who deserve care. It is also a very practical matter to (potential) carers to determine whether they are morally justified in denying care to a specific person. For example, in what cases can doctors turn down a request for help? What are good neighbours supposed to do when neighbours fall ill? Can these neighbours refer all requests for support to professional helpers and next of kin?

Obviously, such questions cannot be answered once and for all. The answers to these questions tend to be socially, culturally and situation specific. This is why a *sociological* approach (i.e. an approach that is able to focus on the moral and organizational aspects of problems in historically, socially and culturally specific contexts) to questions of cure and care will always be relevant.

Sick role, deviance and stigma

The American sociologist Talcot Parsons was the first author to develop a model of the duties and rights of patients. His main question was why it is possible for some people to be allowed to be absent from work (or not to fulfil other social duties) without being punished or blamed for their misconduct, or more precisely how this aversion of blame is regulated. Obviously, just the claim that one is sick is not sufficient. Accepting such claims without further ado would open the door for all kinds of malingering, and then society would collapse because people would stop responding favourably to requests for help. In other words, altruism and therefore society can only exist when there are public mechanisms by which the genuineness of a claim can be judged. However, when someone claims to be sick, how can we know that their claim is genuine? Parsons (1951) developed a model of the 'sick role' for his (American) society in the 1950s, in which the assessment of 'genuineness' is delegated to the profession of medicine. His model consists of the following four elements.

- A person is allowed to take the 'sick role' or patient role (i.e. being absent from work and neglecting other social duties), but they must fulfil the following conditions.
- The patient must seek professional help (i.e. see a doctor).
- They must follow the advice given (i.e. adhere to the medical regimen).
- They must do everything to become healthy again as soon as possible.

Crucial to this model is the fact that the medical profession takes on the social duty of sanctioning irregular behaviour (such as being absent from work). Lay members of society are able to judge whether someone's claim to the patient role is justified by assessing whether they have sought medical help and followed the advice given.

Parsons' model has been criticized on empirical grounds (see, for example, Levine and Kozloff, 1978). For example, there are many illness episodes in which no medical help is sought (e.g. for common flu), but nevertheless the patient role is recognized by others. There are also many patients who do not seek medical help, or who do not follow all of the medical advice that is given to them, or who do not attempt to get healthy again. This applies to many chronic patients, who often only claim a partial patient role (e.g. as a partially disabled worker). However, Parsons' critics have often missed the point of his model, namely that it is not a model of actual, empirical facts, but rather it is a model of the structure of moral reasoning with regard to illness claims. Parsons would not deny that some patients do not seek professional help and/or do not do their best to recover, nor would he deny that some patients who do everything that is expected of them are not recognized as 'real' patients. However, he would claim that in all such cases the model explains how judgements have been made.

Deviance

Parsons' approach implies that some behaviours, such as staying in bed when others are working, require some special interpretation and response. The general term for such behaviours is *deviance*. Other examples of 'deviant' behaviour include taking property from another person, taking someone's life and being violent. However, it is important to understand that 'deviance' is not simply a characteristic of the behaviour itself, but rather it is a characteristic of its interpretation, which itself is contingent on the context. For example, taking property from another person can in some cases be regarded as 'stealing' and in other cases as 'borrowing'. More importantly, parties might have different interpretations. I borrowed your book and kept it for a while without telling you, but you call me a thief. This means that parties are necessarily engaged in interpretative work, always implicitly and sometimes explicitly. The Dutch physician helped the patient to die peacefully; and the UK doctor may call him either a mercy killer or a murderer.

Consider the example of a woman who feels harassed by a man. She might go to the police and report a case of date rape, or alternatively she might decide to discuss the matter with the man. She might deliberately opt for the latter alternative (e.g. because she thinks that this is the preferred way to solve such problems) or she might do it by default (e.g. because she does not know that she could report this to the police). So, after all, was it an instance of date rape? Lawyers and judges might reach a verdict, but this would only illustrate that an event *becomes* an event of a certain type through processes of interaction and interpretation. What happened between this woman and this man *becomes* a date rape only when the relevant parties interpret it as such. The same applies to illness. A patient is someone who is *recognized* as such by relevant parties.

Although Parsons regarded the sick role as a response and a solution to forms of *deviance*, such as sickness absence and other forms of neglect of one's usual duties, the term 'deviance' is seldom used in relation to illness, just because taking on the sick role is a means of *normalising* this neglect. However, the term is used quite widely in the sociological literature on mental illness. It is used mainly to understand the contested nature of much psychiatric diagnosis, and to explain difficult policy issues such as the (moral and legal) grounds for involuntary hospitalization and for being found not guilty of crimes on psychiatric grounds.

Stigma

For some individuals on some occasions it might be helpful to be recognized as someone with a mental illness – for example, if this helps to mitigate the severity of a conviction for a crime, or if it gives access to much needed professional help (or just care). However, many people want to avoid being diagnosed as 'someone with a mental illness'. This reluctance can often be explained by a wish to avoid stigmatization. *Stigma* is a sign (e.g. a visible handicap) or a label (e.g. a psychiatric diagnosis) that signifies to a third party (e.g. a potential employer or lover) that its bearer is in some way morally defective. The effect of this interpretation by others is that the stigma bearer is excluded from normal life opportunities such as jobs, friendships, and so on. According to what by now will be a familiar line of reasoning, the concept of stigma does not refer to an actual relationship between having a handicap (e.g. being wheelchair bound) or diagnosis (e.g. mental illness or epilepsy) and a moral defect. Rather, it refers to a relationship that is *attributed* by others. Stigmatization is therefore usually viewed as a form of discrimination. Instances of actually enacted stigma (e.g. of discrimination against people with a handicap or illness) are documented and discussed in the media almost daily. Of sociological interest is a less frequently discussed but arguably more pervasive phenomenon, which Scambler and Hopkins (1986) have termed *felt stigma*. Their research showed that, in the case of epilepsy, actual discrimination (*enacted stigma*) is relatively rare, but the fear that discrimination might occur (*felt stigma*) influences patients' behaviour to a large extent.

Summary

- The *sick role* is, like any social role, not a description of how people actually behave but rather a model of the structure of moral reasoning with regard to illness claims.
- Similarly, *deviance* is not an attribute of behaviour but rather one of its interpretation by others.
- *Stigma* is a sign (e.g. a visible handicap) or a label (e.g. a psychiatric diagnosis) that signifies to a third party that its bearer is in some way morally defective.
- *Felt stigma* (i.e. anticipated stigma) has the same social effects as *enacted stigma*.

Discussion point 1

Recall an occasion at school when a pupil did not attend an important test due to illness. Describe the response of yourself and the other pupils who did attend. How did you assess the 'genuineness' of the illness? Was this assumed or doubted? On what grounds? *Interpret your behaviour in terms of Parson's model of the sick role.*

Illness behaviour

The concept of *illness behaviour* was coined in the 1970s. Other terms that more or less describe the same phenomenon are *help-seeking behaviour* and *health-seeking behaviour*. The seminal publication from which much later research originated was an article by the American sociologist Irving Zola entitled 'Pathways to the doctor' (Zola, 1973). Zola described his topic as:

> how and why an individual seeks professional medical aid. The immediate and obvious answer is that a person goes to a doctor when he is sick. Yet the term 'sick' is much clearer to those who use it, namely the health practitioners and the researchers, than it is to those upon whom we apply it – the patients.
>
> (Zola, 1973)

To illustrate this statement, he quotes a respondent who had said:

> I wish I really knew what you meant about being sick. Sometimes I felt so bad I could curl up and die, but had to go on because the kids had to be taken care of and besides, we didn't have the money to spend for the doctor. How could I be sick? How do you know when you're sick, anyway? Some people can go to bed most anytime with anything, but most of us can't be sick, even when we need to be.

This respondent's statement contains, in a nutshell, a number of essential elements of a model of illness behaviour that is still relevant today. These elements are as follows:

- the *experience* of symptoms – 'How do you know when you're sick?';
- elements of the *patient role* – going to bed, not doing your usual (paid or unpaid) work, going to the doctor;
- *social circumstances* that determine whether someone is able to take on the patient role – I had to go on because the kids had to be taken care of and besides, we didn't have the money to spend for the doctor. Some people can go to bed most anytime with anything, but most of us can't be sick, even when we need to be';
- *health care system characteristics* – lack of money to spend for the doctor is a determinant of illness behaviour in many countries. It is less important in most European countries, where almost everyone has access to a national health service (as in the UK) or to comprehensive insurance coverage.

Other relevant determinants of illness behaviour that are not mentioned by this respondent include the following:

- *illness career* – patients who have previous experience of illness and of health care will have gained more knowledge about how to interpret symptoms and what to do;
- *culture* – Zola discovered, for example, that US citizens of Italian origin had a lower pain threshold than those from other ethnic groups. Another cultural element is the availability of a network of folk healers and whether it is customary in an ethnic group to heed the advice of such healers;
- *social network characteristics* – the decision to adopt the patient role is often dependent on the advice of other people (e.g. a mother or spouse).

These factors might be schematically represented in the following (simplified) model of health-seeking behaviour (see Figure 4.1).

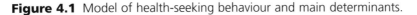

Behaviour   Symptom definition → Lay consultation → Seeing a doctor → Adherence
and referral

Main determinants   Cultural   Social   Characteristics of the health
care system

Figure 4.1 Model of health-seeking behaviour and main determinants.

Note that all elements of this model can be 'discovered' by asking the two questions mentioned at the beginning of this chapter that define the sociological approach.

1. What is the *meaning (significance)* of the symptoms (pain, fever, etc.) to the patient?
2. How is the patient's response to these symptoms *organized* and *co-ordinated*?

Symptom iceberg

The concept of illness behaviour refers to the response of patients and their environment to symptoms. This response is to a large extent invisible to the health care system. For instance, Zola's respondent described above does not go to a doctor, even if she is sick, for the reasons explained in her statement. For these and similar reasons, there are many more people who have serious symptomatic disease and who are not under medical care than there are people receiving treatment. This discrepancy is called the *symptom iceberg* or *clinical iceberg* (see Table 4.1 below for some quantitative examples of this discrepancy).

It is open to debate what this discrepancy means. It means something different for patients than it does for epidemiologists and doctors. For patients it means that they suffer (more or less) but do not consult a doctor, either because they do not want to (because they think that such a consultation is not

Table 4.1 Ratio of symptoms and episodes to consultations

Headache	1:184
Backache	1:52
Emotional problems	1:46
Abdominal pain	1:29
Sore throat	1:18
Pain in chest	1:14

Source: Banks *et al.* (1975).

necessary, or that it is not helpful) or because they cannot (for financial or other reasons). From the perspective of doctors and epidemiologists, the existence of the symptom iceberg means that there is considerable under-reporting. This is not particularly relevant for so-called 'trivial' complaints. However, it is believed that a (by definition unknown) proportion of the complaints that are not reported *should* have been reported (e.g. because they are the first symptoms of a serious disease, such as cancer, early detection and treatment of which is important).

The under-reporting of potentially serious complaints is the result of a pervasive but insoluble feature of health care, namely the *interpretative asymmetry* between professionals and lay people. The latter do not interpret symptoms in the same way that doctors do. They have less professional knowledge and experience, and they apply different standards to the same phenomena. This is logical and understandable, because it is precisely the reason why people go to professionals (in this case doctors) for advice in the first place. More relevant to our sociological approach to illness behaviour is the fact that the interpretative asymmetry between lay people and doctors is not only due to differences in professional knowledge and training but – arguably much more importantly – also due to the application of fundamentally different criteria. Many of these criteria (which are specified in the above model of illness behaviour) have no relation to the objective or subjective condition of the patient, but rather to 'external' factors such as family obligations, the opinion of spouses and other relatives, group culture, social support and other such factors. From the professional medical perspective, such factors are 'contingent' and therefore elusive. (In another context, namely mental health care, the sociologist Goffman (1961) even claims that people are admitted to mental hospitals because of 'contingencies' rather than their illness.) If one wants to decrease the 'under-reporting' of symptoms, much more is needed than just telling people that they ought to consult doctors. One should 'medicalize' the whole social and cultural context in which people live.

The image of a symptom iceberg – and the corresponding notion of under-reporting – captures only one side of the problem of interpretative asymmetry. The other side of the coin is 'over-reporting' of symptoms that, from the doctor's perspective, are 'trivial' or sometimes non-existent. This is the logical result of the fact that the asymmetry between the medical professional and the lay perspective is not quantitative but qualitative. For doctors, it is as difficult to understand why people do not present 'serious' complaints as it is to understand why some people, anxious mothers of very young children in particular, do present 'trivial' ones. Both the 'under-reporting' and 'over-reporting' of complaints – concepts that, as is clear in their formulation, are part of the professional rather than the lay perspective – can only be fully understood through an identification with the life-world of the lay people to whom they are applied. Such identification is not only hindered by the professional perspective (and by the *meanings* it almost automatically implies, such as the notion of 'triviality'). It is also hindered by *organisational* features of the health care system such as the fact that there is no time for doctors to investigate the background of a complaint fully ('Why is this trivial complaint being presented by this patient at this point in time?').

Summary

- *Illness behaviour* – a patient's response to symptoms – cannot only be explained by the type and severity of the symptoms, but is also influenced by 'contingencies' such as the social and cultural context in which the patient lives.
- Both 'under-reporting' of more or less serious symptoms ('symptom iceberg') and 'over-reporting' of trivial complaints can be explained by the different meanings that symptoms have for patients and doctors (*interpretative asymmetry*).

Discussion point 2

Recall the last time you fell ill. Describe how you noticed that something was wrong. How did you interpret these first signs (symptoms)? Did you discuss your condition with other people? With whom did you discuss it? What was their advice? Did you follow their advice? Did you consult your GP or another doctor? Why, or why not?

Interpret your behaviour in terms of Parsons' model of the sick role and of the model of the health-seeking process.

Biography and biographical disruption

One important way of investigating the *meaning (significance)* of symptoms (and illness) for a patient is to locate the onset, treatment and management of symptoms and illnesses as particular types of disruptive events in a patient's life. In an article based on semi-structured interviews with patients with rheumatoid arthritis, the sociologist Michael Bury (1982) coined the term *biographical disruption* for this particular effect of symptoms and illness on a patient's life. The concept of biographical disruption does more than highlight a general approach to the study of the significance of an illness for patients (i.e. as a disruption of a patient's 'biography'). More importantly, it also helps us to understand the *specific*, contingent significance of a particular symptom or illness for each specific patient, by analysing it in the context of the unique biography of that patient.

Being diagnosed with a terminal illness means in an obvious sense that the patient's life is 'disrupted'. A person with a disabling although not terminal disease, who cannot walk or work any more, is the victim of an equally obvious disruption. However, the concept of *biographical* disruption is slightly different in several ways. First, it highlights the subjective rather than the objective impact of a disability – that is, the impact that is determined by the *meaning* which is attributed to the event (e.g. disability, diagnosis) by the patient. In the previous section the attribution of such a meaning to a symptom or illness has been described as 'contingent', suggesting an element of mere chance. The concept of *biography* allows us to qualify and specify that statement. The meanings attributed to symptoms and illnesses by patients, which are 'contingent' from the biomedical perspective, are usually entirely understandable if they are interpreted from within the specific biography of a particular patient. If symptoms, disabilities, etc. are interpreted within the subjective life-world of patients, their behaviour begins to make perfect sense. Secondly, we use the concept of 'biography' (rather than 'subjectivity') because the most important characteristic of the subjective meaning of symptoms and illnesses for a person is its projection on a *temporal* dimension (i.e. as occurring at a specific point in a person's life course). Thirdly, the concept of biography is intimately linked to an idea about personal identity.

In summary, *biography* is the projection of an evolving, continuously shifting idea of self ('identity') on a subjective time-scale. Applied to the patient mentioned earlier, who has just been informed about a terminal diagnosis, it is not so much the announcement of actual biological death that counts as the disruption of an expected or hoped for biographical trajectory. Similarly, the meaning to a patient of being physically disabled and wheelchair bound is dependent on the patient's *biographical work* – that is, the development of an idea of 'self' and an imagined future life course in which the disability 'fits'. For example, Pound and colleagues, when discussing stroke patients, observed that 'their response to the stroke revealed more about the nature and context of their lives than about the stroke itself' (Pound *et al.*, 1998: 503).

Before giving some examples which will clarify the concept of *biography*, two further aspects need to be highlighted. One is the intimate connection between biography and narrative. Because biography is subjective and is connected with notions of 'self' and 'identity', it cannot be conceptualized as just the chronological mapping of events on an objective and linear dimension of time ('calendar'). A biography attributes meaning to a chronological order of events by imbuing it with the notion of *agency*. Events do not just happen in a specific order, but they happen in that order because I wanted them to happen and created for myself the conditions in which they could happen. For example, 'I graduated as a medical doctor and specialized as a surgeon because I am intelligent, worked hard, and became friends with the professor of surgery'. *Narrative* is the theoretical term for adding elements of (subjective) agency to an otherwise 'meaningless' chronological order of events. The other aspect, which is intimately related to the notion of agency, is the inevitable moral character of any narration of events. If some events can be explained by my cleverness, hard work and friendly personality, some (adverse) events or the absence of other (positive) events might be attributed to less laudable personal characteristics. In other words, a biography is a narrative about oneself and one's life that inevitably allocates responsibility and blame.

Illustration

Patient 1: Now I've had a taste of what can happen to someone who is in the stream of life. It's just unbelievable that it happened to me. I was so active, so busy all the time. Then I was laid low, and all of a sudden I was trapped.

Patient 2: If I do exercises, if I go to therapy, then if the arm won't work I'm not going to be mad at myself. I'll say, 'Well, you did everything you could'. But if I don't do the exercises, and I don't do the therapy, then I'm going to be mad at myself. I'm going to say, 'John, you didn't do the right things to improve yourself.'

Summary

- *Biography* is the projection of an evolving, continuously shifting idea of self ('identity') on a subjective time-scale. It can best be viewed as a *narrative* – that is, as a story that one tells about oneself.
- A pervasive aspect of any biographical narrative is its *moral* character. Whatever the character of the events reported in the narrative, the teller attempts to present him- or herself as morally 'good'.
- A biography usually takes for granted the fact that someone's body is functioning well. It is not noticed. Therefore the onset of an illness or handicap is experienced as a *biographical disruption*.
- *Biographical work* must be done to repair a disruption. The aim of this work is to enable a re-telling of the biography in such a way that the illness and its effects are accounted for in the story.

Discussion point 3

Write two short autobiographical statements (a maximum of 200 words each) with two very different types of reader in mind (e.g. one for your personal tutor at medical school and the other for the recruiting officer of staff for a children's summer camp where you would like to work next summer).

Examine the differences between the two statements. Explain these differences. Identify moral elements in both texts (e.g. phrases in which you (implicitly or explicitly) claim a virtue or (implicitly or explicitly) blame other people or things for something less laudable (e.g. a failed examination)).

Narrative reconstruction

The *moral* character of biography is pervasive and is observable in the smallest medical event. For example, consider the statement by Zola's respondent discussed above:

> I wish I really knew what you meant about being sick. Sometimes I felt so bad I could curl up and die, but had to go on because the kids had to be taken care of and besides, we didn't have the money to spend for the doctor. How could I be sick? How do you know when you're sick, anyway? Some people can go to bed most anytime with anything, but most of us can't be sick, even when we need to be.

This is not only an account of determinants of illness behaviour, but also a presentation of self as a morally good person:

> I am a good mother who takes care of the kids even when I feel so bad I could curl up and die. I am not like some people who go to bed most anytime with anything.

There is thus a strong moral element in the response to symptoms and illness. However, illness itself is also seen as a moral event, for which responsibility must be allocated. A person whose illness is self-inflicted must be blamed. The attribution of blame and responsibility is an activity in which we engage routinely when we discuss diet, exercise, smoking and alcohol intake, and particularly when some unhealthy behaviour has led to sickness absence or to the non-fulfilment of some other duty. This is also the reason why people want to know what has caused their illness, even in cases where medicine has no answer to this question.

When patients ask 'Why me?' they are usually not interested in a 'scientific' answer but rather in a moral one in which blame and responsibility are allocated and from which the biographical meaning of the illness for the person can be constructed. Medicine cannot give such an answer in principle. Although causal determinants, such as smoking, are known for specific diseases in general, science cannot usually determine with certainty what has caused a specific case of the disease. Moreover, even if this is possible, such a scientific value-free construction will not be accepted as an adequate answer to the moral question. This is why people 'find' their own answers. They have to do so. The sociologist Gareth Williams has coined the term *narrative reconstruction* for the process by which patients find an answer to the question 'Why me?'. Because different people have different resources that they can use for this reconstruction – related not only to their educational, religious, vocational and political background but also to the 'contingencies' of their personal biography – the result is always profoundly personal and apparently idiosyncratic (Williams, 1984).

Summary

- *Narrative reconstruction* is any biographical work of retelling the biography after a disruption.

- More specifically, the term *narrative reconstruction* is used to describe the process by which patients find an answer to the question 'Why me?'.
- As in all biographical work, people can only make use of the cognitive resources (ideas, theories, ideologies and convictions) which are available to them and which they have accumulated in their life to date. Therefore the new biography that results from a *narrative reconstruction* will reflect those resources.

Discussion point 4

Imagine that you have been involved in a traffic accident which was partly caused by your own drink driving. The result of this accident is that you cannot concentrate on reading and studying, and therefore you are unable to continue your medical training.

Write a new version of one of the autobiographical statements that you wrote for the previous discussion point, with the same reader in mind. Examine and explain the differences between the two versions, with special emphasis on the attribution of blame.

Quality of life

As discussed above, individuals who want to be recognized as *bona fide* patients are obliged to seek and follow professional advice and to do everything in their power to recover. We tend not to see this duty as a special requirement or burden, because we assume that *bona fide* patients behave in such a way in any case, without being urged by others. Furthermore, we tend not to regard this duty as *work* that requires patients to spend resources in terms of physical and mental energy, money, time and management skills. In actual practice, being ill – particularly being chronically ill – requires a great deal of quite heavy work and quite diverse skills. In a seminal text, Anselm Strauss and his colleagues and students (Strauss and Glaser, 1975; Strauss *et al.*, 1984) focused attention on how people manage to live as normal a life as possible in the face of disease and, in particular, on the work involved in this management. They discussed the different forms of patient work, including the following:

- monitoring of symptoms ('symptom control work');
- managing crises ('crisis work');
- adhering to the medical regimen ('regimen work');
- biographical work ('identity work');
- managing uncertainty;
- managing transport;
- comfort work;
- the work of keeping marital relationships repaired;
- the work of preparing for dying.

Scenario

Some examples of everyday problems that are encountered when living with a chronic illness are listed below (from Strauss and Glaser, 1975).

- Can I visit my friend's apartment without having an asthma attack?
- Can I make it to the bathroom quickly enough?
- If I attempt sexual intercourse, will my back pain flare up?
- Do I risk a heart attack if I take on this interesting project at work?
- Can I negotiate the path from my car to the store?

On the basis of more recent research that has been partly inspired by the work of Strauss and Glaser, the following forms of patient work could be added to the above list:

- managing the treatment calendar (keeping appointments, travelling to and from clinics);
- waiting.

Taken together, all of these different types of work can add up to a considerable workload for patients and their carers. However, they must be done if life is to go on, and therefore they must be co-ordinated so that time, energy and other resources are allocated for each type of work. This requires the performance of yet another, higher-level order of work known as *articulation work*. This is:

> The organization and co-ordination of all types of work that are necessary to plan and implement any plan of action. It includes identifying the types of work and the associated tasks to be done, giving priority to tasks in terms of their importance, making arrangements for who will do them and when, calculating the need for resources and obtaining and maintaining them and assuming and delegating responsibility for tasks.
> (Corbin and Strauss, 1988)

This overview of patient work applies mainly to outpatients who manage their lives more or less independently. The work required from patients who are hospitalized is different. Some or all of their management tasks might be taken over by professional staff. However, other patient work is needed in this situation, in particular the work of being a 'good' patient by being cheerful and by dutifully obeying the staff's orders (for an overview, see Porter *et al.*, 1999: 98–9 and Scambler, 1997: 71–4).

The concept of 'quality of life' originated in the 1960s and 1970s as a critical concept. Its main function was to criticize the dehumanizing effects of a technological approach to illness, and medicine's inability to support (chronic) patients in the everyday management of their condition. The concept was not well defined, and it can best be glossed as 'happiness'. Because the concept of quality of life was coined as critical or opposite to the (bio)medical approach, it could be regarded as highlighting those aspects of life that, by definition, were out of reach of a medical approach. However, interestingly, at the same time there was also a tendency to expand the definition of health in such a way that it would incorporate the non-medical aspects of life captured by the concept of quality of life (see, for example, World Health Organization Quality of Life Group, 1991). The subsequent debate about the differences and overlaps between the concepts of 'health', 'well-being', 'quality of life' and 'happiness' has not resulted in clear distinctions. On the contrary, these concepts and their boundaries are now more contested than ever.

It is often believed that the reason for the lack of clear definitions of concepts such as 'health' and 'quality of life' is that these concepts are subjective and therefore 'individual'. This view overlooks the fact that people are quite able to share definitions of these concepts, particularly if they belong to the same family or cultural group. The 'problem' with these concepts is not that they are subjective, but rather that they are irredeemably moral, and therefore political. A consensus (national or international, within the medical profession or inter-professionally) about the 'correct' definition of a concept such as quality of life would presuppose a political consensus between culturally, religiously and politically very diverse groups. The lack of clear definitions is thus an expression of the *social* and *moral* rather than of the alleged *subjective* or *individual* nature of these concepts.

If a concept is not clearly defined, it cannot be measured. On the other hand, a concept can only play a role in policy-making if it is measured and if statements can be made about its increase or decrease over time (or about its differential distribution over groups or conditions). This measurement imperative is overriding in our society and this applies, because of its biomedical tradition and culture, to the health service in particular. The result is that, in this era of evidence-based health care, there are literally hundreds of different 'quality of life' (QoL) measures in use within (and also without) the health service and medical research. Dozens of such measures are added each year. Apart from the label 'quality of life', most of them have hardly anything in common. It is therefore fair to say that there are as many concepts of quality of life as there are measures. Apart from the label (QoL), these measurements have one other common characteristic, namely that they all involve patients' self-reports. Their form is therefore a self-completion questionnaire in almost all cases. Despite the huge differences between the hundreds of QoL measurements, two main approaches can be identified.

First, the most common approach is that traditional *clinical* criteria are redefined as indicators of 'quality of life' (QoL). For example, dyspnoea and fatigue can be two of the symptoms of lung disease. Obviously, patients with lung disease will feel discomfort because of such symptoms, which might actually have been the reason for them coming to see the doctor in the first place. Lack of breath and fatigue are also prominent items of all measures that are used to assess the QoL of patients with lung disease. In this approach, QoL is mainly a new fashionable way to elicit information from patients that signals clinical success. Despite (or perhaps thanks to) its clinical bias, QoL measures developed within this approach have contributed to a new development in clinical practice, namely a growing awareness of the contrary effects ('side-effects') of treatment. For example, a QoL measure for lung cancer patients will include, apart from breathlessness and fatigue, an item such as nausea, which is a (side-) effect of radiation and chemotherapy. This makes it possible that an evaluation of the effects of the treatment will not only assess the (desired) gain in breath but also the (non-desired) increase in nausea and other side-effects.

The second approach to QoL measurement is for well-known and quite obvious *social* effects of illness to be redefined as QoL. For example, people have always known that disease and ill health do not only cause physical suffering, such as pain and other forms of discomfort, but also result in other types of misfortune, such as a decrease in earning capacity, poverty, loss of friends, and depression and anxiety. Conceptually it is an impoverishment if such diverse aspects of (mis)fortune or (un)happiness are brought together into one or a limited number of measures. However, integrating such diverse social phenomena into one measurement has also made it easier for doctors to incorporate them as elements in their decision-making and in the assessment of the effects of their treatments.

The increasing use of QoL measures in medical decision-making and in clinical research therefore involves gains and losses. Lost are insights into what it actually means for the patient (and their relatives), with their specific biography and in their specific circumstances, to be ill and to receive treatment. One can argue that, with this loss of 'meaning', the essence of the patient's viewpoint, and in particular its moral aspects, are lost. On the other hand, it is exactly this neglect of the moral and biographical aspects in QoL measures that makes it possible for the doctor to integrate 'social' effects of the illness and its treatment in decisions about and evaluations of treatments. QoL measures are a means of translating moral aspects of a patient's life (which are incompatible with biomedical reasoning) into amoral but clinically significant numbers. Doctors and clinical researchers are mainly interested in *illness-related* QoL – that is, QoL that is more or less directly dependent on the patient's health. From the patient's perspective it might be less obvious and also less important to what extent an experienced level of 'quality of life' is related to health and illness or to other determinants. For example, a patient with lung disease might experience unhappiness due to family circumstances (e.g. marital problems, which existed before the onset of the disease but have been exacerbated since) which contribute to his experienced lack of breath.

For this patient, it is difficult to tell to what extent his unhappy family life (which is not measured by QoL measures but might be measured by, for example, a social support scale) and his lack of breath (which is measured) are due to his illness and its treatment. Apart from the difficulty in discriminating between 'illness-related' QoL and QoL that is related to other determinants, this example also illustrates another problem that is neglected in the current use of QoL measures, namely that of (relative) relevance. It is implicit in almost all health advice (e.g. about diet, exercise, sex) that health is more important than happiness, and that one should only pursue those forms of happiness that are labelled as healthy by doctors. Similarly, implicit in the clinical use of measures of health-related QoL is that a patient's 'quality of life' can be reduced to the absence of symptoms such as dyspnoea, which might (and in actual practice often does) lead to a neglect of the patient's concerns. Ironically, in such cases the use of QoL measures (which were introduced to support a more patient-centred approach to health care) supports a doctor-centred view of what should matter to the patient.

This can be observed in decisions on treatment programmes in particular. For example, consider the effect of the organization of radiation therapy on the quality of life of cancer patients (Costain Schou and Hewison, 1999). Cancer patients can either refuse therapy (which they sometimes do) or accept it (which they often do), but when they have accepted therapy, patients tend not to have any influence on the way it is given. Because 'conquering' the cancer is assumed to be the only important and overriding interest of the patient, it is taken for granted that the patient has to accept whatever arrangement is 'offered', regardless of its influence on the patient's social life. Thus patients receive a card or letter stipulating times (e.g. three times a week) at which they should make themselves available for therapy, and how they should prepare themselves. Usually no information is requested (or even allowed to be volunteered) from the patient about preferences that might be dependent on travel arrangements, availability of individuals by whom the patient might prefer to be accompanied, birthday parties, regular hobbies (such as a weekly chess or bingo afternoon), and so on.

It is considered to be 'obvious' that organizational imperatives on the part of the hospital or clinic, *and* the 'objective' interest of the patient in becoming cured of cancer if possible, cannot be compared to 'trivial' practical matters such as a patient's travel arrangements. In actual practice this viewpoint is confirmed by the almost total compliance of patients with clinic arrangements as they are presented to them. Because the work that patients (and their relatives) do in order to comply with such arrangements is invisible to them, providers of treatment may regard this work as 'trivial' or at least easy to accomplish. The same invisibility applies to the effects of treatment arrangements, and of the costs involved in complying with them, on the patient's quality of life. These effects are not measured in the usual QoL measures for cancer patients, which tend to focus on symptoms of the cancer, symptoms of psychiatric disease (depression and anxiety), and side-effects of treatment. These QoL measures assess quality of life in terms of clinical criteria, and can therefore contribute to an assessment of the extent to which the treatment has been successful ('quality of treatment'). However, they cannot assess quality of life in terms of other criteria that might be more important to the patient, and may therefore also not contribute to an assessment of the degree to which treatment was arranged in a patient-centred manner ('quality of care').

Summary

- The management of (chronic) illness is hard work.
- Quality of life (QoL) originated as a patient-centred subjective outcome measure complementary to clinical outcome measures.
- Illness-related QoL usually measures the presence or absence of symptoms

(of the disease) and side-effects (of treatment) and, less often, the impact of the illness on the patient's social life (e.g. work, family relationships and income).

• A patient's quality of life is also dependent on the quality of care. Aspects of a patient's quality of life that are related to quality of care are very rarely measured by QoL measures.

Discussion point 5

Interview a patient with a chronic illness or handicap. Try to obtain as much information as possible about what having the illness or handicap means to the patient in terms of their daily functioning and plans for the future. Write a short report summarizing your main findings.

Identify the main indicators of biographical disruption. Identify elements of narrative reconstruction and of other biographical work. Describe the main elements related to the everyday management of the disease and the medical regimen. Identify the main (social, material, etc.) resources used by the patient. Identify the impact of the way in which health care is organized (accessibility, flexibility, 'patient-centredness') on the patient's life. Have you got any information about the patient's main values or criteria by which they evaluate their situation? On inspection of all these different elements of the patient's life, on what basis could an assessment be made of the patient's 'quality of life'?

The burden of care

The issues discussed in the earlier sections of this chapter apply as much to spouses and other next of kin as they do to patients themselves. Family members play an important role in the interpretation of symptoms, in decision-making about help-seeking and in the management of the sick role. As such they also contribute to the management of the *moral* aspects of illness behaviour (e.g. by an intervention such as 'I don't mind what your colleagues will say. You stay in bed because I care about you'). More importantly, they inevitably become affected themselves by the illness of their family member. Their own biographies are often disrupted as much as that of the patient, and therefore they must also engage in narrative reconstruction and other forms of biographical work. This obviously affects their quality of life as well.

The illness of a family member has an immediate impact on how family life is lived. Holidays have to be cancelled or rescheduled. Visits to relatives, friends or clubs that were previously routine events now take more time and effort (if they are not cancelled altogether). Income might be considerably decreased. Because relatively more resources (in terms of time, energy and money) have to be spent on family tasks, the family member's own career, education or social life may be negatively affected. Relationships between couples may change considerably (e.g. when partners cannot continue a formerly active and happy sex life). These are just some examples. Therefore the spouse and other family members will often ask the same question as the patient: 'Why me/us?'. As discussed above, this question requires a morally satisfying answer, as is demonstrated by the following quote from the wife of a stroke patient: 'I get upset to think we've worked hard together to enjoy this time of life and now this has happened. You feel there's no justice sometimes.'

The illness of a relative is as much a black spot on the family member's own moral slate as it is for the patient. It means that the illness of the other person, to whom one is connected, has to be accounted for in one's own biography. It must be integrated into one's own identity. This is explicitly formulated in the following account of the mother of a girl with Down's syndrome:

> I only appreciated later that Sarah had changed everything for every family member. My parents were grandparents of a Down's syndrome baby. Carey was aunt to a Down's syndrome baby, and Tom and Nicholas were cousins of a Down's syndrome baby. New identities for everyone. The ripples were to go on and on.
>
> (Mother of a newly born girl with Down's syndrome, *The Guardian*, 8 February 1999)

The effects of the disruption of a spouse's biography, and of an often considerable loss in terms of quality of life, are similar to those for the patient him- or herself. Negative effects might range from envy of others with healthy partners to depression and (not uncommonly) divorce. Often this is seen as a kind of betrayal, or at least as the breaking of a vow. However, it is important to appreciate that the biographical disruption caused by an illness results not only in changed relationships (between assumedly unchanged individuals) but also in *changed identities or individuals*. That is why we talk about *biographical* disruption. The wife of a stroke patient in the following quote gave her marriage vows to 'my George', not to her current husband: 'He's just not my George, not as he was. His nature has completely changed. You can't get through to him. He's the reverse of what he was.' Similarly, the stroke patient's wife in the next quote was married to a more affectionate and loving husband than she has now: 'He's different to what he was before. He doesn't think of the little things he did before. He was very affectionate; he's not so loving as he was before.'

Family members' biographies can, and usually will, be disrupted by the immediate social and other effects of the patient's illness, even if they do not play a role in the actual care of the patient. However, usually some family members do play an important role in the care of the patient, and the physical and emotional work involved in this imply an additional burden for them. Usually it is still taken for granted that spouses take on the carer's role. Although this applies to women in particular, and it is socially and culturally more acceptable for men to profess lack of appropriate capabilities or willingness to be a carer, it is not the case that only women carry the burden of care (see Table 4.2).

Table 4.2 Percentage of adults who were carers, according to gender, in 1995

	Men	Women	Total
Carers	11	14	13
Caring for someone in same household	4	4	4
Caring for someone in another household	7	10	8
Main carers	6	9	8
Caring for at least 20 hours a week	3	4	4

Source: Rowlands and Parker (1998).

Scenario

Married women find it harder than men to make essential lifestyle changes follow-ing a heart attack – because their husbands refuse to help. While men are often supported by their wives as they adjust their diet and habits after a heart attack, women cannot rely on their husbands to do the same for them. As a result, women may be left more at risk of a second heart attack.

(from *The Times Higher Education Supplement*, 4 July 1997)

The persistence of the social (and moral) norm that spouses, particularly women, should take on the care for each other and, for that matter, that chil-dren (particularly daughters) should care for their parents, can partially be explained by the lack of alternatives. Who else would care? However, it must also be explained by the invisibility of the work that is involved, and therefore by lack of knowledge of what it actually means to be a carer. Back in 1974, an editorial in the *British Medical Journal* entitled 'Stroke and the family' formu-lated this as follows:

> Only those who have experienced it fully appreciate the despair which sometimes overcomes a wife or husband who, without warning or train-ing, has to assume for months or years a responsibility combining the skills of nurse, remedial therapist, psychologist and speech therapist. This role, which calls for unfailing optimism, and the patience of Job, also calls for a measure of sympathetic understanding and support from community services which is seldom forthcoming.
>
> (Anonymous, 1974)

This editorial suggests that professional skills (of nurse, remedial therapist, psychologist and speech therapist), and therefore training and/or support, are needed as well as 'unfailing optimism and the patience of Job'. This combination of competences will only rarely be found, even in professionals applying for similar jobs. Obviously, in practice, carers are not selected but they suddenly ('without warning or training') become carers. They do this out of moral obligation and/or love (between which carers themselves sometimes make a distinction, and sometimes do not). Examples of reasons (or motives or accounts) given by carers on the BBC Radio 2 programme *Why Do We Care?* (transmitted on 10 June 1997) included the following:

- Tony Terret: 'I care for Felicity because she's my wife. You know, that's simply it really. But I don't think of myself particularly up in lights as a carer.'
- Pauline: 'Mum was a damned good Mum, and while I can do everything I can for her I will.'
- Jenny Triptree: 'I think you become a carer because the circumstances are there and you do it. I mean, I don't want to be a carer. I loved my Mum; she'd been a really good Mum. My husband and I had a great relationship. And I cared for them both, because that was it. But I didn't want to care. You know, I wouldn't have chosen that. But I made sure that I did look after both of them, and I will carry on looking after my mother until she dies. But I wouldn't wish that life on any of my children. I couldn't bear to think that my children would go through what I've gone through in the last nine years really.'
- Janet McKay: 'I'm the only daughter, the only child. So the responsibility was mine. When mum had her stroke, seven years ago. You know, I love her very much but I don't like her sometimes. She gets very very nasty on occasions, and very difficult to cope with. I felt that my life was nothing else but caring. I got very angry with her one night. And I was really at the end of my tether. And I put her in the lift and I kept sending her up and down the staircase . . . because I felt that I could have picked her up and shaken her and I thought it was the safest place for her.'

The last quotation is a good illustration of the requirement that carers should have 'the patience of Job', as mentioned in the above extract from the *British Medical Journal* editorial. It also refers to the fact that caring is a two-way relationship, and that the person being cared for must participate in this in an appropriate way. This is also captured by the following quote from the wife of a patient with a damaged spinal cord:

> A lot of the time, I felt a lot of hatred towards him because I felt that he was treating me like a servant, a housekeeper, rather than a wife. I didn't realize he didn't know how to treat me. He didn't know where he was. It could have broken up the marriage if I had let it get to me.

On the other hand, patients often develop feelings of guilt just because they realize that they cannot be the husband (or wife) that they were before. In practice it is very difficult (and for many too difficult) work – in addition to the hard work of caring – to develop or maintain a marital relationship (or, for that matter, one between lovers), which usually assumes some degree of reciprocity. Since 1974, when the *BMJ* editorial quoted above was published, not much has changed. The dominant attitude to caring by spouses (and, for that matter, other relatives) is still mainly one of sympathy and occasional support. The assumption that caring for a loved one is an opportunity to express and even develop one's love of one's spouse or other relative is still dominant. Neither in public opinion nor in care policy is it acknowledged that, in actual practice, caring for the chronically ill is in many respects damaging to the relationship, and therefore often results in the very opposite, namely anger, loss of love, and sometimes violence.

Summary

- The concepts of *biographical disruption* and *biographical work* apply not only to patients but also to their carers.
- Unpaid informal carers provide most care.
- Informal care is regulated by socially, culturally and context specific systems of rights, duties and obligations. This area is therefore a moral minefield.

Discussion point 6

Interview a lay carer of a patient with a chronic illness or handicap, preferably the patient's spouse or partner. (The patient could be the same person whom you interviewed for the previous self-assessment question.) Try to obtain as much information as possible about what caring for the patient means to the carer in terms of their daily functioning and plans for the future. Write a short report summarizing your main findings.

Identify the main indicators of biographical disruption in the carer's life. Identify elements of narrative reconstruction and of other biographical work. Describe the main elements related to the everyday work of caring. Identify the main (social, material, etc.) resources used by the carer. Identify the impact of the way in which health care is organized (accessibility, flexibility, 'patient-centredness') on the carer's life. Have you got any information about the carer's main values or criteria by which they evaluate their situation? On inspection of all these different elements of the carer's life, on what basis could an assessment be made of the carer's 'quality of life'?

Worked examples

Example 1: a woman with an allergy

A divorced woman without children sees her doctor about a terrible itch and hay-fever-like symptoms. The problem appears to be a clear-cut case of an allergic response to cat hair. The doctor advises the woman to get rid of her two cats. Two months later, the woman sees the doctor again with the same symptoms, which are now more severe. It appears that the woman still lives with her cats. She requests some form of anti-allergic medication, apparently with the objective of keeping her cats. The doctor refuses and says that it is not the aim of the health service to provide expensive medication for people who would not need it if they would only live responsibly and follow advice.

COMMENTARY

This woman is – apart from an allergic body – also a *person* whose *quality of life* depends on many other factors apart from being free of itching and sneezing, and it depends particularly on her relationships with other people and with objects. Probably her cats are important beings in her life with which she has meaningful relationships that cannot possibly be severed. For the woman it might be (almost) a *moral* obligation, and/or a matter of *identity*, to keep her cats and to care for them. On what basis could the doctor know that his morality is superior?

Example 2: a complaining patient

A deputy manager with vague but persistent, and sometimes very painful, stomach complaints sees his doctor. He is given a referral to a clinic for internal medicine. When he makes an appointment at the clinic, he hears that he must wait for 6 weeks. Furthermore, the appointment will be on a Wednesday morning, when he has to attend the weekly management team meeting. He can only get an appointment at a more convenient time (for him) if he is willing to wait a further 3 weeks. After some consideration, he chooses the latter option, mainly because he does not want to make things more difficult at work by being absent from the management team meeting. Nine weeks later, after he has arrived at the clinic strictly on time, he must wait more than an hour before being called in for the consultation. The latter is rather short, and basically the same ground is covered as with his GP. The doctor at the clinic advises an endoscopy. The patient is referred to another desk to make an appointment for the endoscopy. Fortunately, there is no waiting-list for endoscopy and he can make a choice between an appointment on the next Thursday or Friday morning. Because he is not allowed to drink or eat anything in the 12 hours before the endoscopy, and because he has his weekly drinking session with his friends on Thursday nights, he chooses the Thursday morning. On Wednesday he is informed by telephone that his appointment has been cancelled and has been rescheduled for Friday morning. He complains, but the caller is not receptive to his view. He does not attend his friends' social evening, and on arrival at the endoscopy clinic he complains again. When he explains why he had initially chosen the Thursday morning (rather than the Friday morning), this is used as an argument for discarding his complaint. Because people with stomach complaints are not supposed to drink anyway, he is regarded as a 'bad' patient who is responsible for his own health problems and who is a nuisance to health care staff because of his demanding behaviour.

COMMENTARY

Although this man wants to get rid of his complaints, he is also a *person* involved in activities such as earning a salary (and therefore carefully trying to avoid doing anything that might damage his career prospects) and maintaining friendships (which in his view is not possible without drinking together). In general, health care organizations and their staff have no idea how important such activities are for a person's well-being and quality of life, and they assume that such activities are by definition less important than their organizational imperatives. Their time, costs and responsibilities are *always* more important than the patient's, and a patient who does not understand or accept this is not 'deserving'.

Example 3: a baby with a rash

The father of a 6-week-old baby calls a GP weekend service on a Saturday night. He tells them that the baby has a rash on her face and shoulders, and that she seems to be uncomfortable. He is not able to explain why he thinks the latter. He requests to see a doctor. Initially he is told that this seems unnecessary but, when he persists in his request, an appointment is made. The father, mother and baby appear within 5 minutes at the surgery, where they must wait for half an hour before it is their turn to see the doctor. They frequently look at the baby with concern and gradually become more agitated. When it is their turn, they behave angrily towards the doctor. The doctor examines the child and cannot find anything alarming. When he complains to the parents that they have taken up his time unnecessarily, the mother starts to cry and says that she just wanted to know for sure whether the baby had some serious illness. The doctor convinces the parents that the baby is not uncomfortable and that the rash is harmless. Reporting to his colleagues on Monday morning, the doctor calls these parents 'folk who think that one can ask doctors to change nappies or whatever comes to their mind'.

COMMENTARY

Illness behaviour depends on many factors, such as experience, knowledge, advice from other lay people, and so on. These parents appear to have no experience with babies, no knowledge of how to interpret the baby's appearance and behaviour, and above all they seem to have no other people (such as their own parents, sisters, friends, etc.) to rely on for advice that they can trust. The fact that these parents lack the resources which most other people have should be part of a diagnosis, and should be used as grounds for an intervention (rather than as grounds for condemnation).

Key text: Bury on biographical disruption

Bury M (1982) Chronic illness as biographical disruption. *Sociology of Health and Illness* **4,** 167–82.

The concept of 'biographical disruption' was coined in this article. Bury conducted semi-structured qualitative interviews with 30 patients who had been referred for the first time to an outpatient rheumatology clinic. By means of the qualitative interview method, Bury was able to capture the meaning that events had had for patients. In the analysis, through comparison of all 30 cases, a common pattern was found.

Onset and the problem of recognition

'The emergence of the condition implied a "premature ageing" for the individual. As such, it marked a biographical shift from a perceived normal trajectory through relatively predictable chronological steps, to one that was fundamentally abnormal and inwardly damaging. The relationship between "internal and external reality" was upset. Commonsense assumptions lose their grip and yet alternative explanations do not readily present themselves.'

Emerging disability and the problem of uncertainty

'On being told that they definitely had rheumatoid arthritis, reactions combined fear and relief. Some said that, as they had known it prior to consultation, it simply confirmed the worst; others were beset with anxiety, especially about the future. The image of rheumatoid arthritis as a crippling disease is strong, and despite attempts by staff to reassure patients that only a small proportion of sufferers become severely disabled, many saw a future of growing dependency and invalidity. Not only this, but individuals also face the limits of medical knowledge and treatment regimens. A realization that the latter (involving periods of rest and activity) are difficult to follow and often less than effective slowly dawns. Doctors unwittingly reinforce this by telling patients that no cause of rheumatoid arthritis is known. Thus, whilst the diagnosis of the disease provides something firm to relate to, and to explain to others, the actual nature of the disease remains elusive and the treatments empirical.'

Chronic illness and the mobilization of resources

'The disruption of friendship and community involvement arises not only because of functional limitations (e.g. restrictions in mobility, problems of fatigue) but also because of the embarrassment which such disabilities create. Maintaining normal activities (e.g. being able to sit in one position for a long period of time at a cinema, or maintaining normal appearances in a social gathering at a club or pub), have to become deliberately conscious activities, and thus frustrating and tiring. In the end the effort simply does not seem worth it. The erstwhile taken-for-granted world of everyday life becomes a burden of conscious and deliberate action. The simplest outing becomes a major occasion of planning and expedition. Thus the handicaps of social isolation and dependency which flow from these disruptions in social intercourse are not simply derived from the ability or inability to carry out tasks and activities.'

Discussion

'In describing the experience of the onset and development of rheumatoid arthritis I have tried to suggest a perspective which conceptualizes chronic illness as a particular kind of disruptive experience. This disruption throws into relief the cognitive and material resources available to individuals. It displays the key forms which explanations of pain and suffering in illness take in modern society, the continuity and discontinuity of professional and lay modes of thought and the sources of variability in experience arising from the influence of structural constraints over the ability to adapt.'

Key text: Williams on narrative reconstruction

Williams G (1984) The genesis of chronic illness: narrative reconstruction. *Sociology of Health and Illness* **6**, 175–200.

The concept of 'narrative reconstruction', which is a companion of the concept of 'biographical disruption', was coined in this article. Williams conducted semi-structured qualitative interviews with 30 patients who had been first diagnosed as suffering from rheumatoid arthritis at least 5 years prior to the study. The aim of the study was to explore how and why people come to see their illness as originating in a certain way, and how people account for the disruption disablement has wrought in their lives. In the analysis, through comparison of all 30 cases, it appeared that patients reconstructed their biographies in very different ways. These differences could be explained by relating their narrative reconstructions to their educational, religious, vocational and political background as well as to the 'contingencies' of their personal biographies.

Bill: narrative reconstruction as political criticism

'I was a working gaffer . . . but, you know, they were mostly long hours and the result was every time I had a session like, my feet began to swell and my hands began to swell. I could not hold a pen, I had difficulty getting between machines and difficulty getting hold of small things. I didn't associate it with anything to do with the works at the time, but I think it was chemically induced.'

'I was trying more or less self-analysis. Where have I got it from? How was it come? And you talk to different people over all ages and you find that they are at a loss. They don't know, nobody knows. And who do we ask? Ask the doctor [who says]: "It's just one of them things . . . and there's nothing to be done about it." But it seems a bit . . . thinking in my mind when I go to bed . . . I can't go to sleep straight away, I have to wait until I get settled and your mind is going all the time, you're reflecting "How the *hell* have I come to be like this?" '

Gill: narrative reconstruction as psychology

'It was stress that precipitated this, the stress perhaps of suppressing myself while I was a mother and wife; not women's libby but there comes a time in your life when you think, you know, "Where have I got to? There's nothing left of me". I'm quite certain that the last straw was my husband's illness. So, I'm sure it was stress induced. I think that while my head kept going my body stopped.' 'I sometimes wonder whether arthritis is self-inflicted . . . not consciously. You know, your own body says, "right, shut up, sit down, and do nothing". I feel very strongly about myself that this happened to me, that one part of my head said, "if you won't put the brakes on, I will". Because I had

had many years of very hard physical work, you know – washing and ironing and cooking and shopping and carting kids around and carrying babies and feeding babies and putting babies to bed and cleaning up their sick.'

Betty: the transcendence of causality and narrative reconstruction

'The Lord's so near and, you know, people say "Why you?". I mean this man next door he doesn't believe in God or anything and he says to me, "You, my dear, why did he choose you?" And I said, "Look, I don't question the Lord, I don't ask, He knows why and that's good enough for me". So he says, "He's supposed to look after . . ." and I said, "He is looking after his own and he does look after me". I said, I could be somewhere where I could be sadly neglected. Well, I'm not. I'm getting all the best treatment that can be got, and I do thank the Lord that I'm born in this country, I'll tell you that.' 'I've found the joy in this life, and therefore for me to go through anything, it doesn't matter really, in one way, because I reckon that they are testing times. . . . He never says that you will not have these things. But He comes with us through these things and helps us bear them and that's the most marvellous thing of all.'

Further reading

Allott M and Robb M (eds) (1998) *Understanding health and social care. An introductory reader*. London: Sage (with the Open University Press).

Armstrong D (1994) *Outline of sociology as applied to medicine*, 4th edn. Oxford: Butterworth-Heinemann.

Bury M (1991) The sociology of chronic illness: a review of research and prospects. *Sociology of Health and Illness* **13**, 451–68.

Helman CG (2000) *Culture, health and illness. An introduction for health professionals*, 4th edn. Oxford: Butterworth-Heinemann.

Scambler G (ed.) (1997) *Sociology as applied to medicine*, 4th edn. London: W.B. Saunders.

Strauss A, Corbin J, Fagerhaugh S *et al.* (eds) (1984) *Chronic illness and the quality of life*, 2nd edn. St Louis, MO: CV Mosby Company.

Epidemiology

5

Mary Jane Platt and Simon Capewell

Introduction
Epidemiological methods
Key text: Doll and Peto on UK doctors and smoking
Epidemiology of common diseases
Further reading

> I keep six honest serving-men
> (They taught me all I knew);
> Their names are What and Why and When
> And How and Where and Who.
> (Rudyard Kipling)

The study of the distribution and determinants of health-related states and the application of this study to control health problems.
(J. Last, from *A Dictionary of Epidemiology*)

Introduction

This chapter aims to provide an introduction to epidemiological methods relevant to the study of medicine. Epidemiology is the study of the distribution and determinants of disease in human populations, in order to improve health. By better understanding how a health problem occurs, strategies to reduce disease and promote health can be developed. The knowledge of the 'what', 'when', 'where' and 'who' informs this understanding. Epidemiology provides the necessary tools and epitomizes Calvin's philosophy that measurement improves understanding.

The topics covered in this chapter include descriptive epidemiology, population transition, and measurement of disease in populations. The major risk factors for disease in the UK will be discussed before considering the epidemiology of a number of common causes of death and disease.

For more detailed information, interested students are referred to half a dozen good epidemiology textbooks and to published and electronic sources of current information listed in the final chapter of this book.

What epidemiology can do

Epidemiological techniques are used to make inferences based on findings from groups of people, or *populations*, rather than from individuals. Clear definitions are needed for *what* is being studied (*case definition*), the population under study (*who*) and the relevant time (*when*) and place (*where*). Variations in person, time and place provide information on the natural history of the disease and clues to its potential aetiology, and also identify possible treatment options. Epidemiological methods can help to assess whether a new treatment option is effective. Analysis of potential risk factors for a disease or condition can also provide opportunities to actively promote health as well as prevent illness. Epidemiological methods are also used to assess whether these strategies are effective, and to measure the effectiveness of health services (*health services research*). Epidemiology techniques are traditionally classified as *descriptive* and *analytical*, and this chapter will follow this convention.

What epidemiology cannot do

Epidemiological techniques are applied to groups of individuals, not to specific individuals. For example, it is possible to estimate the risk of lung cancer in female smokers, but not to predict accurately whether a particular woman will develop the disease.

Epidemiological methods

Measurement in epidemiology

If the event measured is the *new* occurrence of a disease or condition, it is referred to as the *incidence*. The incidence rate of a disease or condition is defined as the number of new cases diagnosed in a specific population in a specified time period.

Box 5.1 Some examples of incidence rates

- 45 new HIV infections per million population per month in Uganda
- 3 heart attacks per 1000 population per year in the USA
- 36.3 cases of stomach cancer per 100 000 population in Liverpool (1990–94)
- 170 per 1 000 000 was the annual number of suicides among males aged over 45 years in the West Midlands

---

Prevalence is particularly useful for chronic conditions. Prevalence rates summarize the *total* amount of disease present, and thus describe the burden of disease in a population.

The principal measures used to assess the amount of disease in populations are incidence and prevalence.

RATES

As epidemiology is looking at events occurring within groups of individuals (populations), quoting the number of events that occur is only useful if it is set within the population and time frame in which the events occurred. For example, the finding of 10 cases of chicken-pox identified in a class of 30 five-year-olds in a single school in a specific week is very different to 10 cases of chicken-pox reported in a year in a town with a population of 30 000. *Rates* are often used within epidemiology to summarize this type of information and put the events in perspective.

A rate has the following general form:

$$\frac{\text{Number of events}}{\text{Population at risk of the event}} \text{ in a specified time period.}$$

The prevalence of a disease or condition is defined as all cases of a condition (new and ongoing) in a specified population at a specified time

Prevalence can be quoted as that at a specified point in time (*point prevalence*) or as that within a specified duration of time (*period prevalence*).

Box 5.2 Some examples of prevalence rates

- There were 450 HIV-infected individuals per million population in Uganda, as of 1 December 1998
- In 1997, the number of pregnant women in London infected with HIV was 1.9 per 1000
- As of 1999, 1% of the UK population had congestive heart failure
- The prevalence of treated asthma in Wales was 69 per 1000 in 1994

Incidence and prevalence are not independent. The prevalence of a disease is related to its incidence and its duration, i.e. the length of time between diagnosis and recovery or death. Provided that neither the incidence nor the duration of the disease is changing, its prevalence can be estimated by the following formula:

prevalence = incidence × duration.

CASE DEFINITION

When measuring health conditions within populations, it is important that there is a shared understanding of the event under scrutiny. Diseases present with a range of signs, symptoms and degrees of severity. For example, arthritis may leave one patient housebound and prevent another from playing sport. Professional and public understanding of health-related terms may also be different. For example, few patients who go to their GP with 'flu' will be suffering from influenza. To overcome these difficulties, the concept of *case definition* is used. Without a clear case definition, different estimates of disease incidence may only reflect different definitions, rather than true differences in the event frequency.

Box 5.3 Two examples of case definitions

- *Stillbirth*: a child which has issued forth from its mother after the 24th week of pregnancy and which did not at any time after being completely expelled from its mother breathe or show other signs of life.
- *Raised blood pressure*: a person with at least three sequential blood pressure readings in the previous 2 years, for whom the average of the last three readings was greater than or equal to systolic 160 mmHg and/or diastolic 100 mmHg.

Descriptive epidemiology

DESCRIBING THE POPULATION

Individuals do not exist in isolation, but are part of a group. Groupings (or populations) can be defined by geography (a country, region or village) or by other shared characteristics (e.g. attending the same school or health centre, having the same chronic disease, or sharing the same occupational income band). Understanding the grouping (e.g. its age and sex make-up) is invaluable for predicting and managing a wide range of health and other problems. An effective method of achieving this is by using a graphical display, known as a *population pyramid*. As Figure 5.1 shows, despite the two practices being of similar size, Practice 2 has a much higher number of older people, whereas Practice 1 has a larger number of children and young adults.

Disease incidence and prevalence can vary within a population, so when answering the question 'who?' about a disease or health state, typically the frequency of the condition is described in terms of the age and sex of its sufferers. Expressing disease frequency by age-specific incidence rates quickly shows whether a person's risk of the condition alters as they age. In a similar manner, disease incidence can vary by sex. Other personal attributes that are used to tease out differences in patterns of disease include marital status, ethnic origin, employment status and social status (see the examples below). It is the differences identified that contribute to the greater understanding of the condition under study, whether by demonstrating an effective intervention, generating a potential causes hypotheses, or simply raising further questions about it.

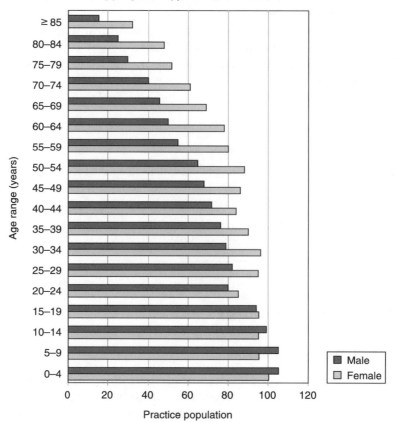

Figure 5.1 Graph of population pyramids from two (hypothetical) GP practices. (a) Practice 1. (b) Practice 2.

Box 5.4 Some examples of variations in health outcomes

Social inequality:
- Coronary heart disease deaths aged < 65 years are threefold higher in deprived men than in affluent ones.
- The stillbirth rate ranges from 5.0 per 1000 births among infants with fathers in social class I to 7.3 per 1000 births among infants with fathers in social class V (England and Wales, 1997).

Age:
- The age-specific incidence of breast cancer in Merseyside and Cheshire for the period 1990–94 ranged from 28 per 100 000 in women aged 30–34 years to 286 per 100 000 in women aged 80–84 years.

Geography:
- Deaths from tuberculosis ranged from 6 per 1 000 000 in England to 10 per 100 000 in Scotland (1997).

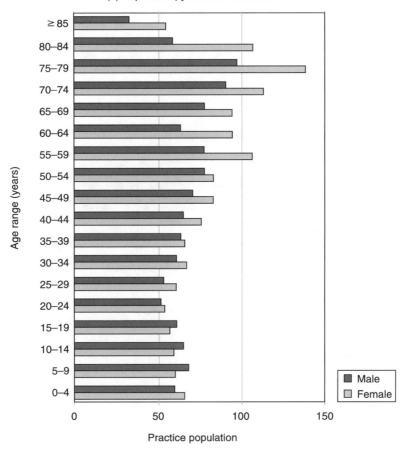

(b) Population pyramid for Practice 2

Figure 5.1 (*contintued*)

Case study

Population changes (including population pyramids) (see Figure 5.2a and b)

The figure illustrates the *demographic transition* – that is, the change in the population profile of England and Wales between 1841 and 1991. The 1841 pattern, which is similar to that still seen in many less developed countries, shows that 36% of the population were children. The triangular shape reflects the high mortality rate seen at all ages. Death rates as high as 1620 per 10 000 were seen in children less than 1 year of age (compared with the 1991 rate of 74 per 10 000). Life expectancy for a child born in 1841 was 41 years for a boy and 43 years for a girl. This contrasts with the life expectancy for a child born in 1991 (73.2 years for a male and 78.8 years for a female). Improvements in survival, reflecting for the most part better social conditions rather than advancements in medicine, have brought about the pattern seen in 1991, with 30% of the population between 25 and 44 years of age. The patterns of cause of death have also changed markedly over the last 150 years. One-third of deaths in the mid-nineteenth century were due

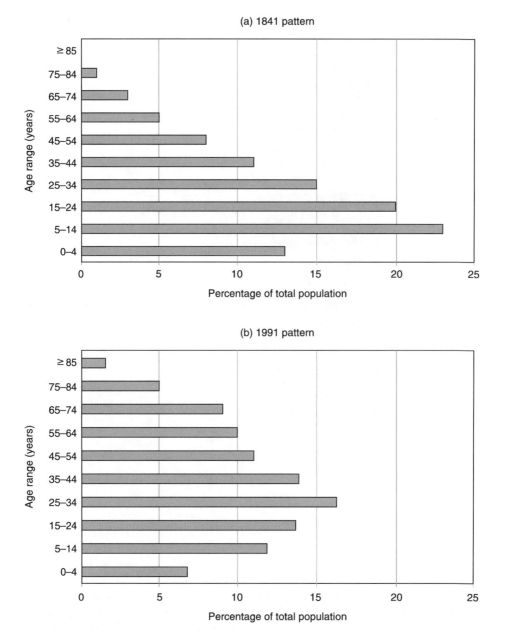

Figure 5.2 Population pyramid showing the change in the population profile of England and Wales between 1841 and 1991. (a) The 1841 pattern. (b) The 1991 pattern.

to infectious diseases, compared with less than 1% in 1991. In contrast, only 6% of deaths in the mid-nineteenth century were due to circulatory system causes, but 45% of deaths in 1991 were attributed to these causes. Deaths due to neoplasm have risen from 1.5% in the mid-nineteenth century to 27% in 1991. This change in causes of death, which is in part a result of the change in the population profile, is known as the *epidemiological transition*.

TIME

In epidemiology, it is often useful to look at the timing of disease incidence and prevalence. By monitoring changes in a disease over time (e.g. over 20 years), clues to aetiology may be identified. For example, increasing prevalence of asthma correlates with an increase in air pollution. Monitoring over time also allows the assessment of the impact of preventative interventions (see the case study on pertussis later in this chapter).

Sometimes it is the timing of the onset of a sign or symptom that provides a clue to its aetiology. This is particularly true in infectious disease, where knowledge of incubation periods can aid diagnosis (e.g. the appearance of a rash 14–17 days after exposure to chicken-pox usually heralds the onset of a new case of the infection). Extrapolating from data collected during the investigation of a food poisoning outbreak can provide clues to both the source of infection and the suspected organism.

Some conditions have a natural pattern. For example, meningitis is more common in the autumn and winter months (see Figure 5.3). Other conditions may have a cyclical pattern over several years, such as measles (see Figure 5.4). Thus declines in the incidence of a disease may reflect a natural pattern rather than changes in the condition or its treatment.

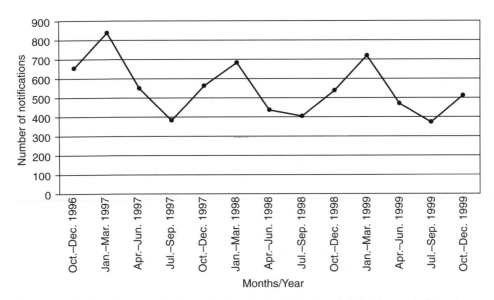

Figure 5.3 Meningococcal disease in England and Wales during the period 1996.

PLACE

Variations in prevalence and incidence according to where a disease is seen can also be a useful clue to the origin of a condition. Differences can be observed both between countries (e.g. the prevalence of malaria) and within

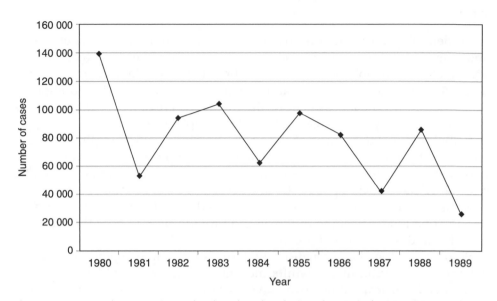

Figure 5.4 Measles cases in England and Wales during the period 1980–90.

countries, with local variations by communities or regions (e.g. higher rates of coronary heart disease in Northern England, and a higher prevalence of breastfeeding in South-East England). A difference in the distribution of a risk (or preventative) factor may offer an explanation for the observed variation in disease patterns, or provide evidence for a hypothesis on the aetiology of a condition.

The classic example of using information about the geographical distribution of disease to prevent illness is the action of John Snow in nineteenth-century London. John Snow was well known as the anaesthetist who administered chloroform to Queen Victoria. He was also an epidemiologist. He noticed that cholera was much more common in people who lived in Broad Street than in those who lived in other streets in the area. This provided him with evidence that the water pump could be the source of the infection, and to test this hypothesis he removed the handle from the pump, and noted that the number of cases in the area dropped rapidly.

Comparison of the rates of disease among immigrants with the rates observed in their country of origin and the rates observed among the indigenous people of their adopted countries can provide a useful insight into the relative contribution of environmental and genetic factors to disease development.

Case study

Routine data on immunization, and disease notification of pertussis (see Figure 5.5)
    The graph shows the changes in notifications of pertussis (whooping cough) over the last 58 years in England and Wales. By superimposing data on pertussis immunization uptake rates, it can be clearly seen that the disease incidence rises

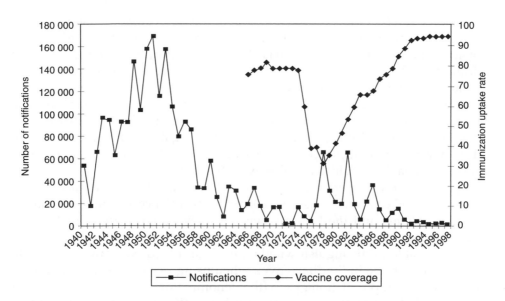

Figure 5.5 Notifications and immunization rates for pertussis in England and Wales during the period 1940–98. Source: Registrar General's annual returns (1940–73), Office of Population Censuses and Surveys (1974–78) and Office for National Statistics (1979–98).

when immunization rates decline. This provides evidence for the effectiveness of pertussis immunization (which can be used in health promotion), as well as demonstrating the effect on the population when large numbers of parents withhold immunization from their children, in this example because of groundless fears that pertussis immunization causes brain damage.

KEY INFORMATION SOURCES

Epidemiological information comes from two main sources, namely routine statistics and special studies. Within the UK, the Office for National Statistics (ONS) collates and publishes the routine statistics (or the Information and Statistics Division in Scotland). The most useful routine statistics for epidemiological use are those relating to the population (e.g. birth, population size, and death) and to disease (e.g. cause of death, cancer incidence, and communicable disease).

Information on population size and subgroup classifications (e.g. occupation-derived social class categories, age, sex and area of residence) are based on data collected at the 10-yearly national census. Errors made in reporting data on the census form compromise the accuracy (or *validity*) of the data. Figures relating to the population size and constitution in the intervening years are estimated on the basis of the annual numbers of births, deaths and migrations. Information on births and deaths published by the ONS is drawn from data reported to the Registrar of Births, Marriages and Deaths at the time when these events are registered, usually by the next of kin. Again, the level of accuracy can by reduced by errors (e.g. in the reporting of personal details or in death certification). Data on cancer and infectious disease incidence are obtained through the regionally based national reporting systems that exist within the UK. The local 'Proper Officer' – usually the Consultant in Communicable Disease Control (CCDC) – is notified of cases of specific infectious diseases, in accordance with legal requirements. The Communicable Disease Surveillance Centre (CDSC) also collates and disseminates further data on infectious diseases. Although it is not a legal requirement, there is in addition a regionally based national system that collects data on all cases of cancer, summaries of which are also available annually.

Apart from the cancer and communicable disease data mentioned above, most published data on disease incidence and prevalence are based on contact between patients and the health service, in either a community or hospital setting. However, this data is often 'episode based', which means that it is not always possible to distinguish whether, for example, three admissions relate to one, two or three individuals. Even when using person-based data, it may not be clear what population group (the denominator) is appropriate, making it impossible to calculate rates. An exception to this occurs when figures are derived from a general practice population, such as the decennial publication on *Morbidity in General Practice*.

The population prevalence of risk factors and health-promoting behaviours can be estimated from data from surveys published by the ONS. The information in these surveys comes from randomly selected samples of the population. These special studies, which are often repeated at regular intervals, can provide useful information, particularly on the prevalence of smoking and alcohol consumption in different areas of the UK and how these have changed over time. Examples of such surveys include the General Household Survey and the Infant Feeding Survey. Individual government departments (e.g. the Department of Health, Department of Trade and Industry and Department of Education and Employment) also publish health-related data. These data are presented at both individual and episode level, and may be based on samples or cover the entire population.

Estimates of the prevalence and incidence of other diseases are often based on estimates derived from individual studies published in the medical literature (e.g. *British Medical Journal*, *The Lancet*, etc.).

MORTALITY AND MORBIDITY

It can be seen that information on disease incidence and prevalence is limited, and is often only available for a highly selected sample. Thus much work describing disease epidemiology is based on data derived from death certification, and mortality (death) is used as a surrogate for morbidity (illness). Using mortality data and cancer incidence data, Figure 5.6 illustrates how useful, and sometimes how misleading, estimates of disease incidence may be when they are based on mortality data. For example, because cancer of the oesophagus has a poor prognosis, mortality reflects incidence and is thus a useful surrogate measure. In contrast, colon, breast and cervical cancer

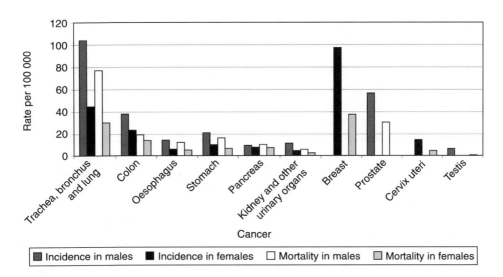

Figure 5.6 Age-standardized incidence and mortality for selected cancers in 1993 in Europe.

mortality is half the incidence and, for such common conditions, using mortality rates as a surrogate of incidence will severely underestimate the frequency of the condition.

Association vs. causation

> 65-year-old man in Essex cottage drops dead (a) an hour after plane flies overhead or (b) a minute after black cat crosses in front of him or (c) a second after his left main coronary artery is totally blocked by a blood clot.
>
> *(Daily Planet news item)*

We live in a world of associations. In medieval times medicine depended on bizarre treatments, including blood letting. The alleged benefit was based on the *post-hoc, propter-hoc* fallacy. That is to say, if something happened after something else, then the two events were thought to be causally related. Fortunately, the evidence-based paradigm has slowly prevailed over the last century.

How do we 'know' that smoking (sometimes) causes lung cancer? Austin Bradford Hill made it easy when he published the following eight very helpful criteria.

1. *Biological plausibility.* Can we see the complete molecular pathway? Yes, tobacco tar contains over 1000 recognized carcinogens. Each stage is now well described – tobacco smoke, lung, lung epithelium, tumour induction and tumour promotion.
2. *Reversibility.* Does the removal of the putative agent(s) reduce risk? Yes, stopping smoking halves the subsequent risk of lung cancer in the first year and decimates it after a decade.

3. *Animal demonstration.* Does an animal model exist? Yes, many of the beagles who were exposed to cigarette smoke in laboratories developed lung cancer, whereas control animals did not.
4. *Dose response.* Was this observed? Yes, the risk of lung cancer in long-term smokers increases progressively with the number of cigarettes smoked per day (5, 10, 15, 20, etc.).
5. *Follows exposure?* Is there a temporal relationship? Does lung cancer always follow rather than precede exposure to the suspected carcinogen? Yes, almost always with a time lag of 20 to 30 years.
6. *OveR time and over seas.* Is the relationship consistently seen in different series of cases and different places? Yes, there are now many reports from across the world.
7. *Design of experiment.* Some study designs are more reliable than others. The evidence from a randomized controlled trial (RCT) is more convincing than that from an observational study. However, for many exposures an RCT is unethical. The two main types of observational studies are *cohort* and *case–control* (see Box 5.5). Evidence derived from cohort studies is considered to be more reliable as the design is less vulnerable to systematic error (bias).
8. *Strength of effect.* How big is the risk? The larger the risk, the more likely it is that the relationship is causal. In cigarette smoking and lung cancer, smokers are over 10 times more likely to get lung cancer than non-smokers.

Look at this list again and you will see a useful mnemonic to remember these criteria: **BRADFORD'S.**

Key text: Doll and Peto on UK doctors and smoking

Doll R and Peto R (1976) Mortality in relation to smoking: 20 years' observations on male British doctors. *British Medical Journal* **2**, 1525–36.

During the 1940s, scientists began to wonder whether smoking might cause lung cancer. In the USA and in Britain two case–control studies suggested that, compared with other hospital patients, lung cancer patients had a twofold or threefold higher likelihood of being smokers. Although this was useful, case–control studies are notoriously vulnerable to bias. Better evidence was needed, so Richard Doll and Richard Peto designed a large *cohort* study. With the help of the British Medical Association (BMA), they forwarded a questionnaire about smoking habits to all male British doctors. A total of 34 440 men replied.

Doll and Peto then painstakingly followed 98% of this cohort prospectively for 20 years. They carefully recorded the certified cause of all 10 072 deaths. Compared with lifelong non-smokers aged under 70 years, the death rate among cigarette smokers was twofold higher.

The extra deaths were mainly due to heart disease, lung cancer, chronic obstructive lung disease and various vascular diseases. Lung cancer mortality was 20-fold higher in the very heavy smokers.

Because this cohort reduced its cigarette consumption substantially during the period of observation, lung cancer became relatively less common as the study progressed, but other cancers did not, 'thus illustrating in an unusual way the causal nature of the association between smoking and lung cancer'.

Box 5.5 Summary of the advantages and disadvantages of cohort and case–control studies

Cohort studies

In a cohort study, study participants are *classified by exposure,* and followed up to determine the outcome.

Advantages	Disadvantages
A particularly useful method of studying rare exposures	Time-consuming and requires large samples
Allows direct calculation of incidence rate, and therefore relative risk can be determined	Follow-up period may be extended and thus expensive, and subjects may be lost to follow-up, compromising study power
Temporal relationships not a problem, because exposure clearly precedes outcome	Not an efficient method for studying rare diseases
Limited opportunity for bias in well-designed study	
Evidence from a well-designed cohort study is strongly suggestive of a causal association	

Case-control studies

In a case–control study, study participants are *classified by outcome* (i.e. 'case' or 'control') and then their exposure is determined.

Advantages	Disadvantages
A useful and efficient method of studying rare and chronic diseases	Cannot estimate risk of disease directly, so estimate relative risk by odds ratio
Requires a relatively smaller sample size, and is thus cheaper than a cohort study	Vulnerable to bias in selection of both cases and controls, and in information collection, particularly recall bias
Shorter time is needed for study, so results are available sooner	Can be a problem in accessing and/or accurately measuring exposure information
	Not efficient for rare exposures

Practical points

THE TRADE-OFF BETWEEN COST AND QUALITY

Case–control studies can be conducted quickly, by just one or two researchers, and are therefore cheap. Although some cohort studies can be undertaken retrospectively, for prospective ones, follow-up is clearly going to be time-consuming and will require a lot of resources. It therefore needs to be a topic which is important and worthwhile.

GENERALIZABILITY

So much for British doctors, but can these findings be generalized to non-medics, or to people from other countries?

There seemed to be no reason why not, and this was confirmed in subsequent cohort studies of other occupations in the UK and elsewhere.

Other outcome measures

Epidemiologists are not just interested in counting dead bodies. Today, a comprehensive lung cancer epidemiological needs assessment would also consider the morbidity (burden of illness) caused, the reduced quality of life of the patients and their carers, their use of health services, and the resources consumed both by the NHS and overall.

Epidemiology of common diseases

Degenerative disease

In developed countries which have undergone the population (demographic) transition (see above), the burden of early death from infectious disease has been replaced by chronic degenerative diseases appearing in middle and old age, such as diabetes, heart disease, stroke and most cancers. This is called the epidemiological transition. Most of these diseases do not have one single 'cause', but have a multi-factorial aetiology. In other words, the risk of a heart attack is progressively increased by the occurrence in one individual of several factors operating additively or even multiplicatively. For example, even in one man, smoking combined with hypertension, a fatty diet and deprivation is seldom enough to cause a heart attack – increasing age is also required.

Understanding the distribution and determinants of health (*risk factors*) is thus a crucial part of epidemiology in the UK and elsewhere. The major risk factors affecting western society include smoking, alcohol, poor diet (and obesity) and hypertension.

SMOKING

Tobacco is the single biggest preventable cause of death and disease in the UK and elsewhere. It can be defined as active inhalation of tobacco smoke from cigarettes, cigars or pipe, or passive inhalation of other people's smoke. Tobacco is legal by historical accident. If cigarettes were introduced today their production and sale would probably be banned (just think about heroin and cocaine).

Smoking is implicated in the deaths of over 100 000 people in the UK every year – six times as many as accidents, suicide, heroin and AIDS put together. Smoking causes 40 000 lung cancer deaths and 60 000 heart disease deaths, as well as thousands more deaths from stroke, peripheral vascular disease, chronic obstructive airways disease and many other cancers (mouth, throat, oesophagus, stomach, liver, bladder and leukaemia).

Although the overall adult prevalence of smoking in the UK has declined from 50% in the 1950s to 30%, it is worrying that smoking prevalence has now begun to rise again, particularly in young people. Smoking rates are highest in the most deprived and least educated social groups. Nicotine acts as a relaxant, but unfortunately is phenomenally addictive and increases blood pressure. Tobacco tar contains over 1000 known carcinogens, as well as increasing blood clottability (and thus increasing the risk of thrombosis formation).

Diseases caused by smoking are difficult to treat, and cure is rare. Thus to improve health, smoking needs to be discouraged both by enabling children to make a positive choice not to smoke, and by helping current smokers to give up. The benefits are immediate, as ex-smokers halve their risk of heart disease within 1 year and halve their risk of cancer and chronic obstructive airways disease within 5 years. However, competing interest from both the government and industry dwarfs the impact of the health promotion strategies currently operating in the UK. At present, tobacco provides 1% of UK advertising revenue and 10% of sports sponsorship. The tobacco industry fights every step, bribing scientists and politicians and cynically shifting to softer targets in the Third World. Each year, the tobacco industry profits run into billions of pounds, with another £7 billion going to the government in tax and over £200 million spent on advertising (to replace the 300 customers lost each day through death). The industry also targets children, and about 20% of 15-year-olds now smoke. However, some countries have demonstrated that it is possible to have a successful, comprehensive tobacco control programme. This incorporates the banning of both advertising and, crucially, all other forms of promotion (e.g. logos on clothing, travel wear, boots, etc.), with aggressive taxation policies, and progressive legislation in workplaces and public places.

DIET AND OBESITY

A healthy balanced diet has been well described. It includes a high intake of complex carbohydrates (e.g. bread, potatoes, pasta) with plenty of fresh fruit and vegetables, and a low intake of fat (particularly saturated fat), salt and sugar. An adult ideally requires only 50–100 g of protein per day and 1 unit of alcohol. Healthy eating is learned at home and reinforced at school. Barriers to healthy eating include poverty, poor education and a deluge of unhealthy dietary messages from the media and advertising, compounded by government failure to use the effective mechanisms of food-pricing policy and subsidies.

Disease or death due to frank dietary *deficiency* is rare in the UK. Protein calorie malnutrition, and vitamin deficiencies such as scurvy and pellagra, rickets and osteomalacia, are very unusual and principally affect the very young, the very old and the very poor. As in other western countries, the main dietary problem that impacts on health is an unbalanced diet compounded by excess calorie intake. Diseases that are associated with poor diet include cardiovascular diseases (e.g. coronary heart disease, stroke and peripheral vascular disease), which are all increased by diets high in saturated fat and salt and low in fresh fruit and vegetables. The effect of diet probably explains much of the observed geographical variation in the prevalence of cardiovascular disease. For example, in countries such as Finland and the UK, there is a huge excess of cardiovascular disease compared with France, Japan or China. The positive time trends observed in recent years, particularly in the USA, reflect progressive improvements in diet. Poor diet also has an indirect effect on cardiovascular disease. Infants born to women with poor diets are smaller than the population average, and have a higher risk of cardiovascular disease in adult life. This has been described by Barker (1997) and others, who have suggested that poor intrauterine growth may result in relatively small babies who are more susceptible to hypertension, diabetes and heart disease as adults. This is often referred to as the 'Barker hypothesis/effect'.

Other diseases that are aggravated by poor diet include osteoporosis (which is more common in small women who smoke, are inactive and have a low calcium intake) and dental caries (which is most common in deprived groups with a high intake of refined sugar, confectionery and fizzy drinks and a low intake of fluoride from toothpaste or drinking water). Diet also plays a major role in several cancers, including those of the large bowel, stomach, oesophagus, uterus, prostate, lung and cervix. As with most risk factors, diet is not the only determinant. The observed effects are compounded by smoking and social deprivation.

Obesity, which is the result of excess calorie intake, is increasingly common in western societies. Around 40% of men are overweight (body mass index (BMI > 25) and 10% are obese (BMI > 30), and about 25% of women are overweight and 7% are obese. Obesity reduces insulin sensitivity, increases blood cholesterol and promotes atheroma formation. Through these mechanisms obesity also increases the risk of cardiovascular diseases, including coronary heart disease, stroke and peripheral vascular disease, and diabetes, as well as other conditions such as hypertension, gallstones, arthritis, depression, subfertility, hiatus hernia and accidents, and some cancers, particularly cancer of the breast, prostate and uterus.

The diagnosis of obesity is usually obvious, and can be confirmed using ideal weight tables based on extensive insurance company evidence. Obesity prevention requires the promotion of a healthy, balanced diet, supported by congruent messages at all levels (community, media and national). Schools, young people and mothers represent particularly important target populations. The prevailing social norms are complex. There is a very striking paradox, with a generally overweight middle-aged population and a young generation obsessed with thinness. Around 15% of adolescent girls suffer from anorexia nervosa, bulimia or an eating disorder with an abnormal body image.

The management of obesity is difficult, and weight reduction tends to be limited and short term. Dietary advice focuses on reducing fat and salt intake, increasing the intake of complex carbohydrates and fibre as well as fresh fruit and vegetables, increasing the level of exercise, and setting a target of one pound weight loss per week. One kilogram excess body weight is equivalent to 7000 kilocalories, so good motivation and long-term effort are required.

HYPERTENSION (HIGH BLOOD PRESSURE)

Hypertension is defined as a systolic blood pressure exceeding 140 mmHg and/or diastolic blood pressure exceeding 90 mmHg. Although blood pressure is observed to rise with age in western countries, this is not seen in less developed societies. The development of hypertension is related to dietary intake of salt and saturated fat, compounded by lack of exercise and obesity, with a small genetic component and an important intrauterine 'Barker' effect (see above). Prevention strategies are based on the promotion of a healthy diet (as defined earlier) and more exercise, the progressive reduction of intake of salt in processed foods, and smoking control as described above.

Hypertension is rarely a disease in itself, but it is a significant risk factor of many diseases. It is estimated that it explains about one-quarter of all coronary heart disease, two-thirds of all strokes, and is a significant contributor to heart failure, renal disease and peripheral vascular disease. It is a common problem, with approximately half of all middle-aged and elderly adults having the condition. It is diagnosed with a sphygmomanometer by taking repeated measurements over several weeks. Simple management strategies include encouraging affected individuals to increase their exercise level, lose weight, improve their diet and stop smoking. These strategies can be followed by medication with thiazide, beta-blockers, angiotensin-converting enzyme (ACE) inhibitors or calcium antagonists.

ALCOHOL

The role of alcohol as a risk factor for ill health and death is ambiguous. It is implicated in over 28 000 deaths per annum in England and Wales, and costs the NHS over £120 million every year, yet people who abstain from alcohol have a higher all-cause mortality rate than those who drink in moderation. Current guidelines in the UK suggest a 'sensible' drinking level of 3 to 4 units per day for men and 2 to 3 units per day for women. A unit is defined as 8 g of absolute alcohol. This is equivalent to half a pint of beer (3.5% alcohol by volume or ABV), a *small* (95-mL) glass of wine at 11% ABV, or 1/6 gill (24 mL) of spirit (40% ABV).

However, excess alcohol consumption is associated with increased mortality from cancer, cerebral vascular disease, accidents and violence. Some occupational groups are particularly at risk of death from alcohol-related disorders. These include publicans and others in the catering trade, as well as doctors and lawyers.

Over 85% of women and 90% of men consume some alcohol every week. Health protection (legal and fiscal) measures to limit excess alcohol consumption include the imposition of taxes on alcohol-containing drink, restricted access to alcohol through licensing laws, and restrictions on advertising. Other protective legislation includes drink-driving regulations. Secondary prevention, using 'brief interventions' in primary care (encompassing the assessment of intake and the provision of information and advice at an individual level) is cost–effective, and can reduce consumption by 20%. The 'CAGE' questionnaire (see Box 5.6) is particularly useful for identifying individuals with excessive alcohol consumption.

Box 5.6 The CAGE questionnaire

Have you ever felt you should **C**ut down on your drinking?
Have people **A**nnoyed you by criticizing your drinking?
Have you ever felt bad or **G**uilty about your drinking?
Have you ever had a drink first thing in the morning to steady your nerves or to get rid of a hangover (**E**ye-opener)?

Source: Bush B, Shaw S, Cleary P, Delbanco TL and Aronson MD (1987) Screening for alcohol abuse using the CAGE questionnaire. *Journal of the American Medical Association* **82**, 231–5.

Common specific diseases

It is beyond the remit of this chapter to provide a detailed analysis of the epidemiology of specific diseases and how this information can be used to prevent disease and promote health. However, we shall present a case study on coronary heart disease, and a summary of the epidemiological profile of several other chronic diseases.

Case study: coronary heart disease (CHD)

DEFINITION

CHD is defined as cardiac impairment due to reduced blood flow in one or more coronary arteries.

MORTALITY

There are about 140 000 deaths due to CHD in the UK annually (equal numbers of men and women), representing about 25% of all male and female deaths. This is still one of the highest mortality rates in the world.

PREMATURE DEATHS

About 60% of male CHD deaths occur below the age of 75 years, compared with 35% of female deaths. This results in about 1.2 million years of life lost (YLL) in men and 1 million YLL in women every year.

PATHOLOGY

CHD results from narrowing or blockage of coronary arteries by atheroma (fatty deposits in the vessel wall) plus thrombosis (the development of a blood clot).

TIME TRENDS

CHD mortality is now falling in the UK and in most other industrialized countries. *(Discussion point: why is CHD mortality increasing in Eastern Europe and developing countries?)* These declines reflect risk factor improvements (a healthier lifestyle, less smoking, a healthier diet, hypertension treatment and increasing affluence) *as well as* medical and surgical treatments for established disease.

CARDIOVASCULAR RISK FACTORS

These act together multiplicatively. 'Fixed' risk factors include age, male sex, and a family history of premature CHD. The major 'changeable' risk factors are smoking, poor diet, high cholesterol, hypertension and deprivation. Many other minor factors have been described, including exercise, obesity, triglycerides, homocysteine, etc.

CLINICAL PRESENTATIONS

CHD can manifest as *sudden death*, a *heart attack* (myocardial infarction; MI), angina (chest pain on exertion or stress) or *progressive heart failure* (shortness of breath, ankle oedema and fatigue). Many CHD patients are chronically disabled with poor quality of life.

ANNUAL INCIDENCE

The annual incidence of new cases of MI and angina is approximately 1–2%, but it is higher in the elderly. A quarter of MI cases die within the first hour, and half die during the first month.

CHD PREVALENCE AND NHS ACTIVITY

CHD affects about 5 million people in the UK. Much of this 'iceberg of disease' is hidden in the community. GPs see approximately 1 million affected individuals annually, and about half a million are seen in hospital (CHD accounts for about 4% of bed days and 4% of NHS admissions). About 40 000 patients undergo coronary artery bypass graft surgery or angioplasty every year. CHD therefore generates an immense burden for patients, carers, the NHS (£2 billion) and the state (£6 billion). Variations exist in diagnostic, admissions and treatment policies. Most CHD patients eventually die of CHD, stroke or peripheral vascular disease.

CHD PREVENTION

This is complex and politically controversial. Prevention is preferred by the Government (because it is cheaper) and by more educated or affluent members of the public (due to prevailing concepts of positive health and avoiding disease). The

Government regularly publishes CHD targets (e.g. to reduce CHD mortality in those over 65 years of age by 40% between 1990 and 2000).

Primary prevention means prevention before atheroma begins:

1. in individuals with risk factor(s);
2. in the whole population. National programmes to lower average levels of risk factors have been successful in Norway, Finland, Australia and the USA. They have a low cost and potentially large public health benefits;
3. high-risk strategies involve identifying individuals at higher risk for CHD (e.g. diabetics, patients with hypertension or previous CHD), mainly opportunistically in primary care consultations. The costs are higher and the benefits are smaller because it excludes the 'fit' majority.

Secondary prevention means acting after CHD has become obvious – that is, targeting patients with angina, MI or stroke. Multiple risk factor reduction is then attempted, including smoking cessation, diet, fish oil supplements, medication (e.g. aspirin, beta-blockers, ACE inhibitors, statins) and exercise. Comprehensive *rehabilitation* programmes are usually only offered after MI or surgery.

Prevention strategies

1. *Smoking cessation.* This is best achieved by highlighting specific cardiovascular risk factors, tobacco advertising, pricing, smoke-free environments and health education.
2. *Diet.* Improvement can be achieved by cholesterol reduction, antioxidants, blood pressure reduction and weight reduction. Lipid-lowering drugs are effective but costly.
3. *Blood pressure reduction.* This can be achieved by diet, exercise, weight reduction and medication.
4. *Exercise.* This is best rated as social activity for all, not for the excellent few. Health education and transport policies are therefore also important.
5. *Deprivation.* Large gradients exist, but can they be decreased? Further research is needed.

Important CHD prevention issues and conflicts

1. Ideology vs. evidence of cost-effectiveness. Conservatives want *individual initiatives* whereas socialists prefer *population initiatives*.
2. Public health vs. powerful vested-interest groups. Tobacco, advertising, dairy and food retail lobbies are rich, powerful and cunning.
3. The media are generally more interested in exciting new treatments for existing patients than in less dramatic strategies for preventing future cases.

STROKE

A stroke can be defined as a neurological impairment due to sudden catastrophic brain damage following blockage by thrombosis or embolus or rupture of a brain artery. It accounts for deaths in about 40 000 men and 40 000 women each year in the UK. Men are usually younger, with almost half of deaths occurring before the age of 75 years. Mortality rates rise steeply with age, and stroke is particularly common in older women. The risk of stroke is increased by hypertension (high blood pressure), smoking, social deprivation and poor diet. However, deaths rates from stroke are falling in western countries as the population blood pressure falls and hypertension treatments increase, diet improves and Barker intrauterine 'programming' effects decrease. The prevention of stroke is mainly achieved by the early detection and effective management of hypertension at all ages. In addition, like coronary heart disease, strokes can be prevented by addressing the other major cardiovascular risk factors, namely smoking, diet, lack of exercise and social deprivation.

The neurological deficit that is commonly seen in stroke sufferers is weakness of an arm or leg or both (hemiparesis), with or without impaired speech. Approximately half of all strokes are fatal, with half of the survivors making a good recovery and half (usually the more elderly) remaining chronically disabled. Between 60% and 80% of stroke cases are admitted to hospital, with the diagnosis being made by history, examination and, ideally, by CT or MRI scan. Initially, treatment is supportive. Active multidisciplinary rehabilitation in stroke units has been demonstrated to improve outcome, with lower mortality and less long-term disability. Stroke accounts for around 2–3% of NHS costs, mainly reflecting the costs of both long hospital stays and the need for long-term care.

RESPIRATORY DISEASES

Pneumonias can be defined by radiological or pathological evidence of pulmonary consolidation, and can be categorized by cause (viral/bacterial, e.g. pneumococcus, other bacteria, atypical organisms) or more usefully by age (childhood, adult and the elderly). Clinical features usually include shortness of breath, fever and cough. Diagnosis is usually by examination, X-ray and microbiological culture of sputum (which assists the choice of antibiotics). The prognosis depends on the severity and on any underlying condition. Death from bronchopneumonia is a common terminal event in a variety of immobilizing conditions such as stroke, cancer and heart failure. Primary prevention of pneumonia in children includes good nutrition and comprehensive immunization. The 'at risk' elderly (those with chronic disease) must receive influenza immunization. Physiotherapy can help by maintaining mobility and preventing pooling of respiratory secretions.

Asthma can be defined as wheezy shortness of breath which varies over short periods of time (episodic). It is a very common condition, affecting up to 20% of children and 5% of adults. It is often associated with atopy (hay fever and eczema) and, intriguingly, is more common in westernized than primitive societies. Clinically, asthma involves recurrent episodes of shortness of breath and wheeze, which are usually relieved by bronchodilator treatment (inhalers or tablets) and reduced by anti-inflammatories such as steroids or chromoglycate. Asthma tends to improve through childhood, but severe cases persist into adulthood. Deaths are rare (about 4 per 100 000 per year) and, like hospital admissions, are mostly preventable.

Chronic obstructive airways disease (COAD) refers to chronic bronchitis, emphysema or both, and is due to airway and lung damage associated with impaired respiratory function. It is prevalent in middle-aged men (about 10% of cases, compared to 5% in women), who are principally smokers. It has an incidence of about 1 per 1000 per year, and is particularly associated with deprivation (a threefold gradient). Both morbidity and mortality from COAD are declining in the UK as smoking and industrial pollution decrease. Clinical features include progressive shortness of breath on exertion over several years, frequent winter chest infections, and chronic cough with the daily production of some sputum.

COAD treatment involves stopping smoking, sensible exercise, medication with bronchodilators (e.g. salbutamol) and inhaled steroids (e.g. beclamethasone), and treatment with oxygen for the most severe cases. Continuing smoking reduces the prognosis and premature death is common. Its primary prevention is obvious – tobacco control, and legislation to promote clean air and abolish industrial pollution.

Pneumonias, asthma and chronic bronchitis together account for about 10% of deaths, 7% of hospital bed days and 6% of GP consultations.

MENTAL HEALTH PROBLEMS

Mental health problems can be defined as any psychological rather than physical problem that causes distress or disability. They are on a spectrum ranging from very common, often mild depression and anxiety, through to rarer but severe conditions such as mania and schizophrenia. Mild mental health disorders can affect up to one in three individuals at some stage in their lives, principally minor depression (prevalence 5–15%), major depression (5%), anxiety (5–10%) and bipolar manic depression (1%). Schizophrenia is much less common (prevalence 0.3% and incidence 20 new cases per 100 000). Schizophrenia has a fourfold variation with deprivation and ethnicity, and is more common in men. Diagnosis is based on 'positive symptoms' (including distorted thinking, perception and personality, hallucinations and delusions) plus 'negative symptoms (including apathy, emotional blunting, self-absorption and social withdrawal). Onset is most common in the twenties. Treatment in general practice involves problem-solving, informal and formal psychotherapy, short-term medications progressing to longer-term treatment, referral to specialists (psychiatrists or clinical psychologists) and, less commonly, short-term or long-term inpatient care. The prognosis for mild forms of mental health problems is generally good. However, recurrence is common and can affect work, family and social functioning. The focus of prevention in mental illness is on education of the public and media about mental health problems. There is also a need for more coherent initiatives to address the underlying causes, particularly poverty, social isolation, unemployment, and alcohol and drug addiction.

Suicide is uncommon but easily measurable, and for this reason it is a government favourite for 'mental health targets'. The epidemiology of death from suicide shows two peaks – the first is seen in early adult life, particularly among men, and the second peak occurs in later life, relating to depression, schizophrenia or chronic disease. Suicidal methods reflect local availability, and they vary by sex. Thus guns are often used in the USA, whereas in the UK men tend to choose hanging or carbon monoxide poisoning, whereas women tend to choose overdosing with tablets.

Dementia is defined as mental disorder of old age associated with physical changes in the brain. There is progressive impairment of higher mental functions, including the memory, with inability to solve everyday problems and the loss of social skills and control of emotional reactions, but without clouding of consciousness. Mild dementia may simply involve forgetfulness and tolerable eccentricities, whereas severe damage can include loss of all effective psychological functioning. The prognosis is poor, with an inexorable downward decline and a median survival of less than 5 years. The dementias can be divided into pre-senile and senile (Alzheimer's, multi-infarct and other). The prevalence of dementia increases with age, from 1% among those aged 60–64 years to 12% in those aged 80–84 years, and 33% in those aged over 90 years. The rates are slightly higher in men. The number of sufferers is increasing, reflecting the progressive ageing of the population. Treatment is palliative, with most care being provided informally by family and significant others. Carers can ideally call on increasing support from social services, the primary care team, and commercial nursing and residential homes. Primary prevention is limited. Intriguingly, a high starting IQ and the continuation of a more active physical and mental lifestyle seem to have a protective effect, reducing the incidence of dementia.

ARTHRITIS AND MUSCULOSKELETAL CONDITIONS

Osteoarthritis most commonly affects the spine, hips, knees and wrists, with an overall prevalence of about 2% in men and 4% in women. There is a steep rise in prevalence with age, reaching 16% in women over 75 years. Overuse is a common feature (e.g. farmers' hips and footballers' knees are more often affected). Treatment involves physiotherapy, orthoses (including walking sticks) and surgical replacement of joints (mainly hips, but also knees). Primary prevention, which involves the avoidance of excessive wear and tear of joints, is obvious but unpopular.

Rheumatoid arthritis is much less common, affecting 0.3% of men and 0.5% of women. It can occur at any age, and is the commonest autoimmune inflammatory joint condition. It can affect hands, wrists, elbows, ankles, feet, knees, hips, shoulders, neck and spine. Other problems are common, affecting the skin, eyes, mouth, gut and kidneys. Treatment of rheumatoid arthritis involves the use of anti-inflammatory agents and immunosuppressants, including steroids, azathioprine and cytotoxic drugs. Physical appliances, physiotherapy and surgical joint replacement are also valuable for improving function and reducing disability. Progressive disability is usual, although premature death is uncommon.

Low back pain is very common. Up to 50% of the population experience one or more episodes of disabling low back pain, and chronic problems occur in about 20%. It is best managed by aggressive pain control and early mobilization.

Discussion points

1. What is behind a variable?

Most epidemiological studies include information on the participants' age, sex and ethnic background, but why? Such variables are included because they are considered to be potential 'confounders' – that is, a third variable that is related both to the exposure under study and to the outcome, but is not in the causal pathway. By including known confounders in a study analysis, the authors are attempting to remove their effect on the relationship under study. While this may be obvious with regard to age (older people are at higher risk for most diseases, and have an opportunity for greater lifetime exposure), why are sex and ethnicity considered to be confounders? In the USA, for example, researchers use the terms 'black', 'white' and 'hispanic', but these racial groups are not distributed equally among the income groups.

What problems could ensue in the interpretation of studies when included confounders do have a relationship to the causal pathway?

2. The prevention paradox

The *prevention paradox* was an expression coined by G.A. Rose, who highlighted the fact that preventive measures which bring large benefits to the community may offer little to the individual. For example, the widespread use of seatbelts has significantly reduced the number of deaths and serious injuries in road traffic accidents, yet most people who wear a seatbelt on a car journey are never involved in a road traffic accident.

Can you think of other examples of the prevention paradox? What effect does this have on an individual's motivation to participate in such preventive measures? What challenges does this pose for the community? To encourage seatbelt use, legislative powers are invoked. In what other situations could legislation be used to encourage appropriate preventive behaviours? What are the drawbacks of using legal measures to promote health?

3. Using epidemiology to inform health care provision

Review again the graph of population pyramids from the two hypothetical GP practices shown in Figure 5.1.

How will the patterns of disease differ in the two communities? What impact will these different disease patterns have on the services that the practice populations need? Will this mean that the way in which the practices function needs be different? What preventative services should each practice provide? Will the nature of the practices vary if they are in a rural area or an inner-city area? What other information about the practice populations would you need to answer these questions more fully?

4. The limits of biological mechanisms as explanations for disease aetiology

Coronary heart disease (CHD) results from a combination of thrombosis and atheroma in one or more coronary arteries (see the description earlier in this chapter). The risk factors that cause CHD seem to be well established. However, recent evidence from the Whitehall studies and elsewhere suggests that the risk of developing CHD decreases steadily up the social pecking order, with the highest CHD rates occurring in cleaners and porters, lower rates occurring in filing clerks, and the lowest rates being found in the permanent heads of each Ministry. Could this all be explained by social class differences in smoking, cholesterol and blood pressure? No, even after adjusting for those factors, the gradients remain. Why is this? Some of the gradient is explained by higher income (and presumably everything that it brings with it, including material wealth, greater freedoms and greater choices), some is explained by higher educational levels (and presumably knowledge about healthier lifestyles). But why do these things matter? And even allowing for income, a gradient between high and low status still remains! Why is this? Much appears to be explained by social factors (including networks, support mechanisms, etc.) and much by psychological factors (including self-efficacy, hopelessness, perceived job stress, etc.). But how could these psychosocial factors have any causal effect on the 'flesh-and-blood' biological mechanisms that result in CHD?

Acknowledgements

We thank Barbara Hanratty and Ann Capewell for their constructive comments.

Further reading

Beaglehole R, Bonita R and Kjellstrom T (1993) *Basic epidemiology*. Geneva: World Health Organization.

Bowling A (1995) *Measuring disease*. Buckingham: Open University Press.

Coggan D, Rose G and Barker D (1993) *Epidemiology for the uninitiated*, 3rd edn. London: BMJ Publishing Group.

Donaldson L and Donaldson R (2000) *Essential public health*, 2nd edn. Plymouth: Petroic Press.

Gordis L (2000) *Epidemiology*, 2nd edn. Philadelphia, PA: W.B. Saunders Company.

Kirkwood B (1988) *Essentials of medical statistics*. Oxford: Blackwell Scientific Publications.

Last J (2001) *A dictionary of epidemiology*, 2nd edn. Oxford: International Epidemiological Association and Oxford University Press.

Rowntree D (1991) *Statistics without tears*. Harmondsworth: Penguin.

Stevens A and Raftery J (1994) *Health care needs assessment. Volume II*. Oxford: Radcliffe Medical Press.

Psychological perspectives

6

Christine Bundy

Introduction

This chapter aims to introduce you to the individual from a range of different perspectives or schools of psychology. Later sections focus on the basic psychological processes thought to be the building blocks of the individual, how we learn, how we remember, how we express ourselves and how we make judgements about others. You will be encouraged to stop and think about each section you have read and to reflect on how this influences the way you are, what you believe and what you know. The key concepts appear as broad headings, and it is these that you could use as your basic framework for studying psychology:

- different types of psychology, including behavioural, psychodynamic and cognitive psychology;
- perception, including the visual and auditory systems, pain and extrasensory perception;
- memory, including the multistore theory, the levels of processing theory and connectionism;
- language development and use for communication;
- social influences on how we perceive the world, including attitude formation;
- individual differences between people.

The important terms you need to understand are shown in italics, as are important thinkers who have shaped our understanding. You will be advised what you could read to supplement this chapter, either later in this book or in other texts. You can take it as read that what is covered in this chapter is what you *need to know*.

Psychology is the study of the individual – his or her thoughts, feelings and behaviour. One branch of psychology, *social psychology*, also researches the way in which an individual may behave in a group, but in general psychologists research what goes on *within* the individual.

The same information can be viewed and interpreted in a range of different ways (see also the next section on the perceived world). This is both the strength and the weakness of psychology. On the positive side it means that the individual's own particular way of thinking, feeling or behaving is viewed as unique. On the negative side, however, some critics argue that there are no generalizable principles in psychology and that it cannot be scientific if it does not have these principles. We shall identify the guiding principles in psychology, how the study of psychology is a scientific process and how the beliefs we have that the other sciences, the natural sciences in particular, are 'harder' (and therefore better) science may be wishful thinking rather than reality.

Individuals differ in their ability to tolerate ambiguity. Some like certainty to the extent that they experience anxiety whenever they perceive any degree of uncertainty. Others are happy to accept that there may not be a right or wrong answer to a question. The A-level system in the UK encourages students to believe that there is a *right* answer to most problems or questions and that if the student studies the curriculum well enough he or she will find it. It can come as quite a shock when the same student on entry to a medical career finds that there are very few right *or* wrong answers, but more a case of weight of evidence for *and* against a particular viewpoint, theory or model. This is especially true of problem-based learning courses. It is this latter view that will help you to understand psychology and its different perspectives.

Scenario

- You can gauge your preference for certainty by noting how irritated you feel when in an interview a politician is asked for a 'yes or no' answer to a question but will only answer indirectly by referring to another issue.
- Alternatively, how easy do you find it to choose a sweet from a packet of about 20 different sorts? If you find that you take a long time to choose, perhaps it is because you are overwhelmed with decisions about which is the *right* sweet!

Types of psychology

The purpose of this section is to demonstrate that there is more than one perspective to any issue, and to help you to find a range of solutions to all of the problems you will encounter as a medical practitioner by seeing the same problem in different ways.

Within psychology, as in medicine, there are specialisms. There are some psychologists who focus on child development (akin to paediatrics) or elderly people (akin to geriatrics), some who study the senses, brain and nervous system (akin to neurology), some who specialize in abnormal thinking and behaviour (akin to psychiatry) and some who study the genetic or evolutionary influences on people (akin to genetics). To continue the analogy, within any of these specialisms there is a continuum of activity from laboratory-based,or basic medical science work through to the more applied or clinical work.

Behavioural medicine and health psychology are branches of psychology concerned with how people think, feel and behave in relation to health and illness, and they are heavily influenced by medicine. In addition, psychology is influenced by other sciences and subjects concerned with the individual, such as biology and philosophy, and by those which are more concerned with the interaction between individuals and between groups, such as sociology and anthropology.

Early psychology

Psychology, like medicine, has to be viewed within an historical context. Around 1870, *Wilhelm Wundt* in Germany was the first person to call himself a psychologist. Wundt used the methods of the natural sciences to try to understand individual behaviour. During this time *Sigmund Freud* and *psychoanalysis* were very influential in psychology. Freud was influenced by his own background of neurology, and he brought the then current medical scientific framework to his interest in the emotional life of people. He attempted to use scientific methods to understand psychology, but by today's standards they were inadequate. He used small samples and over-generalized to the population from these inadequate samples. His observations were *biased* because he tended to see only wealthy female clients, but he failed to recognize his biases, and attempted to generalize beyond his sample, claiming that he had discovered general principles on which he built his theory of psychoanalysis.

Psychoanalysis is based on the belief that all of our behaviour is motivated by instinctive urges of which we are largely unaware. This theory introduces the concepts of the *id* (the unconscious or basic urges), the *ego* (the subconscious urges of which we are partly aware) and the *superego* (our conscious or socially acceptable behaviour). Freudians argue that our behaviour and emotional life are the result of a perpetual struggle between the id and the superego. Crisis occurs when there is some unresolved tension between these instinctive urges, and this crisis may emerge as a mental health or physical problem. Early learning experiences are thought to be crucial to the way in which an individual attempts to resolve his or her inner tension. In psychoanalysis the emphasis is on interpreting the external signs of this inner mental strife.

Psychoanalysis is still practised, but there are very few psychologists who specialize in this area today.

Therapies based on psychoanalysis (known as the psychodynamic therapies) are usually applied to people with emotional and behavioural problems.

Psychodynamic theories assert that the individual, while involved in attempts to resolve their inner tension, becomes 'stuck' in an unhelpful behaviour pattern, usually involving others. The focus of therapy is therefore on the nature of the relationships between the person with the problem and other individuals who are emotionally close to them.

Behavioural psychology grew out of a reaction against the 'pseudoscience' of Freud's work. The American animal psychologist *John Broadus Watson* and the Russian physiologist *Ivan Pavlov* began to assert the view that psychology was the study of behaviour, and that the functioning of the mind was not a legitimate area of objective study, as it could not be studied scientifically. Behaviourism was as influential as psychoanalysis, and its influence is still pervasive.

Behaviourism emphasizes the importance of learning, including how new behaviours are acquired through *operant and classical conditioning*, how they are shaped through *reinforcement* and how they can be changed or eradicated through *extinction*.

Classical conditioning refers to the most basic form of learning and describes the association between a stimulus or event and an unconscious reaction. For example, when we smell food and we are hungry we salivate (see the section on the experiments of Pavlov on his dogs in the recommended introductory psychology text for further illustrations of this).

Operant conditioning, on the other hand, refers to the association between a stimulus and a response that the subject has learned to make (i.e. a conscious response). For example, when we are cold we are more likely to put on a thick sweater rather than a thin one, because we have learned that a thick sweater is more effective. For operant conditioning to occur, the effects of the response have to be reinforced – that is, the *consequence* of putting on the sweater has to be to remove the feeling of cold. If the desired effect is achieved, this *positive reinforcement* will increase the likelihood of that behaviour occurring in the future. However, if the cause of feeling cold was the open window, then removing the cause would be the more effective form of reinforcement, and this is known as *negative reinforcement*. Closing the window will prevent you from feeling cold. The third form of reinforcement is *punishment*. If you are shouted at by your mother for making more washing when you put on the sweater, you will take it off again, and this will be perceived as punishing. However, punishment is not the most effective way of increasing the likelihood that the behaviour will occur.

Although not all psychologists are behavioural therapists, most of them use the principles of learning and the use of reward and punishment for shaping behaviour in their work to a greater or lesser extent.

Of course, most learning occurs within a social context, *Social learning theory*, as its name suggests, is concerned with trying to predict under what social conditions learning occurs, and this area of research has been extended to the health field. In 1966 *Julian Bernard Rotter* argued that the likelihood of a particular health behaviour (e.g. taking exercise) occurring is dependent on the extent to which that behaviour is reinforced, and in particular the role of others in determining behaviour. Social learning theorists focus on how the social environment (including other people) can act as a reinforcer of behaviours. This early work by Rotter and others also laid the foundations for the health *locus of control* concept (more about this later).

More recently, *cognitive psychology* has contributed enormously to our knowledge within psychology, especially with regard to how we interpret information (from sensing to knowing) and how we think. According to cognitive theory, certain beliefs (or *schemas*) about ourselves, other people and events develop and are encoded in our minds from an early age. For example, depressed people encode self-defeating or pain-inducing attitudes which persist even in the face of contrary positive evidence (Beck, 1991) (this will be considered in more detail in the next chapter). Cognitive scientists have broadened our knowledge of what it is to be conscious, and how we solve problems, learn language and remember. The broad scope of cognitive psychology ranges from the study of the structure and function of the brain and nervous systems (biological psychology) to how individuals *experience* the world (humanist or experiential psychology).

Summary

- Psychoanalysis assumes that our behaviour is motivated by instinctive urges, of which we may not be aware.
- Behavioural psychology emphasizes the importance of learned behaviours that are acquired through conditioning and reinforcement.
- Social learning theory focuses on how the social environment reinforces behaviours.
- Cognitive psychology emphasizes the way in which we develop beliefs or schemas about ourselves and the world.

The perceived world

This section will introduce you to the psychophysics of perception, memory and language to help you to understand better how people experience the world. It will also encourage you to think critically about the tests you might perform on patients when they come to see you for investigation of a health problem.

Sensation and perception

We 'look' with the eye but 'see' with the brain. There is obviously some overlap between these two systems, but they are interdependent on each other and on the memory system.

The study of the relationship between physical stimuli and the psychological experience of those stimuli is called *psychophysics*. The main areas of research include the sensitivity of the sensory system, asking questions such as how loud a noise has to be in order to be detected (this is known as the *absolute threshold*), and what is the smallest physical difference between two light signals that can be detected (this is known as the *difference threshold*). Sensation (looking) is the first stage of the process of perception (seeing).

The visual system

The eye focuses light signals on to the retina at the back of the eye. At this stage the physical energy of light is converted to neural energy by the process of refraction by the lens and transduction by the photoreceptors in the retina. The retina is a highly organized system of neurones arranged in hierarchical layers. The light is processed by being spread over a wide surface area, thereby maximizing its detection. After this the signal is inhibited in order to prevent random spread. The eye is not simply a camera – the organized image that reaches the retina and subsequently the visual cortex in the brain is a *representation* or an *interpretation,* not a direct copy of the image.

The function of this first stage in the process seems to be to allow the signal time to 'imprint' on the retina, in order to enable the maximum amount of information to be extracted from it. Once the image that is held on the retina has been transmitted to the primary visual cortex, the process of detecting specialized aspects of the signal, such as colour, lines, edges and curves, distance, texture, etc., is started. The neurones involved in this highly specialized work are found only in this primary visual cortex. From there the signals are transferred to the secondary visual cortex, where further refined detection of these specialized aspects of the signal occurs. The signal then takes two pathways, one to the temporal lobes and the other to the parietal lobes where, in organized modules of neurones, the signals are given meaning and matched with previous experience of the same or related signals. This means that the memory system is activated to 'remind' the perceiver of the last time he or she encountered this event. This system is very highly organized and sophisticated, and there are many factors (e.g. mood and fatigue, as well as disease processes) that can interfere with the interpretation of the signal. We shall examine some of these factors later on.

The auditory system

As in the visual system, the auditory signal is initially detected by the sensory organ, the ear. The changes in pressure that are produced by vibrating air (the sound wave) are transmitted to the ear and the processing of this information begins. The signal moves through the middle ear, where it is transmitted and amplified to the inner ear. Here the signal disturbs the fluid in the cochlea, which is set in wave motion. As the hair cells detect this motion of the wave, they convert the mechanical signal into a neural signal, which is transmitted to the auditory nerve and then on to the auditory cortex in the temporal lobes of the brain.

The absolute threshold and difference thresholds also apply to auditory signals, and form part of one of the psychological properties of sound, namely *loudness.* This is measured in decibels (dB). Just to illustrate the scale, the absolute threshold for hearing is set at 0 dB, a normal conversation at about 60 dB and a loud rock band at around 120 dB. Hearing loss is thought to occur with prolonged exposure to 90 dB of sound. The other psychological properties of sound include *pitch*, which refers to the frequency of the sound wave. The higher the pitch the higher the frequency, and the range that humans are able to perceive is from 20 Hz to 20 000 Hz. Signals at the lower end of the scale may be detected via touch as vibrations rather than sound. The ageing process usually results in some loss of sensitivity, especially in the high-frequency range.

There are two theories of how we perceive pitch. The first asserts that the base of the cochlea contains receptors in the basilar membrane that are sensitive to pitch (the *place theory*), while the other suggests that the high-pitched sounds stimulate the nerve to fire more frequently than the lower-pitched sounds (the *frequency theory*). It may not be the case that one of these theories has to be correct and the other incorrect, as there is good evidence for both of them and they are complementary and not mutually exclusive. It is likely that a complex sensory task such as listening to a variable signal (e.g. a conversation between two people) will require both systems to operate.

We have two ears, and you could be forgiven for assuming that there might be some dys-synchrony in the perception of sound. If your right ear is closer to the noise then it will hear it first. The difference between the sound reaching one ear and then the other is calculated by the brain and used to determine the position of the object that produced the sound. This is known as *sound localization.*

Although it is important to understand the physics of this process, we must also remember that other signals may be competing for our attention, and that psychological processes such as reaction time, memory and level of anxiety can all serve to interfere with the signal that is finally received (more of this later).

The other senses of smell, taste, position and movement (*kinaesthesis*) are all important, although they are sometimes called the minor senses. Of course, this does not mean that they cannot be very powerful stimuli when remembering events (see the section on memory below). The general rules outlined for the process of transition from sensation to perception apply to these senses, too. The other two senses I shall mention briefly are pain and extrasensory perception.

It is not possible to discuss the senses in any further detail in this chapter, but the interested reader is referred to any basic psychology textbook. I particularly recommend *Psychology: a European Text* by Zimbardo and colleagues (1995), details of which are given in the Further Reading section at the end of this chapter.

Pain

Consider the following scenario.

Scenario

Tom and Mary were travelling home after a night out with friends. The car in front of them swerved to avoid a dog that had strayed into the road, and Mary, trying to avoid the car, hit a tree. After the initial bump the car began to smoke, and for a while there was no movement within the car. Four or five minutes later when Tom began to stir he knew that there was something very wrong with Mary, who was unconscious. He felt her pulse and found that she was breathing. He knew that it was only a matter of time before their lives would be in danger from the now burning wreck of the car. He mustered all his strength to get out of the car and pull Mary free from the wreck. He felt very weak and wondered if he could carry her to safety. Some minutes later, as he struggled to help Mary to regain consciousness, he could hear the ambulance siren in the distance. Tom was relieved when the paramedics came to assist Mary and him. When he was taken to the Accident and Emergency department, he was able to recall everything about the accident and gave a very good account of how he pulled Mary from the wreck. Accident and Emergency staff were astonished to hear Tom's story, as he had a fracture of the right femur and also multiple lacerations on his face, but he had not reported any pain on admission. A short time later he collapsed in severe pain due to his injury. He spent almost a month on the orthopaedic ward, but eventually made a good recovery.

Until recently the biological theories of pain were the predominant ones. *Specificity theory* suggests that there are specific nerve endings which correspond to the range of sensations we experience (e.g. heat, cold, sharpness or pressure). The theory claims that nerve fibres called A-delta fibres carry sharp signals to the brain, and they travel on myelinated sheaths that relay the signal faster than the unmyelinated C-fibres, which convey dull or aching signals. There is only limited support for this theory, and one of its main problems is that it does not explain how environmental factors can mask pain.

Pattern theory asserts that pain and touch receptors are shared, and therefore any stimulus can be perceived as painful if the intensity of the signal is great enough. However, this theory also has problems. It does not explain how light pressure over a specific area can induce pain in an individual, nor does it help us to understand how in the above scenario Tom might have not experienced any pain until after the accident.

The *gate control theory* is the only theory that helps us to understand the link between physiological and psychological experiences. This theory, which was developed by a psychologist and a physiologist, asserts that the brain can only process a limited amount of information at one time. When we experience pain, the brain is overloaded with sensory stimuli and, in an effort to preserve some spare capacity for additional information-processing, it 'blocks' some pain signals. This is where the analogy of the gate arises. The gate is open when small fibres from the injured tissue convey pain signals to the brain. When the ascending signals are potentially overwhelming, the brain partially closes the gate in the spinal cord to allow some but not all of the signals through. Similarly, the brain will allow some pain response signals to descend the track, but it closes the gate when the signals become overwhelming. Thus when the person is distracted by alternative stimuli (e.g. Tom's need to escape danger, and the competing demands of the situation on his attention) the gate can be closed almost completely. Information is being processed, but the experience of that event is being carefully controlled and the psychological perception of the stimulus is altered.

This theory is supported by the knowledge that children are easily *distracted* from pain by stories that have a *hypnotic* element to them (i.e. that are repetitive, comforting and dominate attention). Adults can be similarly distracted by the use of hypnosis or by certain forms of sensory stimulation (e.g. massage or heat, as used in physiotherapy), which aim to provide an alternative stimulus that competes for attention with the pain signal. This effectively closes the gate (see also the discussion of techniques used to relieve pain, in the next chapter).

Extrasensory perception

No discussion of perception would be complete without a consideration of the claims that are made for extrasensory perception (ESP). These claims are made for two types of extraordinary psychic energy exchange or *parapsychology*. These are ESP – which includes *telepathy* (thought transfer), clairvoyance (sensory stimulation in the absence of physical signals) and precognition (knowledge of future events) – and *psychokinesis* (mind over matter). There is *no* good experimental evidence to support clairvoyance, precognition or psychokinesis. There is some, albeit controversial, evidence for the existence of telepathy, and this comes from the well-publicized *Ganzfield* experiments. (You can find out more about this area from the work of Professor Susan Blackmore in Bristol; for a brief explanation, see *Introduction to Psychology* by Atkinson and colleagues, details of which are given in the Further Reading section at the end of this chapter.)

There are always methodological problems with research into parapsychological phenomena, not least of which are the small sample sizes that are generally used, the lack of adequate controls and the problem of replicating the findings. However, it is important to remain open-minded about the subject, although many psychologists believe that the pursuit of parapsychological phenomena is based not on the pursuit of scientific knowledge but merely on wishful thinking. This is not to deny that people often believe they have experienced psychic phenomena, but it is likely that there is some altered perception involved which can be explained using the known laws of physics. Perhaps the more interesting psychological area of study is why some people feel the need to believe in telepathy, for example, in the absence of any hard evidence.

Factors that influence perception

We are unable to attend to all sensory information simultaneously, but rather we *selectively attend* to incoming stimuli. It follows, therefore, that if we are attending to other messages from the environment (external), such as listening to a conversation in a room where the television is switched on, or to psychological messages (internal), such as a chronic low-level pain signal, this can influence which signals we give our attention to, and to what extent we do so. Extremes of temperature and drugs that alter consciousness can affect perception and interpretation of the information, especially if that information is ambiguous. Furthermore, the social context (i.e. what others say they see, hear or feel) can influence our perception. Our mood can have a profound effect on perception and interpretation, particularly if we are depressed. Anxious people tend not to 'hear' information, especially new information, accurately. Perhaps the area that has been the focus of most research is the component parts of the stimulus itself. The context of the stimulus gives us cues to understanding it (for a discussion of the importance of grouping, figure-ground, reference frames, motion perception, and depth perception, among other cues, see any introductory chapter on perception). By and large we see, hear or feel what we expect to and/or what we have experienced in the past. Much of what we experience now is dependent on our memory for similar experiences in the past.

Scenario

- It might be useful here to stop and think about how radiologists interpret radiographs or other results of imaging techniques. Are they born to be good radiologists, or do they learn with experience what to attend to and what to overlook? What factors could interfere with the process of interpretation of these ambiguous images?
- Similarly, when you first heard heart sounds through a stethoscope, how easily were you able to differentiate the important sounds from the background 'noise'?

Summary

- Vision and hearing have complex neuropsychological pathways. Importantly, they both involve mechanisms which allow us to represent and then interpret external stimuli.
- The gate control theory of pain is based on the assumption that the brain can only process limited amounts of information at any one time.
- Extrasensory perception is an exciting topic, but there is little firm experimental evidence to support it.
- Perception is crucially dependent on our ability to attend to stimuli selectively.

Memory

Memory is the active process of retaining and recalling information about past experiences. There are two main types of memory. The first is concerned with facts about events in the world and relationships between facts and meanings, and it is known as *declarative* knowledge (e.g. knowing that gravity causes objects to fall). The second type is memory for how to do things, which is known as *procedural* knowledge (e.g. knowing how to ride a bike or tie one's shoe-laces). These two forms of knowing are probably stored as memories in different ways. There are some things that are remembered with an aid or cue (*recognized*) and some that do not rely on a cue (*free recall*). The best-known way of thinking about memory is the *three stores* view of Atkinson and Shiffrin (1971). This describes the process of *encoding* information, *short-term storage*, and then the transfer into *long-term storage. The last part of the process involved in remembering is the retrieval stage.* This may sound very straightforward, but each of the three stages is complex.

Encoding/sensory storage

We select a signal from the range of stimuli surrounding us and are able to hold it for encoding for a very short period of time, around a second or so, before competing input takes up the space. This allows us to work on the trace of the stimulus, giving it meaning, matching it up with past experiences and maximizing the chance that it will be retained.

Short-term memory

The second stage or short-term memory (STM) can hold information for seconds or occasionally minutes, where again we are actively trying to convert it into permanent memory or long-term storage by attending to it in order to extract the maximum amount of information from it. Our storage capacity in STM is limited, and information is usually lost after about 20 seconds unless we actively try to convert it to long-term memory (LTM). Some of the ways in which we can help the processing include rehearsing (repeating it in order to hold it in short-term store), chunking (putting it into meaningful 'bits' in order to compress information like a computer's zip function, usually limited to about +7 or −2 'bits') and elaboration (linking it with something else meaningful). All of these aids to processing assist the transition into long-term memory.

Long-term memory

The third stage or long-term memory (LTM) seems to be a permanent depository for memories. It is well organized and is limited not by one's ability to store the information but by one's ability to recall it. There are three theories of how we organize our LTM. The first suggests that we use a linguistic *system of propositions* (statements about the relationship between two or more ideas, e.g. 'the world is round'). These meaning networks need not be factually based, but could be personal beliefs about the way things are. The second theory suggests that we store information in the form of real (not interpreted) images, known as *eidetic memory*. Those who claim to have photographic memories are using eidetic memory skills. The third position is one of compromise, where the individual probably uses both a verbal code and an image code to store information. This is known as *dual-code memory*.

There are two other competing theories about the way in which memory works. These are the *levels of processing theory* and *connectionism*.

The levels of processing theory proposes that we store the information on three levels. The first is in terms of its physical appearance (the word or event as we 'saw' it), the second level is in terms of its sound (its unique sound which is different to similar-sounding words or events) and the third level is in terms of its meaning. It takes more work to process information at the third (or deeper) level than at the preceding (shallower) levels. While this would instinctively seem to have some validity as a 'true' explanation, we must be cautious, as there is more experimental and clinical evidence for the multi-store model of memory.

The theory of connectionism asserts that the information is stored in inter-connected units rather than in one location, and is therefore more likely to be stored long term if it connects with many other 'chunks' of information or units. These neural networks are strengthened every time the person encounters that or a similar piece of information, and the information is more likely to be recalled if there are many connections rather than just a few. These theories may not be competing but complementary, and they may relate to different parts of the process of storing and recalling information.

In this chapter we are unable to consider all aspects of memory, and in particular the theories of why we forget, so you are reminded to read the chapters on forgetting in the book by Zimbardo and colleagues mentioned earlier. This will help you to understand what goes wrong with memory processes in diseases such as the dementias.

Scenario

Stop and remember your first day at infant school. You may hear the word 'school', see its form in sensory store, and then hold it there to remind yourself that the task relates to infant not junior school (STM). Then you might recall the event in the form of an image (eidetic memory – your first teacher's face, smell or voice) or an event linked to it (episodic memory – warm milk at play-time). You may have other emotive events connected to it in LTM (your first visit to the dentist, a hatred of times tables or examinations), and finally you will have other related concepts stimulated by the task (school = place of learning, education system = organized centrally, state system or locally, public system, etc.). What becomes clear is that the act of remembering is complex and we can use many explanatory frameworks to understand it. We also become aware of how it is inextricably linked to other cognitive functions such as perceiving and the use of language.

Summary

* The commonest theory of memory assumes that three stages are involved, namely selection and encoding, short-term storage and long-term storage.

- Long-term storage may be based on meaning codes, image codes or a mixture of both.
- Other theories of memory emphasize levels of processing, or connections and neural networks.

Language development and use

From a psychological point of view there are two main issues that we study in relation to language – first, how we acquire language, and secondly, what language can tell us about the way we think. The psychology textbooks often put language and thinking together to illustrate the inextricable link between the two forms of cognitive functioning. Language is the primary form of communication. There are others, such as non-verbal communication, written (signs) communication, etc., but the one that differentiates us from our nearest relatives is the ability to use language. Language is meaningfully structured, but the sound that we allocate to particular words is fairly random – we simply share the meaning that we allocate to words. Language is also dynamic, as the meaning that we ascribe to words is evolving over time (the use of the word 'gay' is an example of this). Language is arranged hierarchically, from *speech sounds* through *words* to *sentence units*. It is these sentence units that convey how we use concepts, and they give us the best insight into thinking. However, whether it is language that shapes thought or thought that shapes language is an interesting question, and as you might expect there are different theories on both of these perspectives.

Language acquisition

There is still some debate as to whether we are born with the ability to use language or whether we learn to use it. *Noam Chomsky*, one of the most famous psycholinguists, argues that we possess a *language acquisition device* that prepares us for learning language (Chomsky, 1975). He conceptualizes this as a genetic programme to learn language, rather than an actual device in the brain. This theory also proposes that there is a *critical period* during which language can be acquired. If this is missed because of some external influence (e.g. lack of appropriate stimulation) or internal influences (e.g. general learning difficulties), then language will never be completely acquired.

B.F. Skinner and other learning theorists give us another perspective on language development. They suggest that language does not differ from any other form of behaviour, and that when babies make sounds instinctively, unless those sounds are reinforced they will not be repeated. Thus they argue that cooing and gurgling, the typical sounds made by infants, are instinctive, and over time the parents 'shape' these utterances into meaningful words and sentences.

Once again we find that these two apparently opposing perspectives are in fact complementary, and both theories could be used as legitimate explanatory frameworks.

Why might language be of interest to you as a medical student? The answer is that quite apart from the detailed knowledge you might need to deal with patients who are aphasic (i.e. unable to express themselves clearly by means of speech) after a stroke or head injury, you might want to consider how the everyday use of language can indicate the way in which the patient is thinking when they come to see you.

Consider the following scenario.

Scenario

Jean went to her GP and knew that she would be criticized for not giving up smoking. This made her nervous. She thought about it and resolved to pretend that she had given up. She had a cough and needed some antibiotics for it. She rehearsed what she was going to say:

'I've had this cough that won't go away and I think I need some antibiotics'. However, when she saw the GP, the first thing she actually said was 'I've got this *cancer* and I need some antibiotics to make it *quit*'.

The GP was astute enough to grasp this insight into Jean's thinking and use it to convey two messages. She said 'I will check if you have a chest *infection* and give you antibiotics for it. I would also like you to consider taking part in the trial of my new treatment programme using nicotine patches for helping to quit smoking.' In this way she communicated to Jean that she knew she was a smoker and would not judge her because of it, but instead offered to help her to give up in a very practical way. The GP also communicated to Jean that she could be useful to the health centre, so making the relationship a little more equal.

Summary

- Chomsky considers that we are genetically programmed to acquire language, while Skinner and other learning theorists believe that language develops through behavioural conditioning. Both perspectives may be useful in medicine.

Social influences on the perceived world

We are all social beings, which means that the majority of our lives will be spent with other people. The rules that govern how we perceive the material world also govern our perception of the social world, including both ourselves and other people. This section will introduce you to some of the research areas in social perception, and will encourage you to think critically about how you reach decisions about the type of person someone is and how that guides your behaviour towards that individual.

Attitude formation

Attitudes are likes and dislikes with regard to objects, situations and people. We begin to form attitudes about others as soon as we meet them.

Attitudes have three components – cognitive (thoughts), affective (feelings) and behavioural. The cognitive component is better known as *stereotyping*, the affective component as *prejudice* and the behavioural component as *discrimination*. Although there may be a positive or negative aspect to each of these, psychologists have more often tended to focus on negative attitudes. There is usually some consistency between the three components of attitude, which is why if someone holds a negative stereotype of a person they are also likely to discriminate against them. Indeed, if we experience conflict between our thoughts, feelings and behaviour, this creates anxiety in us, and it is known as *cognitive dissonance*.

Attitudes are influenced by a range of factors, including the following:

- knowledge or beliefs about the person or situation (e.g. all white people are racist);
- a desire to express our values (e.g. it is wrong to be racist);
- a desire to protect ourselves (e.g. I did not get the job because I am black);
- a need to fit in with our social group (e.g. my family and friends have experienced racism and I identify with them – therefore I hold the same attitudes as them).

Many psychologists have demonstrated that there is little consistency between thoughts, feelings and behaviour on many important topics. Furthermore, many of them argue that there is greater inconsistency than consistency demonstrated. What we know is that our attitudes serve many different functions and might be socially constructed – that is, they will depend on the situation we are in rather than on a fixed set of rules about our beliefs.

Attitudes best predict behaviour when they are strong and consistent, based on a person's direct experience and when they relate to the behaviour to be predicted.

Summary

- Attitudes involve thoughts, feelings and behaviours.

Individual differences

There are few areas within psychology that divide people into 'camps' better than individual differences, and the two main aspects of research within this area are personality and intelligence.

Personality

Personality is the generic term for how we express our individual characteristics. We hold what initially appear to be contradictory beliefs about personality. On the one hand, we believe that we are all unique human beings, but on the other hand we also believe that we share common characteristics with others. What we mean by this is that some aspects of our 'character' are shared with others, but the sum of all of those character traits is expressed in a unique way, and it is this which defines our 'personality'. We might think about the common characteristics in terms of being shy or good with figures or typical Cancerians, but we would be loath to agree that all shy or numerically skilled people are alike, or that all Cancerians are identical.

The early work on personality tended to classify people into a limited number of *types*, and then further graded them according to the degree to which they possessed *traits* of that type. *Hippocrates* was one of the earliest personality theorists. He classified people into four types according to the relative proportions of the humours (body substances) – blood, phlegm, black and yellow bile – they possessed. The idea that it is one's physiology that determines personality has a long tradition and is still popular today. The physician *William Sheldon* classified people according to their body shape. Sheldon argued that endomorphic people were soft and round and usually sociable, that mesomorphic people were muscular, strong, assertive and courageous, and that ectomorphic people were thin, long, artistic, introverted and contemplative. Whether you are happy with the types as they are described by Sheldon may be determined by your personality!

More recent work has focused on personality traits rather than types. *Gordon Allport* (1937) described three groups of traits, namely *cardinal traits* (those that would define someone as exceptional, e.g. profound goodness), *central traits* (those major traits you would identify in an individual, e.g. aggressiveness) and *secondary traits* (those you would have to look very closely for, e.g. a tendency to be shy in social situations involving members of the opposite sex). *Hans Eysenck*, one of the century's most prominent psychologists, tried to reconcile the types and traits work when he developed the four quadrants of the personality circle (see Figure 6.1). Eysenck (1947) argued that there are two basic axes – first, that of introversion vs. extraversion, and secondly, that of instability vs. stability.

The most current research in this area highlights the 'Big Five' personality factors. Costa and McCrae (1985) describe these factors as *extraversion* (gregarious, warm and positive vs. reserved and shy), *agreeableness* (compliant and sympathetic vs. quarrelsome and unfeeling), *conscientiousness* (self-disciplined and dutiful vs. irresponsible and chaotic), *neuroticism* (anxious and self-conscious vs. calm and self-assured) and *openness to experience* (creative and intellectual vs. unimaginative and uninterested).

So far, all we have done is to *describe* types or traits, and many critics of this work highlight the lack of any underpinning theory. As one would expect, all

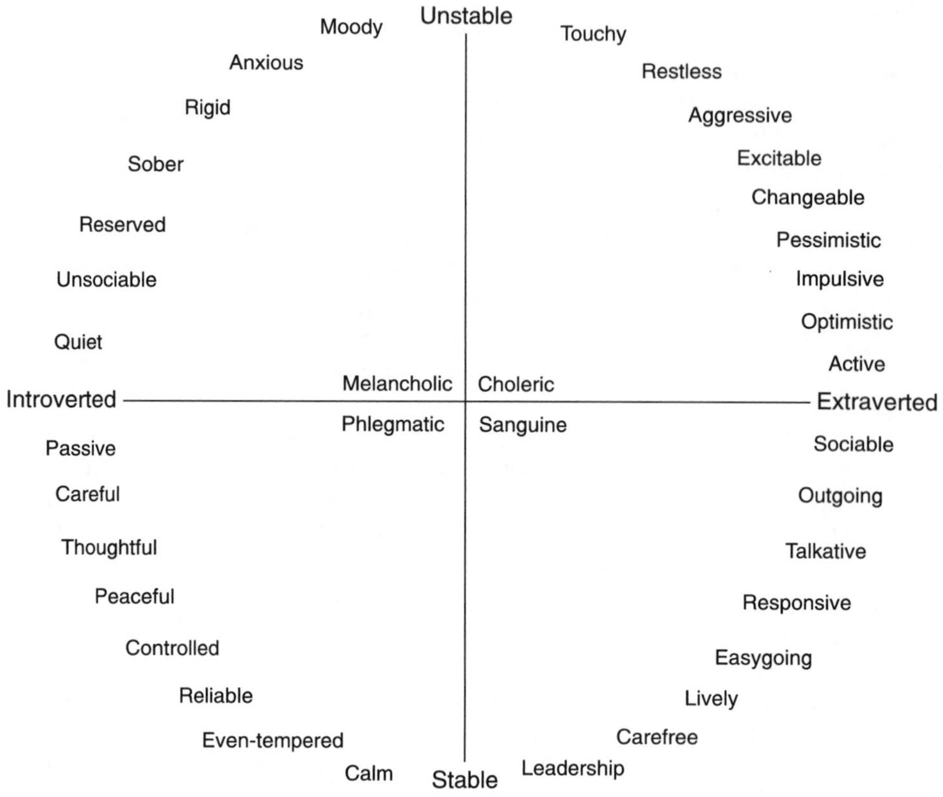

Moody | Unstable | Touchy
Anxious | | Restless
Rigid | | Aggressive
Sober | | Excitable
| | Changeable
Reserved | | Pessimistic
Unsociable | | Impulsive
| | Optimistic
Quiet | | Active
Introverted —— | Melancholic | Choleric —— Extraverted
| Phlegmatic | Sanguine
Passive | | Sociable
Careful | | Outgoing
Thoughtful | | Talkative
Peaceful | | Responsive
Controlled | | Easygoing
Reliable | | Lively
Even-tempered | | Carefree
Calm | Stable | Leadership

Figure 6.1 Eysenck's personality circle: the four quadrants.

of the major perspectives of psychology have a theory as to how these types or traits developed within individuals. This chapter will not explore those theories but, as a useful exercise, you could try to match the main perspectives with the following statements about personality in Box 6.1.

Box 6.1 Try to match the statements about personality in the left-hand column with the perspectives listed in the right-hand column

Personality is the result of a constant struggle between inner forces	Behaviourism
Personality is determined by the contingencies of reinforcement	Psychoanalysis
Personality is determined by the person's genetic make-up	Humanism
Personality is the result of social factors in our environment	Cognitive theory
Personality is the expression of constructs, schemes and encoding strategies	Social learning theory
Personality is the expression of a person's experience of the world and growth potential	Biological psychology

The attempt to measure individual differences systematically is known as *psychometrics*. Psychometrics relies heavily on statistical methods and makes the assumption that traits/types are normally distributed (see the section below on the bell-shaped curve). One of the central issues within the individual differences field is how accurate our measurement tools are. A number of other problems are associated with trying to measure these differences that are best illustrated by the work on intelligence, and this is one of the reasons why the two areas are often linked.

Intelligence

Intelligence is the ability to adapt flexibly and effectively to the environment (Sternberg and Wagner, 1986). Whether intelligence is biologically determined or an acquired or learned set of skills, and whether it is a collection of physical skills or a set of mental processes is hotly disputed. Once again the middle-ground position is probably the most helpful – that is, intelligence is all of these to a greater or lesser extent.

Most psychologists who are interested in intelligence would agree that it probably encompasses three sets of skills:

- the ability to adapt to new situations and challenging tasks;
- the ability to learn optimally from training;
- the ability to think abstractly using concepts and symbols (Phares, 1984).

Early theorists (see, for example, Binet and Simon, 1905) viewed intelligence mainly as the inherent ability to provide accurate solutions to problems. More recent work, such as that by Robert Sternberg (1985) and Howard Gardner (1983), has proposed the idea of *multiple intelligences*. The traditional view of intelligence asserted that it was composed of logical–mathematical ability, spatial ability (being able to rotate and match objects mentally), verbal comprehension, memory and reasoning. The additional factors in the theory of multiple intelligences include musical ability, kinaesthetic ability (athleticism) and interpersonal abilities (being able to identify one's own and others' feelings and use that knowledge to guide behaviour).

Despite these recent developments within the field of intelligence, most of the intelligence tests that are currently used still measure the more traditional aspects of intelligence and do not measure any of the more recently identified ones. This probably explains why we can predict future academic performance from a score on the tests, but we cannot even crudely gauge other achievements, such as success in a career or in relationships.

Intelligence testing

There are problems involved with measuring intelligence that are common to personality testing. Traditionally, the result of a given test will be expressed as a numerical value (the *Intelligence Quotient* or *IQ*), and this value will be compared with those of other people of the same age. If all the scores from the population being measured were to be placed on a continuum, they would form a bell-shaped curve, and this is known as a *normal distribution*. This curve has the same shape as that found in the distribution of other biological values, such as height and weight. The average IQ is 100, and the range of scores is shown in Figure 6.2.

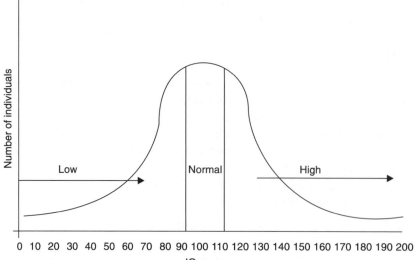

Figure 6.2 The bell-shaped curve of IQ.

One of the problems with IQ testing is that there is controversy as to whether all of the different forms of intelligence can be reduced to a single score. In addition, if we accept that musical ability should be viewed as one of the multiple intelligences and it is not measured, it raises the question of the value of a score that only focuses on aspects of intelligence that do not even correlate very well with musical ability. Once a person has been assigned an IQ score, this can be used to discriminate against them. In the previous section we saw how people stereotype others on the basis of crude schemata or rules based on partial information. Some would argue that the British education system discriminated against a whole cohort of children who were not selected for grammar school on the basis of their IQ scores at the 11-plus examinations.

There is a fiercely fought battle over the 'evidence' that black people have lower IQ scores than white people. The data actually show that African-Americans score 10–15 points lower on standard intelligence tests than do white Americans. This finding is not disputed. However, the reason for this finding is the subject of fierce controversy. Some argue that it is due to genetic differences, and that black people are less intelligent than white people. Others argue that the differences are explained by environmental factors – for example, that black people are not afforded the same opportunities to develop their intellect as are white people, or that the tests used are biased or not culturally valid for black people. Probably the strongest argument against the genetic position is that there are greater differences in the genetic structure within the 'white' population than there are between black and white populations.

Finally, there are doubts about the ability of an IQ test to predict future performance in a work context. In order to obtain a full picture of a person's ability (the IQ plus), *aptitude* (what a person could be good at) and *achievement* (what similar things they can do at the moment) need to be measured. However, that ability is still only a snapshot of the situation here and now. In order to be able to predict future ability, we need to focus more on what social factors (circumstances, opportunities) and psychological factors (motivation and mental health) contribute to a person's whole being.

Summary

* Personality is usually defined in terms of durable dimensions or traits, such as introvert–extravert, neurotic–calm or conscientious–irresponsible. There are many theories to explain how personality develops.
* Intelligence involves the ability to adapt to the environment, learn optimally and think conceptually. Intelligence testing is a controversial subject!

The last section has identified the psychological factors such as intelligence and personality and how we make inferences about people based on what we believe those factors to be. Use your intellectual skill to reflect on situations where making judgements about an individual's attributes could be helpful or unhelpful.

Now consider the relative importance of individual differences in the case of Rob and Tim below.

Case study

Rob and Tim grew up together in the same sleepy village. They were the brightest in their year, and they vied for top place each exam time. Their abilities were uncannily similar – both were good at music, both had an IQ of around 130 and they both played cricket and rugby to a high standard. The boys were equally popular in their class and both seemed to be gregarious. Most of the time they were inseparable.

However, their backgrounds were very different. Rob came from a very traditional middle-class family with two older brothers who were also high achievers. His mother ran the home and his father had a middle-ranking civil service career. Tim, on the other hand, came from a single-parent family with four siblings, all of whom were younger than him. Money was always a problem and his mother had to work to support the family. His father was not around.

When the time came for A-level results and the choice of higher education, no one was surprised to find that the boys had achieved near identical results, having chosen the same pattern of subjects.

At this stage most people would have predicted very similar achievements throughout their lives.

Rob went on to study medicine and achieved a very high position as senior clinician on his own unit. Tim was unable to attend university due to his family circumstances. He trained as a joiner and was now working for a local firm of builders.

Rob played a range of sports and was now captain of his golf club. He was liked and respected by most of his colleagues, who would all rate him as 'well-balanced' and likeable. His own children were achieving well at school and were expected to follow in his footsteps. Tim, on the other hand, gave up sport and became an angry and resentful person. He was in his third marriage and was often in trouble with his employer for being unreliable. His oldest child had behavioural problems and had been excluded from school. His daughter, aged 16 years, had just found out that she was pregnant.

Tim and Rob met up after almost 20 years under tragic circumstances in the Accident and Emergency unit of the local hospital. After all attempts to revive Tim's 16-year-old daughter, who had taken an overdose of medication, had failed, Rob as the senior medical practitioner on the unit had the unenviable task of telling her distraught father that she and the baby had died.

Further reading

Atkinson RL, Atkinson RC, Smith EE and Bem DJ (1993) *Introduction to psychology*, 11th edn. Fort Worth, TX: Harcourt Brace Jovanovich.

Weinman J (1994) *Outline of psychology as applied to medicine*, 2nd edn. Oxford: Butterworth-Heinemann.

Zimbardo P, McDermott M, Jansz J and Metaal N (1995). *Psychology: a European text*. London: HarperCollins.

Psychology and health

Christine Bundy

Introduction

The key concepts in this chapter build on the previous chapter and aim to help you to apply some of the material to your clinical experience. We have used the same format for presentation of the text as in the previous chapter.

The perceived world and health

Memory

Memory is obviously important for its own sake, but it is also crucial for following medical advice – you have to hear, understand and remember such advice. There have been a number of studies examining the factors that influence compliance with medical advice. There are two basic models – the cognitive model and the adherence model.

The *cognitive model* (see, for example, Ley, 1981; Ley and Llewelyn, 1989) claims that compliance can be predicted by a combination of patient satisfaction with the process of the consultation, the degree of understanding of the information given and the accuracy of recall of this information. Memory is therefore one of the key factors, along with whether the patient understands the advice and whether they are satisfied with the consultation. It is easy to make the assumption that if a person is well educated they will necessarily understand the disease and/or its consequences. Studies of how many patients can recall detail from a consultation consistently show that around

25–30% forget crucial pieces of information such as the name of the drug or the duration of treatment. One of the most plausible explanations as to why people forget such important information comes from basic psychology experiments that demonstrate the important influence of mood factors on information-processing. The studies consistently show that when we are anxious we do not absorb information effectively and we are less able to recall information that we 'know' than when we are relaxed.

The second model that helps us to understand the compliance process is called the *adherence model* of communication (Stanton, 1987). This model is similar to that of Ley, but it emphasizes the importance of the social context in which the consultation occurs. The adherence model represents a shift away from *compliance*, which suggests that the doctor is the expert and their advice should be followed, and towards *adherence*, which suggests that there are other factors which might interfere with the process of simply following advice. These factors have now been identified as the patient's locus of control, perceived social support, and the disruption of lifestyle involved in adhering. However, even though this model has a greater social orientation and emphasizes the interaction between the patient and the doctor, it does not emphasize the influence of the beliefs of the health professional on the process.

Some basic rules for improving patient recall are outlined below and incorporate knowledge of basic psychological processes.

1. Tell people the most important thing first (people remember the first thing they are told – this is known as the primacy effect).
2. Make the information short and simple.
3. Be specific.
4. Use repetition (present the important piece of information first and last, as people remember the last item, too – this is called the recency effect).
5. Present the information in a variety of ways.

Look at the information below and use the above rules to rearrange the information sequence and produce a more helpful consultation. See if you can detect the pieces of information that are unhelpful or distracting.

Scenario

Mrs Smith, I have the results of your test. How are you? **You** might **have** a touch of **diabetes**. Your blood glucose level is 11.2. You remember we did some tests last time? Well, one of them was **abnormal**. Have you been feeling thirsty and tired lately? This doesn't mean **you will have to go on insulin** or anything, it just means you will have to be careful with sweet things, not having sugar in your tea or eating puddings and such like **(thinks . . . this is easy, just cut out puddings)**. Make an appointment with the practice nurse. We will have to **take blood** regularly to check the glucose levels, but don't worry; many ladies like you become diabetic in later life.

You may well agree that this is a disastrous consultation. Poor Mrs. Smith is not sure whether she does or does not have diabetes. From this consultation she has no idea what diabetes is and, more importantly, she has little idea what she could do to help to manage it. Phrases such as 'a touch of' are superfluous. Giving numerical results without any explanation of what the actual values mean and the normal range is also unhelpful. The text in bold is what Mrs Smith will probably take away from the consultation. It gives a confused message. Of course, no one conducts this kind of consultation – or do they?

Memory is dependent on how well information is processed. Indeed, memory is a measure of how well we have processed a piece of information. We have already mentioned anxiety, but depression and anger also interfere with all three components involved in the memory process, namely information uptake, storage and retrieval. (For an excellent chapter on memory, see Sternberg, 1995.)

Memory loss due to age

There are many forms of dementia, but the one we associate most closely with ageing is Alzheimer's disease. The well-publicized and devastating effects of Alzheimer's disease probably affect our views of memory and ageing. Because of the publicity surrounding this condition, it is tempting to think that it is far more common than is actually the case. It is true that the prevalence is increased in the over 80 years age group, where it is around 10%, but in the over 60 years age group it is relatively low, at around 1% (Preston, 1986).

Until recently it was believed that general memory decline with age was inevitable, but we now know that this is not so. Whereas a decline in one area, such as short-term memory, might be apparent, this may be accompanied by no changes in long-term memory or recognition memory (Bahrick *et al.*, 1975; Hultsch *et al.*, 1990).

Remember what you read in the section on stereotyping in the last chapter. It might be tempting to put people in well-organized categories (e.g. all old people have memory loss), but this is just a form of shorthand and it will probably not help you to manage individuals effectively.

Language

Good communication is dependent on the skill with which people use language. There are many barriers to good communication, and we have highlighted two of them in the text above. First, anxiety can prevent people (in this case patients) from 'hearing' the message that is intended, and secondly, stereotyping can prevent people (in this case medical practitioners) from hearing individuals' experiences, because they assume that they already know about that patient group.

There is good reason to suspect that health information is processed in the same way as other information, although messages about health may have added weight, especially if someone feels that their health is threatened.

Ley's cognitive approach to understanding how and why people mishear or selectively attend to information has helped us to move away from the simplistic notion that if you tell someone what is good for their health, they will assimilate that information and a behaviour change will be inevitable (Ley and Llewelyn, 1989).

Similarly, Stanton's approach helps us to understand the powerful influence of social factors on the communication process. There are problems at each stage of the process listed below, many of which are related to communication failures:

- the status of the message giver;
- the relationship between the message giver and the receiver;
- *the health message intended;*
- the clarity, accuracy and validity of the message;
- *the health message received;*
- the patient's beliefs;
- the doctor's beliefs;
- the patient's understanding;
- the patient's readiness to change.

Perception, health and pain

Remember Tom and Mary's car accident described in the previous chapter. We feel, see, hear and smell what we expect to, so expectations are central to our experiences. One of the best examples of the interaction between social and psychological factors with regard to the influence of experiences is the *placebo effect*. A placebo is defined as a chemically inert substance that is shown to have a reproducible effect on the phenomenon being studied. A detailed discussion of the very extensive body of research on placebos is beyond the scope of this chapter, but they are a timely reminder that rather than being a supernatural phenomenon, they are natural and an integral part of the social context in which all health care operates. As scientists it is our duty to understand the central role of beliefs about the efficacy of treatment, and not simply to dismiss them as placebo effects.

Summary

- Memory and recall are affected by the ways in which information is presented, and this has implications for the ways in which doctors communicate with their patients.
- Memory loss is not an inevitable part of ageing.
- Placebo effects are important, but they are not yet fully understood.

Health attitudes and beliefs

The social context in which an event occurs also helps to orientate us to it. Therefore the way in which we experience something (e.g. a threat to health) is a combination of psychological factors (thoughts, feelings and behaviours) and social factors (context, cultural and family values, etc.). When we perceive an event, the interpretation of that event is different to the sensation of it. Once the signal has left the retina for the visual cortex, memory imposes meaning on it. All of this suggests that we have an internal representation of the sensation in our brain that we apply to the situation, and we then look for the goodness of fit between our template and the situation.

Recent work on our representation of illness has helped us to understand the processes involved in working out the meaning of a health threat (see Leventhal *et al.*, 1980). In response to a threat to health (either the detection of symptoms or being given a diagnosis), the individual thinks about the *cause*, the *consequences*, the likely duration of the problem (or the *time-line*) and the degree of *control or cure* they might have over it. In response to these thoughts there will be an emotional reaction (either anxiety, depression or anger).

All of these reactions will drive the way in which a person *copes* with the threat. Figure 7.1 shows the components of the three stages of the model and how they interact to produce a response to the threat.

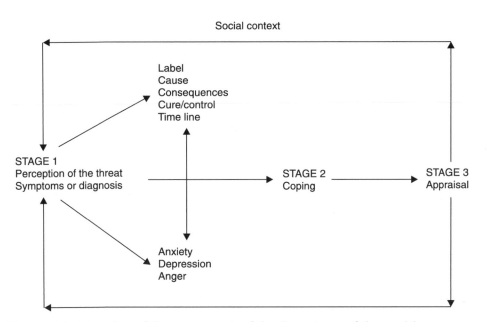

Figure 7.1 Interaction of the components of the three stages of the model.

Things that go bump in the night!

Scenario

Sam was late for work one morning and knew that this meant she would have to stay late at the office to catch up. During a very hurried shower she felt a breast lump. Her first reaction was utter horror. She instinctively felt that it would mean bad news for her, as she was just the type to have cancer, although she could hardly bring herself even to think the word. She knew she was in the 'at-risk' age group (she was 33 years old), and this would mean the end of her career, the end of her independence and possibly the end of her marriage. She could only despair as she thought of her two precious children growing up without their mother. It took 8 weeks and much heart-searching before she plucked up the courage to see her GP, and she knew that day would be the worst day of her life.

Sam had an escalating, catastrophic emotional reaction to the threat. This was based on her many misconceptions about the meaning of the lump, and it drove a very unhelpful behaviour pattern of avoiding the GP visit and becoming immersed in despair (avoidance coping).

Compare this with Sheena's response, described below.

Scenario

Sheena was also in her thirties and found a breast lump by accident one day. She felt very anxious about it and was frightened of the consequences. However, she told herself 'don't jump to conclusions, just find out the facts'. She did a quick search on the Web at work for breast lump sites and found a useful one that was reassuring. It pointed out that she was not in the highest risk category, and that the best course of action was to get a health care professional, preferably a GP, to look at it as soon as possible. After an emergency appointment the same day, Sheena came away with the impression that it was most likely to be benign, but if it was malignant she had done everything that she could so far.

Sheena, too, was frightened, but her fear did not escalate and she was sufficiently motivated to act quickly to gather information (approach coping) and seek appropriate help. These scenarios remind us that people need some degree of anxiety (motivation or stress – the name is not important at this stage) to motivate them to meet a challenge. However, if it rises above a useful level this anxiety demotivates us and encourages us to escape from its unpleasant effects by avoiding it.

Both Sam and Sheena had specific beliefs about health and illness that shaped their thinking. Such beliefs come from a variety of sources, including the television and newspapers, magazines, family myths, cultural values, knowing someone with a particular illness, or particular health education communications (remember the AIDS can KILL campaign). We have all assimilated messages about health and illness, and it is against this backdrop that we act – in other words, our behaviour is the product of our thoughts and feelings. The next time you see someone brushing their teeth, remember that they are giving you a small insight into their beliefs about preventive medicine!

One of the most commonly overlooked reactions to illness is an anger response. When people feel threatened, they may either feel frightened or anxious, depressed or angry. These are primitive responses designed to prompt a fight-or-flight response (see below). We have socialized ourselves into controlling or even completely avoiding (this is sometimes called *denial*) the response we feel in relation to a threat. Women especially are taught from an early age not to express anger. Although it is considered more acceptable for men to show anger, it is still frowned upon. This does not stop us feeling anger, and when it becomes overwhelming we do express it. Most often there will be a trigger to the anger expression, however apparently trivial, and the person on the receiving end will be somewhat bewildered by the magnitude of the response. Health care professionals are often on the receiving end of such a response. Because of the one-to-one nature of the response it is understandable that people take it personally. Very often in their attempts to deal with such anger the health care professional will put it down to personality factors (e.g. he's a difficult person). Sometimes they attribute it to other personal characteristics of the individual (e.g. he's used to getting his way by shouting), rather than seeing it for what it is – an expression by the individual of being under threat. Physiologically the individual who is experiencing the anger is prepared for fight and so has raised stress hormone levels. This adds a further threat to health.

Summary

- The extent to which we will cope with an illness is affected by our beliefs about its cause, consequences, duration, and the degree of control we have over it.
- Anger and denial are common – but often ignored – reactions to illness.

Stress and coping

There is little dispute now that stress can have a major impact on the disease process. Approaches to examining stress have ranged from the biological, such as *Selye*'s general adaptation system (Selye, 1956), through to the more recent models, such as the transactional model of Lazarus (Lazarus, 1966). Selye focused on the strain on the organ systems and the physiological consequences of repeated stress. He regarded stress as a stimulus, and therefore proposed that the frequency, duration and intensity of that stimulus would determine the strength of the response. In 1929, *Cannon* described the fight-or-flight response in physiological terms. Good descriptions of this appear in most basic psychology and physiology textbooks, and we shall not consider them in detail here. Suffice to say the fight-or-flight response is both physiological and psychological, and involves a pathway of responses from the pituitary gland in the brain to the adrenal glands. The result of this hormonal activation is to stimulate all the body systems, putting them on 'stand-by' for fighting or fleeing. Cannon has made a major contribution to our understanding of the physiological pathways involved in the production of the stress hormones. However, his knowledge of the psychological experience of fight-or-flight was minimal. Fortunately, others with an interest in the psychophysiology of stress have mapped the psychology on to Cannon's early work.

Richard Lazarus made us think about stress in a more dynamic way. He argued that whether an event is perceived as stressful or not is dependent on the individual's perceived ability to cope with the stimulus. He helped us to understand that the individual weighs up the stressor (the stressful trigger) and their capacity to cope with it. If the individual's capacity to cope is outweighed by the event, the latter will be experienced as stressful. This helps to explain why two individuals may react to the same event in very different ways. The individual is interacting with the stressor, rather than being a passive recipient of it as Cannon described.

The pituitary–adrenal pathways involved in stress are well documented. There is good evidence that perceived stress results in the release of cortisol, and that this in turn is linked with greater pain, delayed healing time, and delayed recovery and adjustment to a range of health problems. There is still some dispute about the causal role of stress, but for a good overview of the implications of stress see Ogden (1996) and Steptoe and Wardle (1994).

Despite there being little evidence that stress *per se* causes the range of illness that it is supposed to, there is a strong belief among a large proportion of the population that stress causes disease. By now you should understand why it is important to acknowledge the role of these beliefs in guiding illness behaviour.

Coping is usually classified as either approach coping or avoidance coping. Approach coping involves engaging with the problem, actively seeking out information and following appropriate advice. Avoidance coping, on the other hand, involves just what it states, namely avoiding thinking about the problem, and avoiding action related to the problem as a way of managing the emotional distress caused by it. Coping usually refers to the behaviour you can see, but it might be more helpful to think of it as an *approach* to the problem (either mental or behavioural). Although approach coping might seem to be the 'best' coping style, it is sometimes helpful to use avoidance coping. In the short term, especially after an event such as a heart attack, getting over the immediate event may take all of one's resources. Denial at this stage can be helpful. However, if the person is expected to make early lifestyle changes, such as stopping smoking, it is important that they are not using avoidance coping.

Summary of the self-regulatory model

- The cognitive response (the meaning that the threat is given in terms of cause, consequences, etc.) prompts an emotional response (e.g. anxiety, depression, anger).
- These together produce a coping response (approach coping or avoidance coping).
- In the third stage the individual examines how well they have coped.
- If this appraisal is satisfactory, then the meaning of the threat might be modified (e.g. 'I've coped quite well, it can't be all that bad being diabetic').
- If the appraisal is unsatisfactory, then the threat might be increased ('I will never cope with being diabetic, it's ruining my life').

Lifestyle and health

It is well known that certain factors are associated with healthy and not so healthy lifestyles. One of the best studies in this area is the Almeda County Study (Belloc and Breslow, 1972). This longitudinal study examined the lifestyles of all 7000 residents of a state in California. The authors followed the residents over 15 years and found that seven factors were associated with longevity and health. These were as follows:

- sleeping for 7–8 hours a day;
- having breakfast every day;
- not smoking;
- not eating between meals;
- not being overweight;
- consuming only moderate amounts of alcohol;
- taking regular exercise.

These findings might appear to be self-evident, and psychology is often accused of being 'just common sense', but this series of studies was the first to provide us with evidence that lifestyle is predictive of health status.

As a result of this study, psychologists became interested in what factors predict whether or not someone will adopt *health-protective* behaviours (exercising, eating well, etc.) or *health-threatening* behaviours (smoking, excessive drinking, etc.). A number of influences have been identified, and these include the following:

- social factors, such as learning, modelling and cultural norms;
- emotional factors, such as anxiety and fear;
- beliefs – both beliefs of patients *and* beliefs of health professionals.

Assessing the person's *readiness to change* (and coping style) is crucial in deciding how to advise him or her. Prochaska and DiClemente (1982) have identified a cycle of change that they call the transtheoretical model or the *stages of change* model. They suggest that behaviour change is dependent on where people are in this cycle. The stages are as follows.

1. The first stage is called *precontemplation*, when a person is not intending to change.
2. The second stage is *contemplation*, when a person is considering making lifestyle changes, but these still remain an intention.
3. The next stage is called *preparation*, and people often begin by making small changes at this stage.
4. The *action* stage occurs when a person is actively engaging in new behaviour.
5. The final stage is the *maintenance* stage, when a person is using strategies to reinforce the new behaviour.

The stages are not (as their name might imply) straight linear stages, but rather they form a cycle that people go round, sometimes many times (e.g. in cases of smoking relapse), before they actually reach the maintenance stage.

Using the stages of change model, consider which stage the following people are in according to their statements, and see whether you could match up a suitable intervention at each stage.

Stages

Shelly: I have started to look at my mastectomy scar, but I can only manage about once a week.
James: I haven't touched cannabis since 1987.
Ralph: My wife now uses olive oil instead of animal fat.
Tom: Smoking is my only pleasure left, Doc.
Joan: Each time I think about it I leave the room.

Interventions:

Well done! That must be hard, being a DJ. It's a tribute to your strength of character and hard work.
Have you thought about working as a 'Buddy' to help others?
Think about this statement: 'I deserve more pleasure in life after all I have put in.'
This is the first step, and it can be the hardest. Give yourself a reward.
Leave 'Post-It' notes on the mirror to prevent you avoiding seeing yourself.
How can I help you to do it every day?

Quality of life

We considered the principles and issues underlying the concept of quality of life in some detail in Chapter 4 on patients and carers. Here we shall recap briefly and examine the value of this concept from a psychological perspective.

There are many definitions of quality of life. Some of these are very brief. For example:

a state of complete physical, mental and social well-being and not merely the absence of disease or infirmity.

(World Health Organization, 1958)

Others are less brief but more realistic. For example:

an individual's perception of their position in life in the context of the culture and value systems in which they live and in relation to their goals, expectations, standards and concerns. It is a broad-ranging concept affected in a complex way by the person's physical health, psychological state, level of independence, social relationships, and their relationships to salient features of their environment.

(World Health Organization Quality of Life Group, 1991)

What these definitions have in common is the belief that there are three overlapping dimensions to quality of life, namely the physical, the psychological and the social. In addition, they emphasize the importance of the *subjective experience* of quality of life. There are two broad types of quality of life measures, namely the generic and the condition specific. Generic measures allow us to compare between diseases or conditions, whereas the condition-specific measures do not. However, some of the condition-specific measures are more sensitive (see below) than the generic ones. A number of good generic measures of health-related quality of life are available, but the most commonly used one is the Short Form(SF)-36 (Ware and Sherbourne, 1992). The SF-36 assesses these three dimensions and is considered to be *valid* (it measures what it claims to), *reliable* (it measures consistently over time and conditions), *sensitive* (it picks up small changes) and *specific* (it measures the condition accurately). These are the important four elements of any good measure

Health-related quality of life is partially dependent on the reactions to the health threat, as we have seen earlier. In this sense we use it as a *process measure* – that is, we assess the process of thoughts through the stated quality of life. Quality of life is also, and increasingly, used as an *outcome measure* to determine the success or otherwise of an intervention.

However, caution is needed here, because the relationship between disease state and quality of life is not straightforward. Some people with apparently appalling illnesses still manage to achieve a good quality of life, and some of those with apparently minor conditions suffer a greatly impaired quality of life.

Quality of life is something you as potential medical practitioners need to know about, not least because the quality of life of doctors in practice, especially those with 'on-call' duties, is a hot topic and one that will interest you in the future!

Summary

- The factors associated with a healthy life are well known.
- Our willingness to adopt health-protective behaviours depends on our current position in the 'stages of change' model.
- Quality of life issues are important when considering health outcomes.

Psychological problems and therapy

Theories of depression

We have seen in Chapter 5 on epidemiology that mental health problems, particularly anxiety and depression, are very common. Indeed, a report commissioned by the World Bank predicts that by the year 2020, depressive disorders will be the second largest contributor to worldwide morbidity and disability (Murray and Lopez, 1996).

There are many different theories of how psychological problems occur, and these include genetic, biochemical, physiological and social explanations. It is important to consider such perspectives in order to gain an overall understanding of the subject, and if you wish to do so you could consult a standard textbook of psychiatry, or read a personalized account, such as Lewis Wolpert's *Malignant Sadness* (for details of the latter, see the Further Reading section at the end of this chapter). In this section we shall consider the most common psychological explanations for mental illnesses, in particular depression, and relate these where possible to the theoretical models described in Chapter 6.

Psychoanalytical theory views depression as closely related to bereavement. Freud believed that the characteristic depressive features of self-reproach and loss of self-esteem are really expressions of hostility towards another person (who might be dead, absent, or simply not behaving towards us as we would wish), but turned inwards onto oneself. Depression and anger are therefore closely linked. Bowlby combined these ideas with social theories developed from working with children, and animal studies, to emphasize that our experiences of early interpersonal relationships are crucial for our psychological development (Bowlby, 1981). His *attachment theory* assumes that in order to experience ourselves as separate individuals who are comfortable with the world, we must have experienced adequate early caring and be able to internalize that experience. Brown and Harris (1978) have taken this work further. They found that depression is linked to low self-esteem, which in turn relates – in women at least – to the loss of the mother at an early age, the lack of a confidant, the lack of full-time employment and the presence of three or more children at home. They relate recovery to the presence of 'fresh-start' events, described as those which represent 'an important change in the subject's life . . . and that appear to herald new hope – an indication that there may be a way forward' (Brown and Harris, 1989).

On the behaviour side of psychological theories, Seligman (1975) coined the term *learned helplessness* and developed a model to explain depression as resulting from past experience of inability to influence adverse events. According to this model, psychological distress arises from the belief that our actions are futile, and that we can do nothing to restore the losses linked, for example, to bereavement, financial problems or chronic ill health. Our feeling of loss of control can also be due to receiving positive rewards for activities or events to which we have made a negligible contribution (e.g. winning the lottery), since it is essential to our well-being that we feel in control of our own lives. Beck's theories about cognitive *schemas* (Beck, 1991), which we noted in Chapter 6, have also been used to explain depression in terms of the creation and maintenance of distorted cognitions (negative thoughts about ourselves). These include reaching negative conclusions on the basis of a single event (e.g. 'I failed this exam, so I must be completely useless and will never make a good doctor'), focusing on negative rather than positive events in one's life, and describing particular events in extreme, catastrophic terms (e.g.'This is the most awful thing that could ever happen to anyone').

Psychological therapy

There are many reasons why an individual might consider entering therapy. Usually the person has reached a point in their life where they feel that they are no longer able to tolerate a particular situation. In the context of someone with a health problem such as heart disease, diabetes or arthritis, therapy is often entered into reluctantly. Many people feel stigmatized by being told that they should consider seeing a psychologist or psychiatrist. Asking for help with a psychological problem is still viewed as a character flaw by many people. Patients might fear that they are not being taken seriously by the medical profession, or that their problem is regarded as psychosomatic. Hopefully, by now you will realize that the term 'psychosomatic' is not helpful and might be past its 'sell-by date' as a concept. All illnesses are psychosomatic in the sense that they involve the body and mind. *Try to imagine a serious health problem that does not have some social and/or psychological consequences.*

Many more enlightened medical teams now regularly refer patients to a clinical or health psychologist or liaison psychiatrist, and in some more specialized units or health care teams there is often a psychologist on the team. The role of the psychologist in a physical health setting is to identify unhelpful thought processes, address emotional distress and help patients to adjust their behaviour in a way that will improve their quality of life. There are many types of interventions based on the different schools of psychology (look back to Chapter 6 and remind yourself of the different psychological orientations). The cognitively based interventions are by and large the ones with the firmer evidence base. All interventions begin with a thorough assessment. You would not consider giving someone a drug without doing some investigations first and, in the same way, matching a person's problem with the intervention requires some investigative work.

Obviously different problems will require different interventions, but most common psychological reactions to illness can be treated within the cognitive–behavioural therapy (CBT) framework. This involves a thorough assessment of the problem – not just how it presents on the surface, but what the patient thinks about the problem and what they have tried to do to change it. The CBT therapist is interested in patterns of thought, feelings and behaviour. For example, they might ask questions such as 'When you get the headaches, what do you think triggers them mostly?', 'When the headaches begin, how do they make you feel?', 'When you feel . . . what do you usually do?'. In this way any obvious patterns can be detected and the patient feels that what previously seemed like a mess actually has some logical structure. This makes any problem more manageable. CBT therapists also work by challenging the automatic negative thoughts and schemas that patients may have, unravelling distortions in thinking and helping them to learn alternative, more realistic ways of formulating and dealing with their problems. CBT has been shown to be of particular value in helping people to recover from depression (Gloaguen et al., 1998).

People whose psychological difficulties appear to relate to problems in their daily lives are likely to benefit from a different form of psychological help, known as problem-solving therapy. This is based on the observation that emotional symptoms are generally induced by problems of living, and has its theoretical roots in cognitive–behavioural approaches to mental disorders. Problem-solving treatment (PST) has been developed as a specific, collaborative treatment with three main steps:

1. patients' symptoms are linked with their problems;
2. the problems are defined and clarified;
3. an attempt is made to solve the problems in a structured way.

By starting to tackle their own problems, patients can begin to reassert control over their lives, and it is proposed that it is this regaining of control which lifts mood. This therapy has been shown to be valuable in primary care for the treatment of emotional disorders (Catalan et al., 1991), and is effective in reducing the severity and duration of depression in a variety of community settings (Dowrick et al., 2000).

Using the self-regulatory model (SRM) as a framework, we can begin to deconstruct a problem which often seems insurmountable to a patient into its constituent parts. One of the strengths of the SRM is the ability to integrate the physical component of the patient's problem (the symptoms) with the thought processes and emotional reactions that follow the meaning they attribute to the symptoms.

Summary

- Psychological problems such as depression are very common.
- Psychological explanations for such problems can be drawn from psychodynamic or behavioural perspectives. They may focus on our reactions to loss or on our mental representation of the world.

- There is good evidence that psychological therapies, such as cognitive–behavioural therapy and problem-solving treatment, are effective in managing a wide variety of health problems where emotional or psychological factors are present.

Below is an example of a patient with angina, as an illustration of the type of therapeutic intervention we can offer someone with a chronic health problem.

David's angina gets him down

David had minimal coronary vessel disease on the coronary angiogram, and he was on medication that was considered 'optimal'. However, he made repeated visits to the doctor complaining that his angina woke him at night. David's quality of life was poor, he had left his job and would sit at home for most of the day anticipating an angina attack. After the cardiologist had assured himself that David's angina was not worse, he referred him to a health psychologist.

ASSESSMENT

This involved three 1-hour sessions of talking with David about the angina, discussing what he understood about the mechanism, and his knowledge of the heart and blood vessels. To access the illness cognitions, David was asked to talk about what he thought caused the angina, what the consequences were and how long he thought it was going to last. He was asked to demonstrate how he felt when he had an angina attack and exactly what he did about it.

THE PROBLEM

It became clear that there were three main issues. First, David had some very basic misconceptions about angina (he thought each attack was a mini heart attack). Secondly, he was very anxious about dying in his sleep, and when he had an attack he thought the best thing to do was not to expend any energy, as this would precipitate a heart attack. Thirdly, he was physically deconditioning himself by not exercising.

THE TREATMENT

The psychologist recognized that the first important step was to reduce the background level of arousal, as this was perpetuating a demand on the heart even at rest. David was taught relaxation training first over 5 weeks, and then deep relaxation (self-hypnosis) over the next 4 weeks. He was encouraged to practise this prior to sleep at night as well as during the day. After a while his nightmares of running for a bus and inducing an angina attack stopped. Then the misconceptions were addressed. As his work was as a librarian, he was encouraged to make a list of his beliefs about the angina and research them on the Internet and at his local library.

The outcome

After a few weeks David had altered his beliefs about angina. Finally, he was offered physical training at the local hospital's cardiac rehabilitation classes. Although his progress was slow to begin with, he was back at work as a librarian within 4 months. He was no longer troubled by the nightmares, and he now attended an unsupervised exercise class twice a week at the local leisure centre. He reported that his quality of life was better than it had been for a number of years.

Further reading

Ogden J (1996) *Health psychology. A textbook.* Buckingham: Open University Press.

Steptoe A and Wardle J (eds) (1994) *Psychosocial processes and health. A reader.* Cambridge: Cambridge University Press.

Sternberg RJ (1995) *In search of the human mind.* London: Harcourt-Brace.

Wolpert L (1999) *Malignant sadness: the anatomy of depression.* New York: Free Press.

Health economics

8

Cynthia Iglesias and David Torgerson

Introduction

Humans use resources to live and to derive pleasure or utility from life. However, resources are always limited. Economics as a discipline seeks to study the best possible use of the *available resources* within society. To aid this, economists attempt to understand and explain individuals' behaviour in relation to the production, distribution and consumption of goods/commodities. Formally, economics has been defined as follows:

> the study of how men and society end up choosing, with and without the use of money, to employ scarce productive resources that could have alternative use, to produce various commodities and distribute them for consumption, now or in the future, among various people and groups in society. It analyses the costs and benefits of improving the pattern of resource allocation.
>
> (Samuelson, 1976: 5)

The vast majority of the concepts underpinning economic theory have their origin in everyday situations, and for this reason many economic paradigms appear to be merely common sense. A key concept underpinning economic study is the notion of 'opportunity cost'. Scarcity of resources implies that by using resources in one way individuals have to make a 'sacrifice' and renounce the benefits that they could have had by using the resources in another way. For instance, the purchase of a new car may be reflected by forgoing the opportunity to take a foreign holiday. Similarly, increased investment in rail safety will reduce the resources available for improvements in road safety.

Resources are used efficiently if there is no alternative use that is of greater utility to society. For example, at the level of a general practice, if a practice nurse could be used to provide antenatal care for pregnant women rather than to undertake health checks for patients over 75 years of age, and this produced more utility, then switching the resource (i.e. the practice nurse) from health checks to antenatal care would be efficient.

In this chapter we shall explore some of the key economic issues affecting the delivery of health care. First, we shall examine how health care is delivered and the economic rationale behind using market and non-market solutions. Secondly, we shall consider the issue of whether the UK spends enough on health care. Finally, we shall examine the role of economic evaluation in assessing the efficiency of individual health care procedures.

Summary

- All resources are scarce.
- Health economics seeks to maximize the benefit from these scarce resources.
- Efficiency in health care is achieved when the maximum benefit or utility is obtained for any set of resources.
- Health economics is not about saving costs.

Market or state provision of health care

In general, among industrialized nations, health care is not left entirely to the free market even within countries such as the USA. To understand why this is so, we need to examine the concept of market provision of ordinary goods and services.

The free market

For a market to be efficient – that is, to provide the maximum utility (or benefit) within society's resources – two conditions must apply. First, there needs to be a large number of suppliers to the market. Secondly, consumers must be knowledgeable about competing products and services.

In a perfect market, suppliers engage in competition to win a market share for their goods. All other things being equal, they either reduce costs or improve quality. When the price of a product or service falls, the supplier sells more and gains a market share. However, competitive suppliers to the market will endeavour either to reduce their prices, by cutting costs, or to improve quality in order to justify retaining their price differential, otherwise they will leave the market. Thus suppliers are in a constant state of competition as they try to improve their goods and services relative to those of their rivals in order either to retain or to increase their market share and thus their profits.

The second condition for a properly functioning market requires consumers to be well informed about the different goods on offer and their respective prices. Thus a rational consumer will always purchase a product which has either a price advantage or a quality advantage compared with any alternative.

To maintain a properly functioning market, the number of suppliers must not decline in the long term. Thus as some suppliers leave the market because they can no longer compete, they need to be replaced by new suppliers entering the market to maintain competition. Similarly, consumers need to be fully informed about new rival goods and services on offer.

Although most of the economic systems in the developed world are based on the 'free market', it is true to say that all markets fail. The natural tendency is for firms to try to develop monopolies and exclude other suppliers from the market, and then, without the spur for competition, there is little incentive for them to reduce their prices or improve quality. Thus the consumer pays a monopoly price for an inferior product. Governments often intervene in the market to prevent this undesirable situation from arising by preventing one or two suppliers from dominating the market. The process of monopoly development is not restricted to firms. Groups of workers also endeavour to form monopolies. As a result, professional or trade associations are formed, and one of the consequences of this is to prevent members from undercutting each other on price and try to exclude non-members from the labour market.

The second key feature of perfect competition is that consumers are fully informed. However, the consumer is rarely fully informed about different products. Even in a competitive market, consumers often do not have 'perfect' knowledge of the quality and prices of all of the competing products. Consequently, they often purchase products which are more expensive than or of inferior quality to an alternative. Indeed, when confronted with a choice of very similar products, consumers will often regard price as a marker of quality and buy a more expensive item than is necessary.

Although the free market does have its failures, in general it operates sufficiently well to provide most goods and services. However, for some specific services, such as health care provision, it is deemed to fail dramatically.

Health care as a market failure

Health care has a number of features that tend to make it a market failure. First, among industrial nations the provision of health care is largely a monopoly under the control of the medical profession. There is a tendency for all professional or trade groups to become monopolies and put up barriers of entry. However, for medicine, in contrast to most other trades, this tendency is reinforced by the state, which makes it a criminal offence for people to offer a range of medical services (such as prescription medicines) without being licensed by the state. The licensing of the medical profession is under the control of the profession itself. Thus the numbers of medical students are carefully controlled in order to maintain sufficiently low numbers, which will in turn tend to keep medical salaries high. Finally, the medical profession's code of conduct often contains anti-competitive strictures, such as seeing other doctors' patients, or preventing patients from seeing specialists directly, or frowning on advertising and recommending standard fees for services, all of which will further erode any competitive pressures between individuals or groups of doctors.[*]

Some economists argue that the main reason why health care cannot be provided efficiently through the market system is because of this government-sanctioned monopoly. The counter-position is that unless medical practice is closely regulated, more inferior medical services will be consumed by patients, for a given cost, than would otherwise be the case – which is inefficient.

As well as being a monopoly, the complexities of medical care make the average consumer ignorant of which care is best for a given price. As with other market failures, if consumers are ignorant about the merits of a service or product, they tend to equate price with quality. Whereas for other goods and services consumers can learn from experience, by trying a less expensive product, because health care is consumed infrequently and the consequences of having an inferior service are rather more severe than with other products, there is a natural tendency to choose the most expensive treatment that can be afforded. Thus an efficient supplier who reduces costs and prices but maintains quality will be at a disadvantage compared to the inefficient supplier who maintains or increases their price or reduces quality. The incentive, therefore, is for medical suppliers to increase the prices of their services, which is the opposite of what should happen in a functioning market. Furthermore, when doctors are paid in a fee-for-service manner they have an incentive to provide health care that is not necessary in order to increase their incomes. Thus doctors who are paid by fee for service perform more tests and treatments than similar doctors who are paid a fixed salary. Systematic reviews of the way in which doctors are paid clearly demonstrate that the medical profession is strongly influenced in the quantity of care it delivers according to the level of remuneration. For instance, prior to 1991 general practitioners were encouraged to undertake cervical smears as part of their normal duty of care. However, when part of overall GP income was changed such that a proportion of it was dependent on achieving a certain uptake of smears, there was a dramatic increase in the number of smears. This demonstrated that many GPs would not provide cervical smears to women of the required age range unless they were specifically rewarded for doing so.

In summary, the two key requirements of a properly functioning health care market are either absent or severely deficient.

State intervention in health care

In the UK, state provision is viewed primarily as a way of achieving equity of access to health care. Thus a health care system funded from general taxation will provide equal access for equal medical need rather than on the basis of

---

[*] The legal profession has similar anti-competitive practices, such as needing to see a barrister via a solicitor, which is analogous to not being able to see a consultant unless one is referred by a GP.

ability to pay, although the wealthy can still afford to supplement their state provision with private health care. However, for equity of access there is no a priori reason why the state should be a provider of health care. A simpler solution to inequality based on differential incomes is to provide extra payments to the poor such that they can buy their own health care. For example, society allows the poor access to food by taxing the wealthy and transferring (by transfer payments) money to buy food from private suppliers. Other countries (e.g. the USA) go even further and provide food vouchers that are redeemable for food. Thus the market provides food, which is more important than health care for good health – there is no question of a National Food Service. If unequal access, due to unequal incomes, was the only problem with health care delivery, this could be addressed using either transfer payments or vouchers. The main economic rationale for state provision of health care is to address market failings – not equity.

Although state-provided health care purports to address some of the market failings, it is not without problems that threaten efficiency (and equity!). As noted previously, the medical profession, in common with most other trades and professions, responds to financial incentives. The problem with linking payment with output in medical care is obvious, and has been noted for a long time.

> That any sane nation, having observed that you could provide for the supply of bread by giving bakers a pecuniary interest in baking for you, should go on to give a surgeon a pecuniary interest in cutting off your leg, is enough to make one despair of political humanity.
>
> (Shaw, 1946: 7)

Indeed, a number of studies have shown that if doctors are paid in a fee-for-service manner, they will provide more services. Although this may be efficient if the services that are being provided are worth the cost, often this is not the case. Therefore doctors in the NHS are usually paid a sum which is only at best indirectly linked with their output. Hence general practitioners are normally paid an allowance that is dependent on the size of their practice, although some income is linked to performance (e.g. childhood immunizations). Similarly, hospital doctors are paid a salary. However, a salary unrelated to performance gives doctors no incentive to deliver more than the minimum amount of health care. Furthermore, because within the medical monopoly there has traditionally been little or no competition, there is no incentive to reduce costs and improve quality. Thus state-delivered health care can be unresponsive to the needs of the patient and can be inefficient, as there is no incentive to produce the best health care within a given budget.

In an attempt to make state health care delivery more efficient, competition has been introduced into the UK health care system. Thus purchasers of health care – general practitioners in the form of either fundholders or, more recently, primary care groups – can choose between different secondary care suppliers. The idea behind the 'purchaser–provider' split is that the GP will act as an 'agent' for his or her patients and purchase the most clinically effective and cost-effective health care on their behalf. This will introduce the spur of competition between providers, but will only allow agents who have sufficient knowledge to make informed choices about what different suppliers offer.

The purchaser–provider split is not without its critics. An 'internal market' introduces a number of costs, which need to be recovered by improvements in efficiency. This might not occur, and the costs are incurred with little or no corresponding improvements in efficiency. Furthermore, for many areas competition is an illusion, as the local provider is a monopoly and other providers are too geographically distant to offer serious competition. In addition, for rare conditions there will only be two or three specialist centres in the whole country – not enough for meaningful competition. Although it is often difficult to measure the costs of various health procedures, it is even more difficult to measure the effectiveness of output, and both are necessary requirements for purchasers to make an informed choice with regard to different suppliers of health care. Hence the poor quality of paediatric cardiovascular surgery undertaken in Bristol in the late 1980s and early 1990s was not apparent (one assumes) to local purchasers of such procedures. The purchasing of paediatric heart procedures from this hospital at this time was therefore likely to have been inefficient. Clearly, then, even well-informed purchasers (e.g. GPs) may be ignorant of the quality of the service that they are buying. Moreover, in the free market the ultimate sanction of leaving the market (e.g. through bankruptcy) is not, for most providers, a credible threat. Indeed, if budgets are exceeded, managers and doctors can indulge in 'shroud waving' for extra funds to cover the deficit, rather than losing their jobs. Thus in practice there may be little relative reward for a hospital which keeps within budget and is efficient compared with an inefficient provider who squanders their budgetary allocation, as the latter can be fairly confident that the state will bail it out.

In summary, there is no consensus among health economists as to which is the most efficient method of delivering health care services. Furthermore, it is difficult to evaluate novel changes to health care delivery, as these are often politically driven. Thus extensive evaluation of fundholding was not undertaken and so the lessons of this type of purchaser–provider split could not be applied to different forms of the 'internal market'.

Although there is debate as to which is the best structure for delivering health care in the UK, the medical profession and political parties (when they are in opposition) all generally agree that the UK spends too little on health care for a country of its size and comparative wealth.

Summary

- Market failure is a feature of health care.
- State intervention is primarily about improving efficiency, not equity.
- Doctors treat patients partly on fiscal incentives and not completely on clinical need.

Does the UK spend enough on health care?

It is common practice to compare the amount that the UK spends on health care with the amount spent by other countries, and the usual conclusion is that the UK spends too little. Whether there is an economic case for increasing spending on health care or not, informing such a decision by referring to what other countries spend on health is both naive and meaningless.

Health care expenditure is influenced by many factors. First, there is the age structure of the population – older populations generally require more health care. Thus a country with a high proportion of elderly people will tend to spend more on average than a similar sized country with a younger population. Even if the age profiles of the populations of different countries are similar, their health status may not be. Smoking, alcohol consumption and diet are major determinants of ill health and differ substantially between nations, requiring different levels of expenditure. Health care spending may be influenced by cultural factors. For example, some countries have a strong tradition of caring for older relatives within the family (e.g. Ireland), and will tend to spend less on health care than similar countries with no such tradition. Furthermore, different countries have very different accounting procedures and comparisons are therefore unreliable, as some countries will include social care spending as health care while others do not.

Another reason for direct comparisons of health care expenditure being unreliable is due a simple mathematical problem. Consider two similar sized nations, A and B, each of which has a national income of £100 billion and spends 10% on health care. Now let us suppose that country A suffered a severe recession and its income dropped to £90 billion, but health care expenditure was kept at £10 billion. Thus the proportion of national income devoted to health rose by 11% despite no real difference in expenditure. In contrast, over the same period the income of country B rose to £120 billion and its health care expenditure rose to £11 billion, but because health care expenditure did not increase as fast as national income, the proportion of the latter devoted to health fell from 10% to 9%. Clearly it is nonsense to assume that the inhabitants of country A are better off because their country spends a greater proportion of its national income on health care compared with those living in country B. An example of this situation occurred in Finland in the early 1990s, when income fell sharply due to loss of trade with the former Soviet Union, but health care expenditure fell only slightly.

A more sophisticated approach to arguing that the UK underspends on health care is to plot the amount of national income per person against the proportion of income spent on health care per person. Figure 8.1 shows the typical regression line that is obtained when this happens. The graph shows that as a country increases in wealth, a greater proportion of that wealth is spent on health care services. This relationship has been shown a number of times, and generally two countries appear as outliers, namely the UK and the USA. Thus the UK falls well below the regression line whilst the USA falls well above it, implying that the UK spends too little on health care and the USA spends too much.

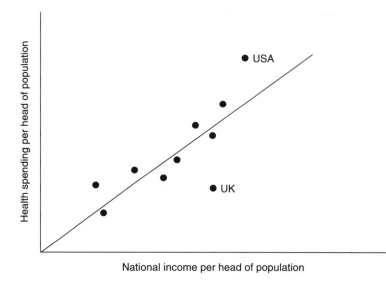

Figure 8.1 Regression of expenditure against income.

The regression line shown in Figure 8.1 is described in statistical parlance as having a good fit, with nearly 90% of the variation explained by per capita income alone. Thus one interpretation of such a relationship is that other factors associated with health care expenditure, such as the age profile of the population, are relatively unimportant. However, the above analysis is flawed because it does not take into account the relative price differences that exist between countries. A crucial factor in the equation is the actual amount of health care that can be purchased for any given amount of expenditure. For example, let us suppose that all salaries in the NHS were doubled at midnight. Because salaries account for about 70% of total expenditure, this would have the effect of increasing the amount of national income by 40% spent on health care, which would easily bring the UK up towards its rightful place on the regression line shown in Figure 8.1. However, doubling salaries with no requirement to do anything extra would not increase the actual volume of health care delivery. Thus the same number of treatments would be performed. Different countries pay medical workers at relatively different rates of pay compared with the National Average wage. For example, in the USA medical workers have a more favourable wage rate relative to the average than their counterparts in the UK. To adjust for these problems, cross-country comparisons are better made with a unit of account known as purchasing power parities (PPPs). For example, if £1 bought the same amount of health care in the UK as $2 does in the USA, the PPP is 2.0. If comparisons are made between countries using PPPs rather than straight exchange-rate comparisons, then the relationship between income and expenditure disappears.

In summary, there are many pitfalls when comparing UK expenditure with that of other countries, which probably make such comparisons meaningless.

However, because these comparisons put the UK's expenditure under the spotlight, they are unlikely to stop just because they are methodologically flawed.

Summary

- The UK is usually perceived as spending too little on health care.
- Cross-country comparisons are so fraught with difficulty that their results are usually meaningless.
- When health care expenditure is adjusted for exchange rate volatility and wage differentials, there is little evidence of UK underspending on health care.

Economic evaluation of health care interventions

Although different in many respects, health economics, like any other speciality of economics, pursues the efficient production and allocation of goods within the health care sector and with respect to the rest of the economy. Because many aspects of health care (e.g. health itself) are difficult to value, health economics faces some unique challenges not encountered by other economic specialities. In this section of the chapter we shall consider the economic evaluation of specific health care interventions. It is this area of health economics with which most medical practitioners will come into contact during their career.

Efficiency

As we have already noted, the aim of health economics is to identify and encourage efficient choices with regard to health care expenditure. There are three types of efficiency – technical, productive and allocative. *Technical efficiency* refers to the relationship between resources and health outcome. Thus a technically efficient position is achieved when the same or a better outcome is achieved for the minimum use of one set of resources. For example, a trial of antibiotic prescription for uncomplicated sore throat has shown no benefit of treatment compared with no antibiotics. Therefore the technically efficient position is for no antibiotic prescription of uncomplicated sore throat, as fewer resources are used for the same outcome (indeed, if one included side-effects of antibiotics, such as allergies, then the outcome is superior). However, technical efficiency cannot compare different interventions that have a different pattern of resource use but produce similar or better outcomes. Consider a comparison of Down's syndrome screening using amniocentesis based on maternal age alone with biochemical screening. Depending on the age cut-off value for screening, biochemical screening may use less of one resource (amniocentesis) but more of another (biochemical tests). Whether one is more efficient than the other will partly depend on the relative costs of these different inputs (i.e. amniocenteses and biochemical tests). *Productive efficiency* is achieved when health output is maximized for a given cost or cost is minimized for a given effect. Biochemical screening will be productively more efficient if the same or a greater number of affected pregnancies are identified for the same or lower cost than with maternal age screening.

Finally, *allocative efficiency* attempts to make a comparison between different health care programmes. For example, should we extend breast screening to older or younger women, or should we purchase more hip replacement operations? Ideally, allocative efficiency is achieved when resources are allocated in such a way as to maximize the total welfare of the community or, in the context of health, the pattern of health care expenditure means that no health gain can be achieved through a change in the pattern of expenditure.

In the following subsections we shall describe a number of different economic techniques which are used to improve efficient resource utilization.

Summary

- Technical efficiency refers to the relationship between the same type of resource and health outcome.
- Productive efficiency refers to the relationship between different patterns of resources and health outcome.
- Allocative efficiency attempts to measure the relationship between costs and outcomes at the societal level.

Cost analysis

In economic evaluation the definition of costs is much broader than merely a financial one. An economic evaluation should include an economically consistent estimation of costs – that is, a measure of the benefit forgone by having used the resources in one particular way and not another. Ideally, opportunity cost evaluation requires comprehensive, disaggregated data at the individual patient level. However, difficulties in obtaining such information necessitate the use of accounting cost data, which are often poor estimators of the true opportunity cost.

The viewpoint of the analysis is a key element in the identification of all relevant costs related to the implementation of any health care programme. Suppose a new drug which delays the admission of patients with Alzheimer's disease to hospital wards or any other specialized institutions is being evaluated for implementation in the NHS. In an analysis with a health care provider perspective only, direct costs, such as the new drug's retail price, and the 'hotel costs' which are prevented by delaying the admission of the patient to a specialized institution, would constitute the main components of the cost analysis. However, from the societal point of view the estimation of costs would need to include not only direct costs associated with the interventions, but also an estimation of the associated indirect cost, such as all of the costs borne by the patient's relatives.

A cost analysis is not usually very helpful in deciding how to make the best use of scarce resources, as it does not consider the benefits of any health care intervention. Clearly, a very inexpensive treatment is inefficient if it does no good at all. Thus it is necessary to prioritize resource allocation quantification of the benefits of a health care intervention, as well as its costs.

Cost–benefit analysis

Cost–benefit analysis (CBA) is the oldest and theoretically the best evaluative method. However, it is also the least widely used method in the health care field. The main distinguishing feature of cost–benefit studies is the measurement of health consequences in commensurate units (money), thus enabling analysts to make comparisons between innovative technologies/programmes from a wide variety of disciplines. Furthermore, the monetary evaluation of both the costs and the consequences of a programme provides information about whether that programme is worth pursuing. In fields other than health, measuring the benefits of resource utilization is less problematic. For instance, in the field of public expenditure on irrigation or flood prevention, the costs of any anticipated action, such as building a dam, can be relatively easily estimated in financial terms. The benefits in terms of reduced flood damage, hydroelectricity generation and increased crop yields can similarly be described in monetary units. Thus if the costs of construction of a dam were outweighed by the monetary benefits accruing to the dam, then it should be built. However, even in this simplistic example one can see how the CBA approach begins to run into difficulties. For example, how does one put a monetary value on the loss of the scenic beauty of the flooded valley due to the presence of the dam? In the health field the application of CBA is particularly fraught with difficulty, given the problems involved in valuing health and life in monetary terms. However, CBA has been used in the health care field, and there has recently been a reassessment of its role. Therefore in the following account we shall describe some of the methods which have been used to attach monetary values to health and life.

The simplest method of putting a monetary value on the number of life years gained is known as the human capital approach. This method, which has fallen into disuse, views human beings as being similar to cart-horses in that an estimated monetary value of their life is derived by estimating the value of their lifetime production in the formal labour force, usually on the basis of wage rates. The problem with this approach is that it tends to discriminate against women, who often spend periods outside the formal labour force, and who earn less then men. It is also biased against retired people who no longer contribute to the formal economy. In addition, it equates the utility of being alive merely as a function of work. Finally, the human capital approach does not quantify the benefits of health care which relieves suffering but has no effect on the capacity to work. For instance, the utility of having a tooth extracted with the benefit of local anaesthetic would be very difficult to capture using a human capital approach, and one might conclude – erroneously – that it was not efficient to use anaesthetic for tooth extraction. It was partly for the reasons outlined above that CBA fell into disuse as a method of health economic evaluation.

More recently there has been an upsurge of interest in CBA by using different methods of monetarizing the benefits of health care. One such method is known as 'willingness to pay' (WTP). In this technique a health care procedure is described to a sample of the population along with its estimated benefits, and people are asked how much of their income they would be willing to pay in order to obtain the benefit of the treatment. This converts the non-monetary benefits of health care into a monetary value which can then be compared with its costs. For example, a recent WTP study among women with severe menopausal symptoms who were using hormone replacement therapy (HRT) to treat the condition showed that the women were willing to pay 12% of their income in order to have HRT, which was far higher than the cost of treatment; thus indicating that this treatment was efficient. However, the technique of WTP is not without problems, not least because many people refuse to answer what they regard as esoteric questions. Furthermore, there is a tendency for people to guess at the cost of the procedure and cite that estimate as their WTP value, which may be more or less than the actual value of the procedure itself.

Cost-effectiveness analysis

Because of the problems of CBA, economists sought to duck the thorny issue of valuing health by using the technique known as cost-effectiveness analysis (CEA). In CEA, health benefits are primarily measured in natural units (e.g. survival rates, mortality rates, pressure sores prevented, etc.) or more preferably in terms of final clinical outcomes (e.g. life years gained, disability days averted). Thus when comparing different methods of screening for cancer, one might estimate a cost per cancer detected, or better still a cost per life saved or life year gained. The use of intermediate clinical outcomes (e.g. cancers detected), although widely used, is only admissible if a clear link between these and a final health outcome is well established, or the intermediate clinical outcome itself is proved to have some value. For example, any study which attempts to investigate the cost-effectiveness of alternative osteoporosis therapies should use a cost per fracture averted rather than a cost per change in the intermediate measure of bone mineral density, as a number of drugs increase bone density but either do not reduce fractures or, in the case of sodium fluoride, increase bone density *and* fractures. Similarly, a cost per cancer detected is a poor measure if all of the cancers detected are so advanced that treatment offers little advantage in terms of survival or quality of life gains.

Although the evaluation of health benefits in clinical terms tends to facilitate the analysis, it imposes significant limitations on the versatility of the results. Comparisons between very different therapies, as well as those between programmes of different types, are literally impossible. For instance, a programme that prevents cancers cannot be compared in the same terms with a programme that increases the number of hip replacements. This limits the use of CEA to disease area comparisons.

Cost-minimization analysis

Cost-minimization analysis is often classified as a particular type of cost-effectiveness analysis in which the health programmes being evaluated happened to produce an equivalent level of clinical outcomes, which in turn allows the measurement of the effectiveness of either intervention only in terms of their difference in costs. Among the alternative economic evaluation techniques, cost-minimization analysis is recognized as the least best method, although it is rarely appropriate since in practice such equivalence in terms of clinical outcomes rarely exists. Cost minimization is often used as the default method of evaluation because there are no data to suggest any differences in effectiveness. For instance, there is no good evidence that one form of HRT is any more effective than its alternatives. Therefore, until there is evidence to suggest otherwise, it is assumed that the most efficient prescription is the cheapest preparation with which a patient will comply.

Cost–utility analysis

Because of the problems associated with CEA and CBA, a third technique, known as cost–utility analysis (CUA), has become widely used over the last few years. CUA combines the qualitative and quantitative aspects of the measurement of health care outcomes into a single measure of utility. The most widely used approach is to estimate quality-adjusted life years (QALYs) to set against the cost of an intervention. For example, if we consider a treatment that lengthens life by 10 years, but at only half the quality of normal life, this would produce 5 QALYs. Thus a QALY captures not only any survival advantage of a treatment, but also the quality of that survival. Figure 8.2 shows a diagrammatic representation of QALY or utility calculation.

The use of a common unit of health output in cost–utility analysis has the advantage of allowing comparisons between different programmes. For example, a comparison could be made of a programme to implement a new drug in the treatment of patients with HIV, where health outcome was measured in QALYs, with a vaccination programme to prevent hepatitis B, where health outcome was measured in the same units.

Incremental analysis

Of key importance in economic evaluations is the notion of incremental or marginal costs and benefits. When deciding whether to expand or contract a health care programme, the decision should be made on the basis of an assessment of the *extra* costs or *extra* benefits of any action. Although this may seem obvious, a common error is to describe the *average* costs and benefits of any action, which can give misleading results. For example, consider a health care

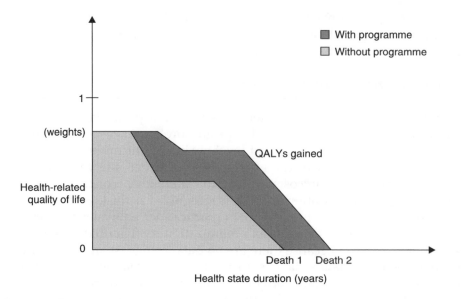

Figure 8.2 Diagrammatic representation of quality adjusted life years (QALYs) or utility calculation.

programme costing £100. If this produces 10 units of output, the cost per unit is £10. Now let us assume that we are going to expand the programme by £20 and this produces 5 more units of output. The incremental cost is £20, the incremental benefit is 5 and the marginal cost-effectiveness ratio is £4 per unit (i.e. £20/5). However, what often happens is that analysts divide the total costs of the new programme, in this case £120, by the total benefits, namely 15 units. This produces an average cost-effectiveness of £8, which is twice as much, in this instance, as the marginal cost-effectiveness ratio.

Consider another example. An evaluation of biochemical screening for Down's syndrome that was published in the *British Medical Journal* estimated that it would cost £38 000 to detect one affected pregnancy. However, the authors had made the error of adding together the existing programme and the new programme. If they had used the more correct approach, the actual marginal cost per pregnancy averted would have been nearly £48 000. Table 8.1 shows a simple worked example of marginal analysis for the prevention of hip fracture using calcium and vitamin D supplementation among residents of a nursing home.

Table 8.1 shows that around 75% of hip fractures occur among women who are in the low body weight category. Therefore, if one had a budget of only £27 500, one could obtain the most benefit by treating the women of lowest weight. However, if the budget was to be expanded, it can be seen that the marginal cost-effectiveness ratio increases by a factor of three, but this sharp jump in cost-effectiveness ratio is disguised by reference to average cost-effectiveness ratios in the last column of Table 8.1. Thus on the basis of the marginal ratios in the table, rather than offering preventive treatment to lower-risk women in residential care, it might be concluded that it would be best to offer such treatment to higher-risk individuals in the community.

Table 8.1 The cost-effectiveness of preventing hip fractures among women in nursing homes

	Fracture incidence in 1000 women aged 85 years and resident in nursing-home accommodation		
	Low body weight	High body weight	Total
Number of hip fractures annually	20	6	26
Number of hip fractures prevented	6	2	8
Cost of prevention	£27 500	£27 500	£55 000
Cost per hip fracture averted	£4583	£13 750	£6875

Discounting and time preferences

In many economic evaluations the different health care programmes have different cost-and-benefit time profiles. In other words, cost and benefits from the programmes occur at different points in time. For example, a vaccination programme to prevent malaria requires an immediate investment resulting in expected benefits which will occur in the future, whereas a programme to implement a new technology for the treatment of breast cancer would also require an immediate investment, but the expected benefits will occur immediately. Since economic evaluations require a comparison of the total costs and benefits of the programmes at one point in time (usually the present), variations in the time profile of costs and benefits must be included in the analysis.

There are two reasons why it is necessary to adjust the value of future benefits and costs to present-day values – a process known as discounting. For costs, discounting is required because an investment in a health care technology in the present rather than in the future results in an opportunity cost of lost interest. For example, if a health care project costing £100 was to be delayed for 1 year and then given a 5% return on the money there would be £105 available for investment after 12 months. Therefore this needs to be taken into account. The other reason why future costs and benefits are valued less than those which occur at the present time is because of time preference. In general, individuals in society prefer present benefits and resources to future ones (i.e. immediate accessibility to resources will invariably be preferred to the uncertainty associated with future events occurring). For example, if there is a choice between saving 1000 lives in the next 12 months and waiting to save 1000 lives in 5 years' time, most people would prefer to save 1000 lives now, which would generate 5000 extra life years.

In economic evaluation analysis, time preference can be accounted for by applying discount rates to both future costs and future benefits. In this context, a positive discount rate is a quantitative measure of individuals' preference for benefits today rather than in the future. Thus the higher the discount rate, the stronger the aversion of individuals to deferring benefits. Examples of people discounting future health effects abound. For instance, smokers will discount the future health effects of their habit in order to enjoy the pleasure of cigarette smoking in the present.

The application of discount rates to future costs is common practice among economists, and there is little disagreement with the practice. However, with regard to the discounting of health benefits there is some controversy. Because health, unlike money, cannot be invested to yield a real rate of return, this is cited as a reason why future health gains should at least be discounted at a lower rate than wealth. Furthermore, research into discount rates tends to show that individuals actually discount future health gains at a greater rate than they do future wealth gains.

With regard to the choice of an appropriate discount rate for public projects, there are two main alternative approaches. The first is to measure the *social opportunity costs* (the real rate of return that is forgone in the private sector), and the second approach is to attempt to measure the *social rate of time preferences* (the societal opportunity cost of giving up financial resources today in exchange for future health benefits). However, in countries like the UK the choice of the discount rate applied to public projects is a government decision. The current discount rate in the UK is 6%, in the USA it is 5%, and for other countries it ranges from 3% to 8%.

Sensitivity analysis

Uncertainty is present at every stage in the process of estimation of costs and health outcomes in all types of economic evaluations. For example, the price of a given resource will vary geographically or over time. Even estimation of the quantity of resource use may involve uncertainty if the data is stochastic (i.e. gathered at the patient level as part of a trial).

The way of dealing with uncertainty is through sensitivity analysis. For example, if the patent on a pharmaceutical product is likely to expire in a couple of years, one might undertake an analysis making the assumption that once patent protection has expired the cost of the drug will fall dramatically. Similarly, the cost of experimental machines, such as CAT scanners, is likely to fall once the technology has been proven and full production is under way.

Sensitivity analysis involves a systematic analysis of the impact of each variable in the study outcomes. This analysis can be performed using different approaches. Depending on the number of parameters being simultaneously varied, they are classified as follows.

- *One-way sensitivity analysis*: only one variable is allowed to vary in a set of plausible values, while the rest remain constant.
- *Extreme scenario analysis*: the worst and best possible values per parameter are calculated and tested simultaneously to estimate the most optimistic and pessimistic scenarios.
- *Multi-way sensitivity analysis*: more than one parameter is varied simultaneously over a feasible set of values, while the others remain constant.
- *Probabilistic sensitivity analysis*: the uncertainty related to each parameter is described using probability distribution functions.

There are various issues regarding the robustness and reliability of a sensitivity analysis. For example, the selection of the parameters on which sensitivity analysis should be performed, as well as the determination of their plausible range of variation, should be clearly justified. In this context, of all the different sensitivity analysis methods, the rarely used probabilistic sensitivity analysis emerges as a powerful tool. The introduction of predefined probability distributions for the whole set of parameters is expected to produce a more realistic estimate of the uncertainty associated with them.

The role of modelling

Lack of information represents a major obstacle to the performance of any economic evaluation study. For instance, most clinical trials are at best conducted for only a few years, whereas the typical patient lives for many decades. Ideally, we would like to have some idea of the costs and benefits beyond the length of a typical clinical trial. Furthermore, for some interventions, such as the introduction of an air ambulance service, trials are simply not possible – hence the increasing relevance and popularity of modelling as a tool to explore the behaviour of unknown relevant variables in economic evaluations. Models are a way of representing a complex reality in a more simple and comprehensive way by utilizing mathematical and statistical techniques. Their applicability in the area of economic evaluation of health technologies is multifold. As well as extrapolating beyond a clinical trial, modelling helps to establish links between intermediate clinical end-points and final outcomes. For example, with regard to osteoporosis, changes in bone density have been linked to rates of fracture. In a study of the effects of oestrogen treatment on fractures, the relationship between treatment and bone density and between bone density and fracture was used to design a model to estimate the cost-effectiveness of the therapy in different age groups.

Modelling has also been used to investigate the generalization of the results obtained from clinical trials. The task is twofold – first generalizing the trial results to the real practice, and then generalizing the results to different settings (e.g. hospitals, regions, countries). The process of generalization has mainly focused on the exploration of all the possible sources of heterogeneity of the information obtained from clinical trials and that observed in real practice, either in the same setting where the trial was performed, or in different settings. Further applications of modelling include performing comparisons of relevant treatments with an appropriate alternative where no trials exist, and providing a secondary source of information when it is not possible to obtain information from primary sources.

Having briefly discussed the various ways in which modelling can contribute in the performance of economic evaluations, it is important to highlight the fact that modelling techniques, rather than providing information about the cost-effectiveness of interventions, are one of the most powerful ways of investigating the high levels of uncertainty surrounding the results obtained from such studies. Through the characterization of the uncertainty, probabilistic modelling can provide information about the value of acquiring further information, as well as facilitating the identification of the key parameters in the study, and determining the appropriate sample size.

Summary

- Cost analysis by itself is rarely useful.
- Cost-minimization analysis makes the heroic assumption that clinical outcomes are equivalent between two treatments, and therefore that the best treatment is the least expensive one.
- Cost-effectiveness analysis measures costs in monetary terms and outcomes in clinically meaningful units (e.g. cancers avoided). Because of this it is difficult to make comparisons across health care programmes.
- Cost–utility analysis compares outcomes in utility units such as quality-adjusted life years (QALYs), and this facilitates comparison between different health care programmes.
- Cost–benefit analysis compares costs and outcomes in monetary terms and is therefore difficult to use in a health care setting.

Discussion and conclusions

Resource scarcity is a fact of everyday life. The implications of this in medical care are that inevitably some patients will die or have poor health because there are insufficient resources to provide effective treatments. It is the role of the economic analyst to ascertain which pattern of resource use minimizes avoidable suffering and mortality. The aim of economic appraisal is not cost containment or cost reduction. Rather it is about improving utility. In this chapter we have given a necessarily brief overview of some of the main issues and techniques that will confront medical practitioners throughout their careers.

Discussion point

The use of health economics has increased substantially in recent years. Indeed, before the 1960s the Department of Health did not employ any economists! Although there has always been resource scarcity in health care, it has only been relatively recently that expenditure on health has been greater than that on other public services (e.g. education and defence). Despite this historical trend towards increasingly large health expenditure, health technologies are costing more and difficult rationing decisions need to be made. A challenge for the future is to ensure that resources are used more efficiently, and one method may be to integrate more economics into undergraduate teaching.

Further reading

Gold MR, Siegel JE, Russell LB and Weinstein MC (eds) (1996) *Cost-effectiveness in health and medicine*. New York: Oxford University Press.

Palmer S, Byford S and Raftery J (1999) Types of economic evaluation. *British Medical Journal* **318**, 1349.

Torgerson DJ and Spencer A (1996) Marginal costs and benefits. *British Medical Journal* **312**, 35–6.

Torgerson DJ and Raftery J (1999) Economic note: discounting. *British Medical Journal* **319**, 914–15.

Torgerson DJ and Raftery J (1999) Economic note: outcomes. *British Medical Journal* **318**, 1413.

Health promotion

9

Alan Beattie

What is health promotion?

Health promotion has become an increasingly prominent item in public policy in the UK and other countries in recent years, and an increasingly important aspect of the work of doctors, nurses and other health professionals, as well as of people in several other sectors beyond the health service. A useful first definition is as follows: 'Health promotion is the process of enabling people to increase control over, and to improve, their health' (World Health Organization, 1986).

An older approach, often equated with 'health education', has been to give people information in order to enable them to take action to improve their own health. However, recent developments have led to the concept of 'health promotion'. This is understood to include not only information-giving, but also other ways of strengthening individuals, as well as action directed towards changing the social circumstances of people's lives – by enhancing supportive community structures, alleviating detrimental economic conditions or reducing environmental hazards.

A framework that summarizes these strategic options in conceptualizing and planning health promotion activities is shown in Figure 9.1.

The four modes of health promotion (Beattie, 1991) can also be summarized as shown in Table 9.1.

This table draws together the principal aims and typical areas of activity that characterize each different mode of health promotion. Practitioners are sometimes attracted to one particular mode because of the distinctive personal and social values it is seen to embody – which may be partly a matter of ethical standpoint, partly to do with political views, and for some people

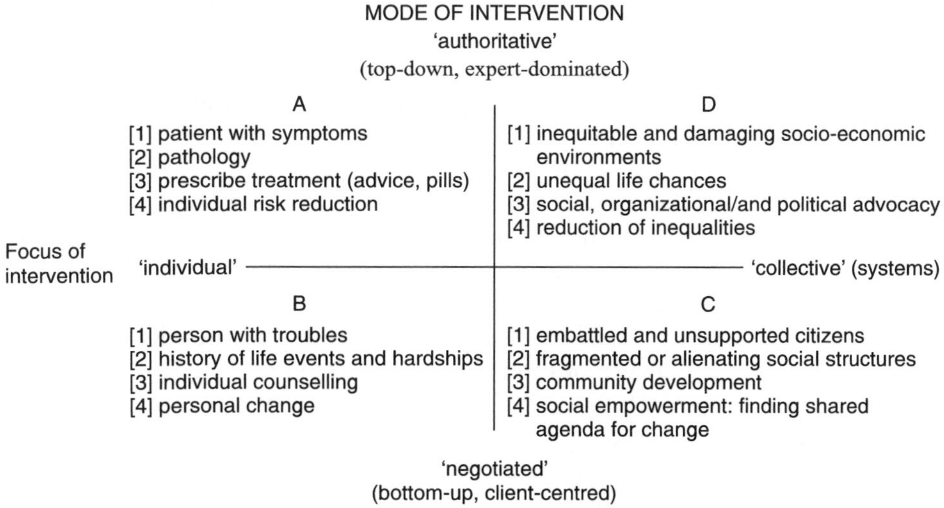

MODE OF INTERVENTION
'authoritative'
(top-down, expert-dominated)

A	D
[1] patient with symptoms [2] pathology [3] prescribe treatment (advice, pills) [4] individual risk reduction	[1] inequitable and damaging socio-economic environments [2] unequal life chances [3] social, organizational/and political advocacy [4] reduction of inequalities

Focus of intervention   'individual' ———————————————————————— 'collective' (systems)

B	C
[1] person with troubles [2] history of life events and hardships [3] individual counselling [4] personal change	[1] embattled and unsupported citizens [2] fragmented or alienating social structures [3] community development [4] social empowerment: finding shared agenda for change

'negotiated'
(bottom-up, client-centred)

Key

[A–D] = four broad approaches to health promotion, each with a characteristic:
[1] way of seeing the core problem;
[2] explanation of the problem;
[3] main recommended line of action;
[4] intended outcome.

Figure 9.1 A four-quadrant framework for reviewing health promotion strategies.

Table 9.1 Four modes of health promotion: aims, practices and underlying philosophies

	Mode of health promotion	Aim	Practice	Philosophy
A	Individual risk reduction	To protect client and to reduce risk of disease	Vaccinate, test, monitor, advise, persuade	Conservative-positivist, functionalist
B	Personal counselling	To help client to take control of their own life	Listen, clarify, reflect focus, resolve, support	Humanistic, liberal, permissive
C	Community development	To support groups in their own agenda of change	Listen, join in, debate, debate, bring together, network	Communitarian, radical-humanist
D	Social advocacy	To lobby official agencies to achieve equity	Report, liaise, appeal, persuade, expose	Radical-positivist, materialist

perhaps more concerned with what types of knowledge they deem to be most trustworthy (e.g. whether it is oriented towards the positivist and 'objective', or towards the humanist and 'interpretive'). These positions (here termed 'philosophies') are summarized in the final column of Table 9.1, although it should be pointed out that many practitioners nowadays try to judge the merits of different modes on strictly pragmatic grounds.

Some insights that arise from scrutinizing this framework (as shown in Figure 9.1 and Table 9.1) are listed below.

1. Medical education has until recently most obviously prepared doctors for the ways of thinking and types of practice that are summarized in quadrant A – what some call 'medical model' health promotion. However, successive waves of reform have opened up medical thinking and practice in the directions A → B and A → D, such that doctors are better equipped for working in partnership with clients to improve their health (a shift from top to bottom on the vertical axis), and better able to appreciate the need (often) to take action to change the social institutions that limit the scope for clients to improve their health on their own (a shift from individual to collective on the horizontal axis). Both of these axes entail value shifts that may in different ways challenge not only the academic knowledge base but also even the self-concept of the medical practitioner.

2. The current organization of medical work means that many doctors specialize (e.g. in hospital-based medicine and surgery) in ways that may encourage a 'mode A' way of seeing the health promotion task. Others may find mode B more convincing as an approach to health improvement, and may move into psychological medicine and psychiatry, or may bring this perspective to bear on specialized hospital practice or on general practice. Yet others may find that mode D offers the most persuasive logic for health improvement, and may move into public health medicine; or may deliberately make time within or beyond their clinical practice for the types of advocacy work that this approach involves – perhaps simply as citizens who happen to work in medicine. Those who find social empowerment and community development (mode C) the most compelling ways of going about the health improvement task are unlikely to find a major medical specialism that exclusively or even predominantly uses such an approach, but can bring it to bear significantly in work with lay community groups or voluntary organizations within general practice, psychiatry, public health – or indeed potentially in any area of modern medicine where listening to 'local voices for health' is an important part of the job.

3. The most important train of thought arising from the framework presented in Figure 9.1 and Table 9.1 may be that in the future every doctor should be able to understand and appreciate all four of the distinctive ways of seeing and ways of doing, and the values that lie behind them – in all four 'modes' – and to recognize that all four of them may have a part to play in a comprehensive and 'whole-systems' approach to the improvement of health. Even for medical practitioners who choose to work within only one mode, it is becoming vitally important to be able to enter into dialogue with other practitioners and agencies who may be using a different approach to health promotion to themselves, and when occasion demands to be able to contribute to shared tasks within a wider team, or to negotiate a division of labour, or to delegate and support those colleagues whose work in different modes of health promotion may need to come into the picture in a multi-strand programme (or may even need to take the lead for a time in some phases of a complex project).

The World Health Organization's approach to promoting health

A major influence in shaping up-to-date strategies for health promotion has been the World Health Organization (WHO), especially in the work it has undertaken since the 1970s. A series of key concepts were formulated by the WHO as part of its work in developing the *Health for All by the Year 2000* framework, and these are being further pursued in the *Health 21* programmes which are now under way. A classic statement of the WHO approach can be found in the *Ottawa Charter* (World Health Organization, 1986), which identifies as the basic tools or 'building blocks' of health promotion the following 'famous five' priority areas for action (Nutbeam, 1986, 1998).

1. *Building healthy public policy (HPP).* This is characterized by an explicit concern for health and equity in all areas of policy, and by accountability for the 'health impact' of all areas of policy. The aim of HPP is to ensure wider social policies that make healthy choices feasible and easier for all citizens.
2. *Creating supportive environments for health (SEHs).* These are environments that offer people protection from threats to health, and that enable individuals to expand their capabilities and develop self-reliance in health. SEHs encompass where people live, their homes, their local neighbourhoods, and where they work and play. Action to create SEHs may include direct political action to develop and implement relevant policies and regulations, and economic and social action (e.g. to foster sustainable environments).
3. *Strengthening community action for health (CAH).* This refers to collective efforts by communities that are directed towards improving health by increasing community control over the determinants of health. CAH is one particular type of social empowerment, in which local people come together to define their own health needs, then work through the conflicts that emerge during this process of participation, and provide mutual social support for each other in meeting their own agreed needs.
4. *Developing personal skills for health (PSHs).* These are the skills whereby individuals manage to deal with the demands and challenges of everyday life. They are life skills – the means of adapting to and surviving adverse life events and social hardships. PSHs are typically seen in people's capacity to live with change, but also in their ability to generate change – to control and direct their own lives. They involve both cognitive and emotional capacities – creative as well as critical thinking, decision-making and problem-solving, self-awareness and empathy, and skills in communication and interpersonal relationships and in managing stress and emotions.
5. *Reorienting health services (RHS).* This is characterized by a concern to emphasize explicit health outcomes in the way that health services are planned, funded and managed. RHS seeks a higher profile for health promotion and disease prevention in balance with diagnosis, treatment,

care and rehabilitation services, and a better appreciation of the needs of each individual as a whole person, together with the needs of all population groups. It also highlights the importance of the contribution to health outcomes of all of the health professions, and of other institutions beyond the health service itself. It therefore involves a call for intersectoral action for health across all government departments.

The WHO continues to emphasize that 'multi-track' approaches to health improvement are far more effective than 'single-track' ones, and that all opportunities must be seized for the implementation of comprehensive combinations of all five of the 'building blocks' defined above. This will require new investments in partnership working and new infrastructures for delivering health promotion.

Box 9.1 The World Health Organization's five key concepts for health promotion

- *Healthy public policy* is the process of trying to ensure that all areas of policy (not just health services) are favourable to health.
- *Supportive environments for health* occur where action to improve health is directed at the settings of people's everyday lives, such as homes, neighbourhoods and workplaces.
- *Community action for health* occurs where local people come together to share their health concerns and support each other in improving their own circumstances.
- *Personal skills for health* focuses on what it takes for individuals to deal with the changes and challenges of their lives, and to manage stress and emotions in creative and adaptive ways.
- *Reorienting health services* is about achieving services that bring practitioners together with a focus on the needs of the whole population and an emphasis on positive health gain.

Health improvement strategies in the UK

In the UK, the policies and strategies brought forward by the WHO at both global and European level have helped to inform or support a great deal of local activity in health promotion since the early 1980s. However, although UK governments have been signatories to the WHO charters, concerted policy development for public health and health promotion at national level was slower in coming, and has sometimes taken a lukewarm and selective approach to the WHO precepts. The *Health of the Nation* strategy introduced in the 1980s was the first attempt by a UK government to establish a coherent and systematic policy for health promotion, and although this avoided direct reference to the context of social inequalities in health, it did highlight a number of key concepts with origins in the WHO approach. The successor to *Health of the Nation* was brought in by a new government in 1999, and was entitled *Our Healthier Nation*. It reflects an approach that is much closer to that of the WHO and places a great deal of emphasis on a wide understanding of the 'health field' and of the need for multi-level, 'joined-up' action for health promotion. This – and related research and development work in the Health

Education Authority – has put firmly on the agenda for planning and action a number of further key concepts that advance the lines of thought seen earlier in WHO policies. The following five concepts seem to offer new 'building blocks' (along similar lines to the WHO's 'famous five' listed above).

1. *Healthy alliances*. One of the key principles of the WHO's strategies for *Primary Health Care* and for *Health for All 2000* since the late 1970s (World Health Organization, 1986) has been to encourage interagency collaboration, to work to improve health by co-ordinating activities across different sectors (health, social services, housing, employment, education and environment). By the end of the 1980s, many towns and cities in the UK were the sites for considerable efforts to strengthen joint work on public health issues. In 1992, as a way of making its *Health of the Nation* strategy work, the UK Department of Health encouraged the setting up at all levels of the service of 'healthy alliances' – that is 'active partnerships between the many organizations and individuals who can come together to help improve health' (Department of Health, 1992: 5). Each of the Key Area Handbooks for *Health of the Nation* that were subsequently published (on HIV/AIDS and sexual health, coronary heart disease and stroke, accidents, cancers and mental health) incorporated a section on healthy alliances that illustrated local examples and approaches to finding 'likely partners' for multi-agency preventive work in each of these five areas. More recently the term has been amended to 'health alliances', but the principle of creating new allegiances between the work of separate agencies in order to deliver health improvements at local level remains central to the 1999 *Our Healthier Nation* strategy. This observes that successful local partnerships will require the development of 'a culture in which learning and good practice are shared' across boundaries.

2. *Healthy settings*. We saw earlier that 'creating supportive environments for health' was a concept brought in by the WHO. This connects in turn to a broader concept of 'settings-based health promotion' and the idea of 'healthy settings' – another area where WHO and UK government policies have increasingly begun to converge. The settings approach tries to make a reality out of the wider, less compartmentalized, 'ecological' view of health, by taking action within the everyday habitats within which we all 'learn, work, play and love'. *Health of the Nation* (Department of Health, 1992) advocated action at the level of healthier homes, health-promoting schools, health-promoting hospitals, healthy workplaces and healthy cities, and subsequent work has pursued the same idea in projects on 'healthy prisons' and 'health-promoting universities'. Concepts such as healthy schools and healthy workplaces continue to be an important element of *Our Healthier Nation*. However, three new instances of this concept are introduced. *Healthy living centres* are recommended as places which bring together a new and creative mix of ways of providing help towards better health (e.g. health screening and advice, dietary information, smoking cessation support, exercise, child care and training, and employment skills development). All of this may be housed in a single building, or it may be

a new network of facilities, and it is regarded as essential that local users are fully involved in the planning of such centres. *Healthy neighbourhoods* are proposed as a focus for improving health by promoting social cohesion and strengthening social networks: 'people relate closely to their neighbourhoods and are likely to be healthier when they live in neighbourhoods where there is a sense of pride and belonging' (Department of Health, 1999: paragraph 4.34–4.35). This is seen as a point at which health improvement must link up with wider 'regeneration' initiatives, such as the 'New Deal for Communities' and 'Single Regeneration Bids' which aim to improve the most deprived local authority areas, and 'Local Agenda 21' plans, which aim to promote sustainable development through environmental projects such as community gardens, new allotments, city farms, new public transport schemes, etc. *Health action zones* have been introduced as a way of encouraging local organizations to co-operate in improving health in the most deprived areas of the country. Their three broad strategic objectives are to reduce health inequalities in a local area, to increase the efficiency, effectiveness and responsiveness of local services, and to 'create alliances for change' that 'add value' by 'breaking through current organizational boundaries', by 'creating synergy between the work of different agencies' and 'by harnessing the dynamism of local people and organizations'.

3. *Healthy citizens. Our Healthier Nation* (Department of Health, 1998) signals an important development in conceptualizing the way in which health promotion practice addresses the individual. As we saw above, it is not new for governments to ask people to take responsibility for their own health – to suggest that there are actions that we can each take to improve our own health. However, the 1999 policy framework goes some way towards incorporating more recent understanding of the extent to which each individual's scope for decision-making and choice is socially constrained, acknowledging that 'better health opportunities and decisions are not easily available to everyone. For example, membership of a gym may not be an option for someone in a poor neighbourhood, or a single mother' (Department of Health, 1999, paragraph 1.34). Local health improvement programmes are therefore called upon to deliver information and programmes that can enfranchise people in matters of health, can combat 'social exclusion' and can help to 'create the right conditions for individuals to make healthy decisions'. This kind of shift in thinking is registered in the idea of 'healthy citizens' and 'expert patients', whereby we are all encouraged to be active agents in helping ourselves and improving our own health, with the support of information from magazines, radio and television programmes, telephone helplines, websites and other electronic media resources.

4. *'Contracts for health'*. A key tool of thought in *Our Healthier Nation* (Department of Health, 1998) is a series of 'national contracts' on each of the major health priorities for which targets are defined in that policy (cancer, heart disease and stroke, accidents, mental health). Each contract lists four dimensions in which action can be taken to improve a particular aspect of health (services, personal behaviour, social and economic, and

environmental), and then describes *which* of the various players in the national and local 'health partnerships' should be doing *what* in each of these dimensions (individual citizens, 'local players and communities', and 'government and national players'). This type of scheme (see Table 9.2) can be a useful device for planning, consultation and review, and has for example been taken further in a series of National Service Frameworks (e.g. for mental health and coronary heart disease) which place health promotion firmly at the heart of mainstream health care development and management. Action guides along these lines bear the unmistakable stamp (and show the benefits) of the 'structures and systems' thinking outlined above, as a crucial way of keeping in mind the 'bigger picture' – the new balance, the 'third way' – linking individual and institutional action on health.

5. *Social capital for health*. This receives only a brief mention in *Our Healthier Nation*, but it is a concept that is clearly helping to drive much of the new thinking that underlies the commitment to 'inclusive and integrated, comprehensive and coherent' ways of tackling poor health. Social capital refers to the invisible fabric of social trust at grassroots level, the formal and

Table 9.2 A contract for action on health improvement

Who does what and why?	Front-line medical/health practitioners can:	Individual citizens can:	Community groups can:	Statutory agencies local and central government can:
Enhance clinical repair and risk-reduction services	Conduct screening and risk assessments; offer information and/or advice; run prevention clinics	Make use of screening and advice services; engage in well-informed active health maintenance	Support complaints about unsatisfactory services; advertise and protect valued services	Modernise services; ensure efficiency, effectiveness and equity; monitor and audit standards and/or frameworks
Strengthen individuals	Offer counselling services; support healthy living centres	Take charge of their own lives; take opportunities for learning and training	Protect vulnerable members; help them to move on and find their own voice	Offer link and liaison services; offer protection or respite if necessary
Strengthen communities	Support and enable deprived groups; challenge social exclusion; work with other local agencies	Exchange experience and information with local people; participate in local networks; provide social support	Maintain local networks; provide social support	Act as statutory enabler; create or maintain supportive infrastructures
Improve wider social economic and cultural environments	Pass on complaints and concerns to statutory agencies responsible officers or higher authorities ('blow the whistle')	Complain about unsatisfactory policies, environments, etc.	Lobby and campaign to transform environments, laws, regulations or policies	Ensure health-promoting policies, laws, regulations, standards, social norms and plans

informal systems for exchanging information, ideas and practical help – the horizontal and 'egalitarian' networks of relatives, friends, neighbours and mutual aid organizations. Evidence is growing that the numbers of deaths in infancy and from stroke, heart disease, accidents and suicide are lower (and longevity is higher) in areas with high social capital, and that public health initiatives generally are more likely to succeed in such areas. The basic idea was seen above in connection with 'healthy settings' – 'social capital' is what regeneration schemes are aiming to build or repair or replace, by increasing social cohesion, strengthening social networks and reducing social stress and divisions. It is clearly a concept that can have far-reaching implications for the future planning and delivery of health promotion, and it helps to pull together and make sense of several of the other key understandings described in this chapter.

Box 9.2 Five key concepts in recent UK government health promotion policies

- *Healthy alliances* is about active partnerships to improve health by co-ordinating activities across sectors (health, social services, housing, employment, education and environment).
- *Healthy settings* is concerned with taking action to improve health within the major 'institutions' of modern life (schools, hospitals, workplaces, prisons, neighbourhoods and cities).
- *Healthy citizens* involves providing much better information and support to the public, in order to make opportunities and decisions for better health more readily available to everyone.
- *Contracts for health* is a methodical way of setting out the range of actions that may usefully be taken with regard to a particular health problem, and who should be doing what across this range.
- *Social capital for health* is a term that refers to the fabric of local life at the grassroots – trust, support, networks of exchange – that makes for cohesion and supports positive health action.

Key concepts applied in clinical practice

Preventing accidental falls among older people

Every year in the UK more than 3000 people aged 65 years or over die as a result of falls, and there are many other statistical indicators that flag up the huge toll of injuries and disabilities due to the high incidence of falls in the later years of life (Downton, 1993). How to reduce this burden of illness most effectively is a typical challenge in orchestrating several different and parallel strategies for health promotion (Oakley, 1996).

1. There is often a great deal of clinical work that can usefully be done. For older people who have already fallen at least once and have received treatment, an in-depth assessment of risk factors can be made before they return home. Older people newly entering hospital or nursing homes, etc., can be assessed in terms of 'falls risk scores', and case management policies (or

care plans) can be developed accordingly. Older people living at home can be assessed and fitted (if appropriate) with body-worn alarms, backed up by staff training and regular checks. Careful guidance can be given on the risks of unsteadiness and falls associated with certain drugs, especially 'polypharmacy'. Specialist falls clinics can be set up to give guidance on this problem.

2. Older people living at home can be provided with education, information and/or advice on how to reduce the risk of falls, what to do in the event of a fall, how to get up after a fall, etc. They can be encouraged to attend sessions of dance and other forms of exercise that are known to enhance the balance, strength and mobility of older people (as well as yielding benefits for psychological well-being, alertness, self-confidence and social interaction).

3. Older people's own homes can be checked for accident risks and hazards, and modified as appropriate (by negotiation!). Where necessary, aids and adaptations can be put in place, as well as other socio-physical and socio-economic elements of domiciliary care and support. Similar reviews can be conducted in hospital wards and day units and in nursing homes, and the ideas associated with 'healthy settings' can be brought to bear to prompt a broader managerial effort to clarify and monitor operational policies and practice protocols, and to involve and update all relevant staff and encourage teamwork and liaison (across agencies where necessary).

4. Local groups (e.g. Age Concern, Help the Aged, tea-dance groups, etc.) can be used as forums to run discussions and debates with older people on concerns about risk and safety, and on achieving a balance between protection and independence in older people's lifestyles. In local schools, adult education institutions or community centres, 'learning and outreach' networks can be set up for older people (and other sections of the community) to engage in discussion about the meaning of 'safety as a community value', 'the competent community', etc. These discussions could draw on techniques of community development and empowerment education to explore the possibilities for local citizen action on 'safe community projects', etc.

Action on stress and emotional disorders

At any one time, around 1 in 6 adults of working age are experiencing mental health problems (e.g. anxiety or depression), and 1 in 250 adults will experience a psychotic illness (e.g. manic depression or schizophrenia) (National Service Framework, 1999). Mental health problems result in the greatest burden of premature death and number of years of reduced quality of life. However, dealing with mental health problems is well known to be a controversial field. Different viewpoints and schools of thought coexist, which recommend what sometimes appear to be starkly different guidelines for practice, and they are frequently the focus of intense dispute (Clare, 1976; Tudor, 1996). Although these different approaches may indeed sometimes be in conflict and incompatible, increasingly they can be used to complement one another as successive phases in an unfolding programme of mental health development work, or as alternative emphases within a comprehensive strategy for mental health, running as parallel strands – with one or another of them being given particular attention from time to time as appropriate. It is another challenge in orchestrating multiple strategies for health promotion.

1. One of the more surprising developments in mental health promotion has been the increasing recognition that service users (current or former psychiatric patients or 'survivors') can provide crucial insights into the planning and delivery of services. Moreover, mutual aid groups formed by survivors can have a beneficial impact on individuals with or at risk of mental health problems. They give clients the opportunity to share their experiences (sadness, frustration or anger prompted by their social circumstances) with others who have 'been there', and they can thereby find – with the support of the peer group – a common agenda and possibilities for empowerment and action to change their lives. For clinicians, liaison with other appropriate agencies may offer an essential entry-point to such support networks – often a local community development worker, or a local voluntary group or agency.

2. For some clients, some of the time, prescribing psychoactive medicines may be best practice in order to cope with an immediate crisis or to alleviate distressing acute symptoms. There are many cases of long-term psychiatric patients who welcome regular or occasional medication that helps to keep crises at bay, and enables them to maintain their independence and autonomy, and to continue to work to resolve underlying problems. Often, however, this focus on the illness or the symptoms can lead to neglect of wider opportunities for promoting mental health.

3. Some clients can best be helped by in-depth counselling that explores feelings and the origins and meanings of symptoms, and can thereby be helped towards a greater sense of control and ownership of their lives. In such cases, referral to other practitioners may be essential. In other cases it may be appropriate to refer a client to adult education or similar 'tailored' education services, where life skills and coping strategies can be learned (or relearned), and new horizons with regard to personal capability and social interaction can often open up. In such cases, relaxation, stress management and exercise seem to be beneficial. In addition, creative and performing arts projects (in hospital or community settings) can give access to individual and group activities that enhance self-esteem and self-confidence, as well as offering new personal insights.

4. Recent policy directives have encouraged clinicians to make themselves aware of the wider socio-economic and socio-cultural contexts that contribute to the burden of mental health problems, such as long-term hardship or abuse (notably of women) or discrimination (notably against black people and those from ethnic minorities). Such awareness can guide action of the types already mentioned here, but can also suggest other interventions (e.g. professional or citizen advocacy to improve local and national policies on inequity in mental health). Other examples of a

broader agenda to which health professionals can contribute significantly are the challenging of the negative stereotypes of mental illness that are portrayed by the media, fighting discrimination against people with mental health problems and promoting their social inclusion (National Service Framework, 1999).

Action on coronary heart disease and cardiovascular health

Coronary heart disease (CHD) is the single commonest cause of premature and avoidable death in the UK. In England every year over 1 000 000 people die from heart disease, three times that number are victims of heart attacks, and nearly five times as many again suffer from angina. The risk of CHD is closely associated with social disadvantage, unskilled men being three times more likely to die from CHD than professional men (and their wives being twice as likely to die from CHD). There is much that can be done to transform this situation (National Service Framework, 2000), but it will require action at many different levels simultaneously (Calman,1991).

1. Clinical interventions are one vital starting point for action. Primary care staff can ensure that coronary risk factors are brought into the conversation (when appropriate) during individual consultations (e.g. smoking, body mass index, eating patterns, exercise). It is important to raise these topics in a personalized way and to link them to individualized care planning. A team approach to monitoring and advising on these risk factors needs to be agreed.
2. Cardiac health promotion needs to go beyond a narrow focus on behaviour change related to the major coronary 'lifestyle risk factors', and to encourage a 'whole-person' approach. This can include support through personal counselling with regard to problems with relationships, alcohol and substance abuse, stress or lack of control in the workplace, etc. Recommendations for personal change (e.g. taking up opportunities for exercise and physical activity at local facilities) can be made more vivid and memorable by linking them to current themes in the media (e.g. news items, or incidents in popular soap operas).
3. Practice nurses and other primary health care team members can arrange to ensure that a higher profile is given to issues related to personal and workplace stress and lifestyle among the practice population, and this can be supported and followed up by primary health care facilitators. This in turn can be linked to the provision of advice, information and advocacy on occupational lifestyles and health, including liaison between workplaces and GP surgeries, etc., with regard to financial and benefits advice. Primary care teams can work with other local agencies to initiate coronary prevention programmes in workplaces, to include both individual attention (clinical checks and advice, personal counselling) and, where appropriate, directives to redesign the physical and psychosocial aspects of the work environment and working regimes. In this way health can be established as

a key dimension in organizational learning, human resource management and corporate development – if necessary across consortia of firms or businesses. It may also be helpful to contribute to local campaigns to improve cycling facilities, and to use other opportunities to encourage more 'physical activity-friendly' policies and environments.

4. Many local community education and community development programmes encourage initiatives to 'look after yourself', such as 'shop smart for your heart', food co-operatives and other community nutrition schemes; and it may be helpful to support and work with such schemes. The same applies to other self-help groups that are linked to active lifestyle or community sport initiatives (e.g. local 'quit-smoking' action groups or local 'heartbeat' support groups), which can benefit from liaison and networking with health professionals (e.g. in a healthy living centre).

Action on teenage pregnancies and sexual health

There are increasing rates of unplanned teenage pregnancy in many countries, and the UK has the highest rate in Europe. The reported incidence of sexually transmitted diseases (STDs) among young people is also increasing. There is a strong link between teenage pregnancy and STD rates and social disadvantage, and young people growing up in the poorer parts of the UK are exposed to some startling risks to sexual health. Strategies in this area of health promotion need to be multi-level and multi-agency, as well as imaginative, flexible and responsive (Allen, 1991; Health Education Authority, 1993).

1. There is a strong case for supporting the development of young persons' drop-in facilities that can offer advice (and probably a freephone helpline) on contraception and sexual health. This should guarantee confidentiality – the single most important factor in services designed for young people, who often have little faith in confidentiality in their dealings with professionals and official agencies. Similar points of access to contraceptive advice and counselling services can be provided at key sites in priority neighbourhoods. It is helpful to extend sexual health promotion services 'vertically' beyond schools and youth agencies, to ensure that sex education and contraceptive advice reach the older male partners of sexually active teenage girls

2. Every school, college and youth centre should be encouraged to develop structured, well-informed and published sex education policies. Sex education programmes should start early, and build up a stage-wise and sustained progression of learning, to allow open discussion of sexual matters and to enhance self-awareness, personal social skills, and the widening of 'life options'. All of this can be linked to a planned health-promoting school/college policy. There need to be rolling programmes of training (on sex education policies and methodologies) for school and college teaching staff, as well as for governors and parents. These should provide participants with access to appropriate information and materials, and with opportunities for review and discussion, as well as to address the

possibility of 'lack of confidence' being a barrier to effective communication. Schools should be helped to maintain sex education resources that can be borrowed by parents for use in the home.

3. New local alliances and coalitions at neighbourhood level can be established in order to improve liaison and co-ordination with regard to sex education between clinics, youth clubs, schools and the staff who work in them (e.g. school nurses, health visitors). Front-line clinicians (e.g. GPs) can be trained to gain a better understanding of what leads to approachability and trust in one-to-one work with young people. In schools, colleges and youth clubs, projects can be set up that focus on messages about sexuality and pregnancy in the popular media (e.g. in television programmes, films, newspapers and magazines, pop/rock music and dance, etc.) and that use creative methods to examine, expose and, where appropriate, challenge the images of love, romance, desire and fantasy which are portrayed by these sources. The settings that are most popular with and accessible to teenagers themselves (e.g. discos, night clubs, 'raves', music stores, and other local events) should be targeted by specially created publicity and outreach projects that highlight positive health messages (e.g. 'I'm a condom carrier', 'safer sex', etc.).

4. There should be investment in 'peer-led' teaching and learning initiatives about teenage pregnancy and sexual health, and other efforts should be made to listen to the voices of young people themselves on matters of sexual health. Local community forums can be developed through schools, youth services, adult education, etc., as vehicles for the discussion of aims and values with regard to prevention of teenage pregnancy – to encourage debate and to share ideas, especially about the dilemmas posed by religious and cultural pluralism.

Action on health in relation to homelessness and housing poverty

The numbers of people sleeping rough ('roofless') in the UK has been growing alarmingly for over 20 years, as has been obvious in city-centre shop doorways, multistorey car parks, cardboard city, etc. However, the traditional stereotype of the destitute 'down-and-out' is misleading, and needs to be replaced by a broader and more fluid concept of homelessness. Young adults and families with children represent a growing proportion of this population, and in addition to street-level homeless people there are many others who drift through a succession of short-term accommodation (e.g. bed-and-breakfast hotels, overcrowded flats in houses in multiple occupation, or living 'care of' someone else). Sleeping rough is just one stage in a continuum of housing poverty. Homeless people are extremely vulnerable. Many have a past history of mental health difficulties, or are at risk of violence and harassment, and their nutritional status, sexual health and self-esteem are often poor. Effective action in addressing these issues requires energetic co-ordination between disciplines (Fisher and Collins, 1993).

1. Health agencies and health professionals need to ensure that local populations of the 'new homeless' have adequate access to primary care. Some services may need to be provided on a more flexible or outreach basis. Difficulties in getting registered and/or retrieving records need to be tackled. Partnership working can be encouraged between primary health care staff and other community teams (e.g. mental health, rehabilitation, child health and welfare).

2. Special programmes of health education can be established for homeless people that extend beyond 'information-giving' on narrowly defined illness topics, and provide access to learning opportunities that encourage the development of broader social and life skills, as well as restoring self-esteem.

3. It is helpful to set up a post of 'health advocate for the homeless', the aim of which is to provide specialist help and advice for the local homeless population, and also to go beyond crisis working and be pro-active in achieving more accessible and better co-ordinated services. Such a post-holder may find it essential to network with local multi-agency resource centres based in the voluntary sector to ensure that clients' inter-connected problems of health, housing and deprivation are dealt with in a seamless manner.

4. Health professionals and their employing agencies should work alongside local authority housing and other departments to champion and deliver healthier housing policies – especially to improve the stock of local housing and the ways in which it is allocated. It may be important to take the lead in linking health and homelessness activities to wider 'anti-poverty' strategies and to joint planning for environmental renewal and social regeneration.

Key text: the Lalonde Report

The publication entitled *A New Perspective on the Health of Canadians*, usually known as the Lalonde Report, appeared in 1974, just on the threshold of the last quarter of the twentieth century. It was an official report of the Federal Department of National Health and Welfare in Ottawa, Canada (it is named after Marc Lalonde, the then Minister of National Health and Welfare). The report is the first example of a national government committing itself to a major investment in developing a policy that gave a central place to disease prevention and health promotion. It led to the setting up of the world's first 'Health Promotion Directorate' (in the Canadian Department of National Health and Welfare in 1978), and much of the work that subsequently emerged from that agency has been a shaping influence in the development of the World Health Organization's *Health for All 2000* and *Healthy Cities* policies and guidelines, and in the testing and formalization of key concepts such as 'healthy public policy' and 'supportive environments for health'. The sustained body of practice that has been built up in Canada since the Lalonde Report has in itself proved highly impressive.

However, the seminal influence of this Report probably derived mainly from the new theoretical model that it introduced, which continues to have many resonances for all those who occupy themselves with policy and practice in public health and health promotion. This new model was 'the health field concept', which argues that access to medical care systems is not the only (or even the most important) determinant of health, and that there are three other determinants, namely human biology, lifestyles and environment.

A diagrammatic formulation of this concept is shown in Figure 9.2.

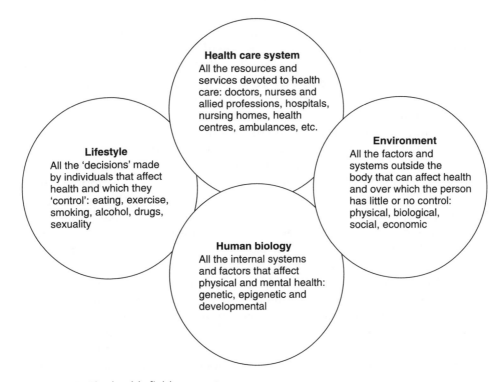

Figure 9.2 The health field concept.

The Lalonde Report uses the health field concept to draw attention to the urgent need in contemporary developed societies to expand our official and professional discourse on health decisively beyond the narrow scope of medical services or the health care system. It argues that 'future improvements in levels of health [will] lie mainly in improving the environment, moderating self-imposed risks, and adding to our knowledge of human biology – rather than in the availability of physicians and hospitals'. An understanding of the pathways through which health and illness are produced in the interplay between biology and environment had been available for some time, and more recently a similar understanding had become available with regard to the interplay between lifestyle 'risks' and medical interventions. However, the health field concept pulls these insights together, juxtaposes them in a vivid phrase and a memorable picture, and provides a salutary stimulus to new thought – beyond the study, out in the worlds of policy and practice. In some respects it can be seen as an early example of the 'whole-systems' thinking in health that has come to prominence very recently. It high-lights the significance of individual lifestyles both as a major source of risks and as a focus for practical action in working towards improved health, yet at the same time it firmly introduces a socio-ecological view of health to set alongside the individual model. In fact, it prefigures one of the main themes in recent policies for health promotion, in proposing that the 'health field concept' offers a tool for inquiry and action in several 'domains' or 'sectors' simultaneously, and indeed that it is only by getting started in several parts of the field at one and the same time (at both the individual level and the systems level) that really effective progress will be made in improving health. It may be said to offer a key new metaphor that helps us to see health more clearly as a landscape stretching away in several directions, rather than as a finished object or a finite commodity – as a complex open system rather than a closed container.

Most commentators acknowledge that, in the event, for the first decade or so after the Lalonde Report was published, national governments in Canada and then in the USA and the UK all drew from it selectively and chose to give priority to action on lifestyles as the new direction for developing health promotion. This is in part an example of the way in which the values that lie behind different approaches to health promotion appeal to particular stake-holders. It is often far more attractive to governments to try to bring about change at the individual level – in people's lifestyles – than to embark on change at the level of wider social systems and environments. It may also be partly a limitation in the health field concept, inasmuch as it separates the lifestyles domain from the environment domain, and implies that individuals have freedom of choice, rather than regarding lifestyles as being closely inter-twined with the physical, socio-economic and socio-cultural environments in which people live and work. It is only since the late 1980s that this dimension of interplay has come to be better understood and taken more fully into account in planning health promotion programmes.

However, the Lalonde Report showed how a fundamental recognition of the 'systems and structures' that determine health (and of which medical care is only one part) can lead to new insights and new approaches to planning. The WHO's key principles enshrined in the 1986 Ottawa Charter and seen in action in the primary health care approach in less developed countries, in *Healthy Cities* projects, and in *Health for All 2000* and *Health 21*, all exemplify the idea that health is best promoted by intervening at several levels (in several parts of the 'field') at the same time. Public health policies in the UK – first *The Health of the Nation*, and then especially *Our Healthier Nation*, and successive reports on inequalities in health – likewise illustrate the multi-level approach to health promotion.

Many theoretical frameworks for reviewing and planning health promo-tion (an example of which is given in Figure 9.1 and Table 9.1) also inherit and take forward the legacy of the Lalonde Report and the health field concept. It is this way of working with a 'whole-systems', open-ended model of health and its determinants, and with a flexible and creative (multi-faceted, multi-level and 'joined-up') approach to intervention, that holds the most promise for improving individual and community health in the future.

Discussion points

1. With the recent rise of concern in health promotion to pay attention to 'lay perspectives', to listen to 'local voices' and to encourage the involvement of local communities in their own health, is the power of decision over disease prevention and health matters shifting from doctors (or other health professionals) to clients? How similar or different is this to other recent trends in the health world, such as patients who 'shop smart' for their health (e.g. in terms of complementary therapies, on the Internet, etc.) or patients who insist on full explanations and evidence for medical advice before they comply with it? What new challenges does this pose for the professional practitioner? On balance, are you in favour of such developments?

2. Contemporary theories and policies for the delivery of preventive medicine and health promotion emphasize the importance of teamwork and interagency collaboration. What are the benefits of working with others in this context? How well are doctors prepared for working to promote health alongside colleagues from other professions and other agencies? What implications do such ways of working have for the boundaries between medicine and other health professions? What are the difficulties or dangers of these lines of development in health promotion? On balance, how enthusiastic are you about moves in this direction?

3. Increasingly, the basis for planning and implementing health promotion programmes both for the general public and for the individual patient is the assessment of risks to health. What dilemmas arise in defining the term 'risk' in different areas and aspects of health today? How well do you think most health professionals and/or health agencies perform the job of communicating about risk with the public? What could usefully be done to ensure a balance between protection of the public interest (or the public purse) and infringements of individual freedom?

Further reading

Ashton J (ed.) (1992) *Healthy cities*. Milton Keynes: Open University Press.

Davies JK and Macdonald G (eds) (1998) *Quality, evidence and effectiveness in health promotion*. London: Routledge.

Perkins E, Simnett I and Wright L (eds) (1999) *Evidence-based health promotion*. Chichester: John Wiley & Sons.

Scriven A and Orme J (eds) (1996) *Health promotion: professional perspectives*. London: Macmillan.

Sidell M, Jones L, Katz J and Peberdy A (eds) (1997) *Debates and dilemmas in promoting health*. London: Macmillan.

Health and social care

Stephen Abbott and Elizabeth Perkins

Introduction

The present welfare state, and our expectations of it at the beginning of the twenty-first century, are very different from the model which grew out of the post-war settlement on welfare. The factors that have influenced these changes are crucial to understanding the current delivery of heath and social care services.

Few policy decisions involving health and social care policy have occurred for abstract philosophical reasons. Major changes in the structure and delivery of health and social care services have at different times served a number of different purposes, not always related to the promotion of health or the needs of service users. Changes in the provision of health and welfare occur when the external or internal conditions, either alone or together, dictate it. In this chapter we shall examine some of the factors which have driven change in health and social care policy. We shall also identify the major differences between health and social services and provide some practical examples of the ways in which these differences have been accommodated.

In the first half of this chapter we shall examine some of the key stages in the development of the NHS. These include the following:

1. public health measures up to 1948 and the emergence of the National Health Service;

2. the beginnings of the National Health Service until 1979;
3. the reforms to the National Health Service since 1979.

This is not intended to be an exhaustive account of the development of the National Health Service. Rather it is intended to identify the way in which health and social care policies have diverged over time, and may now be coming together again.

Public health measures before the National Health Service

Although the Elizabethan Poor Laws of the sixteenth and seventeenth centuries are often regarded as the first significant attempt at welfare provision, it was not until the growth of urban centres in the nineteenth century that there was a truly concerted attempt to improve the health and welfare of the poor. The spread of diseases such as cholera was at this time largely attributed to the expansion of towns and cities and the overcrowded and insanitary conditions that resulted. It was in these circumstances that the sanitary movement led by Edwin Chadwick (the secretary of the Poor Law Commission) was begun. Engels, writing in 1844, noted that:

> The streets are generally unpaved, rough, dirty, filled with vegetable and animal refuse without sewers or gutters, but supplied with foul stagnant pools instead. . . . Heaps of garbage and ashes lie in all directions, and the foul liquids emptied before the doors gather in stinking pools. Here live the poorest of the poor, the worst paid workers with thieves and the victims of prostitution indiscriminately huddled together, the majority Irish, or of Irish extraction, and those who have not yet sunk in the whirlpool of moral ruin which surrounds them, sinking daily deeper, losing daily more and more of their power to resist the demoralising influence of want, filth, and evil surroundings.
>
> (Engels, 1844)

In touching the lives of people who were previously able to afford to keep disease at bay, the cholera epidemics of the nineteenth century created the necessary impetus for a series of public health measures. A number of towns instituted private bills to establish their own sanitary authorities and, in 1847, Liverpool led the country in appointing the first Medical Officer, Dr William Duncan. The first Public Health Act was passed in 1848, resulting in the creation of Local Boards of Health to oversee public health measures such as the purification of water and the cleaning and maintenance of pavements. Sanitary authorities were created in 1872, with the appointment of Medical Officers of Health becoming obligatory.

Running alongside these public health developments was the development of public institutional care for the sick. Voluntary hospitals and workhouse infirmaries were the basis for public hospital care. As the voluntary hospitals, at first provided by religious orders and subsequently funded by charitable donations, became more specialized, the workhouses developed their own infirmaries to care for the 'poor sick'. After the passing of the 1867 Metropolitan Poor Law Act, Poor Law hospitals were developed outside the workhouse, and specialist institutional provision for infectious diseases and asylums for the mentally ill alongside dispensaries for those not in need of inpatient care were instituted. At this time the provision of social care was tied up with the provision for destitution, treatment or control.

Throughout the late nineteenth century the importance of the general health of the population was repeatedly reinforced. The Boer War (1892–1902) highlighted the poor health and physique of enlisting men, and shocked the ruling classes into a recognition of the need for social and political reforms to improve the health of the whole nation. In a letter to the *Morning Post* in 1900, H.M. Hyndeman, a Marxist stockbroker, wrote: 'Lack of good food, good clothes and good air in children is the main reason why some 50 per cent of our working population is unfit to bear arms. Even from the new "Imperialist" point of view this is a serious matter'(quoted in Tsuzuki, 1961: 148).

The election of the Liberals in 1906 heralded the beginning of a new welfare era. A raft of legislation was introduced producing, among other things, entitlements to school meals and a school medical service. In 1911, the National Insurance Act was passed. Part 1 of the Insurance Act provided a system of unemployment compensation for certain industries, while Part 2 of the Act set up national health insurance to provide medical care, maternity benefits and sick pay. Each individual's insurance consisted of compulsory contributions from the employer, the employee and the state. However, access to this insurance scheme was limited to the employee, family members were not covered and entitlement was restricted to general practitioner services (Marshall, 1975).

Despite initial resistance to the insurance scheme among workers who found themselves unable to opt out of the insurance deductions, by 1913, a year after the Act came into effect, there was widespread recognition that the provisions of the Act were not wide enough.

Six years later the provision of a much more comprehensive scheme of hospital and primary health care was recommended by the Dawson Committee. This included the following:

- domiciliary services from doctors, pharmacists and local health authority staff;
- primary health centres with beds for general practitioners, diagnostic facilities, outpatient clinics, dental, ancillary and community services;
- secondary health centres for specialist diagnosis and treatment;
- supplementary services for infectious and mental illnesses;
- teaching hospitals with medical schools;
- promotion of research;
- standardized clinical records;
- establishment of a single authority to administer all medical and allied services with medical representation and local medical committees.

Although the Dawson Committee's recommendations did not find expression until 1948, there were a number of significant developments before then.

The Ministry of Health was formed in 1919 with responsibility for roads, national insurance, planning, environmental health and local government as well as health services. Ten years later, the 1929 Local Government Act marked the end of the Poor Law and resulted in the transfer of workhouses and infirmaries to local authorities, bringing them under the control of the Medical Officers of Health.

In June 1941 the first major enquiry into the provision of welfare and the abolition of want was commissioned and undertaken by Sir William Beveridge. The Beveridge Report provided the basis for the post-war welfare settlement. Published in December 1942, the report was heralded by the newspapers and the war propaganda machine as the charter by which to abolish poverty. To the public mind, it offered the promise of substantial improvements in benefits and services, 'a clean sweep which challenged the previous niggardly provisions of the twenties and thirties when the country had been under Tory rule' (Foot, 1963).

Taking existing services as his starting point, Beveridge aimed at a redistribution of income and the establishment of a national minimum standard of living: 'bread for everyone before cake for anyone' (William Beveridge, speech on *The Pillars of Security*, 10 March 1943). The Beveridge Report recommended that the state should protect the individual not by a system of doles, but by ensuring that everyone could support themselves in times of illness and old age (Bruce, 1968: 306) through social insurance. Central to this was the idea that health, as well as health care, should be available to all regardless of ability to pay – in other words, a National Health Service.

The wartime coalition government was divided over the question of how, and in what form, the Beveridge Report should be implemented. Consequently, it was not until July 1948 that the report was implemented and the first National Health Service was created.

> You provide when you are well, for a service that will be available if, and when, you fall ill. It is therefore an act of collective goodwill and public enterprise and not a commodity bought or sold . . . the claims of the individual shall subordinate themselves to social codes that have the collective well-being for their aim, irrespective of the extent to which this frustrates individual greed.
> (Nye Bevan, 1952, quoted by Barbara Castle in the *Nye Bevan Memorial Lecture*, December 1975)

For much of the nineteenth century it had been held that the 'good society' was best achieved by the state interfering as little as possible in economic and social affairs. It was believed that there was a meeting point between individual self-interest and the greater public good – a natural harmony and balance created, in the words of Adam Smith, by an 'invisible hand' (Smith, 1776: 325). From the latter part of the nineteenth century onwards, as the effects of epidemics and wars took their toll, it had become clear that individualistic, non-interventionist policies only helped certain individuals. The need for coherent national strategies was recognized and a trend in popular social planning towards national state intervention in poor relief, public health and education was established.

Summary

- The first major inquiry into the provision of welfare and the abolition of want was commissioned and undertaken by Sir William Beveridge in June 1941. The Beveridge Report provided the basis for the post-war welfare settlement.
- Beveridge aimed at a redistribution of income and the establishment of a national minimum standard of living.
- The Beveridge report was eventually implemented in July 1948 and the first National Health Service was created.

The National Health Service: 1948–1979

The National Health Service (NHS) was the first major attempt to widen access to medical care by removing all financial and organizational barriers. The structure designed to deliver this service built upon what had gone before (see Figure 10.1).

Key elements of the NHS

While general practitioners retained their independent contractor status they were under contract to a central medical board and paid on a per capita basis.

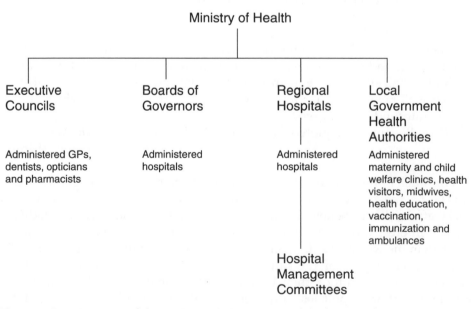

Figure 10.1 Structure of the NHS: 1948–74. Source: Klein (1989: 94).

NHS hospital consultants were allowed to continue private practice in NHS hospitals and a system of distinction awards was introduced. Local authorities lost their control of hospitals, resulting in both voluntary and local authorities being administered by Regional Hospital Boards. The medical profession argued that the local government areas were not suitable for the administration of the hospital service. However, under the National Assistance Act and other legislation, local authorities remained responsible for old people's homes and social work provision.

By the end of the 1950s and early 1960s a consensus on the importance of welfare provision had been reached by both Labour and Conservative ministers. This resulted in the 1962 Hospital Plan, which promised a significant investment in hospital beds over a 10-year period, funded from public monies (Digby, 1989). However, by the mid-1960s it had become apparent that despite the expanding economy, expenditure on health was growing faster than the national income. The Beveridge Report had been based on the assumption that there was a fixed quantity of illness in the community, which the NHS would gradually reduce over time. The report had not taken into account the speed of scientific and technological development. As one Conservative MP of the time stated:

> To apply the Beveridge principle in 1960 is to swallow the drug after the disease has gone. For primary poverty has now almost disappeared. Full employment has lifted the mass of our working population to a level of affluence unprecedented in our social history.
>
> (cited in Marshall 1975: 102)

Expenditure on health had started to increase for several reasons. Progress in medical technology meant that there was an increasing range of conditions for which a form of medical intervention existed. The more services that there were available, the greater was the demand. As Enoch Powell wrote, 'the appetite for medical services *vient en mangeant*' (Powell, 1966). The age structure of the population was also changing. The decline in perinatal mortality meant that many more people reached old age. Once in old age, people also lived longer. Finally, within the Health Service, workers who had for years been among the most poorly paid began to assert their power in a struggle for better pay and conditions. Wage rises boosted the NHS expenditure, making it even less popular with the government of the day.

The Seebohm Committee was set up in 1965 to review the organization of personal social services and consider the changes which might be needed to deliver an effective family welfare service. The recommendations of this committee resulted in the Social Services Act (1970). As a consequence, new social services departments were created. These departments assumed responsibility for those aspects of the old local authority health services such as social work, home help and residential care. The responsibility for services involving medical skills, such as vaccination and immunization, and health education was retained by the health departments of local health authorities and remained under the control of the Medical Officer of Health (Ham, 1992: 21).

In 1974 there was a major reorganization of the Health Service. Increasingly concerns were being expressed about a fragmented service that lacked co-ordination and good management. It was argued that 'there has been no identified authority whose task it has been...to balance needs and priorities rationally and to plan and provide the right combination of services for the benefit of the public' (Secretary of State for Social Services, 1972).

Regional and area health authorities were introduced, and Family Practitioner Committees were developed to administer the contracts of GPs, dentists, pharmacists and opticians. A total of 90 area health authorities were established in England, in the majority of cases with coterminous geographical boundaries with those of the metropolitan and non-metropolitan counties established under the Local Government Act (1972). Just 2 years after the introduction of the reforms, widespread dissatisfaction provided the political impetus for the launch of a Royal Commission on the NHS under the Chairmanship of Sir Alec Merrison. His brief was to consider 'in the interests both of the patients and of those who work in the NHS, the best use and management of the financial and manpower resources of the NHS' (Royal Commission on the NHS, 1979).

The 1970s were characterized by the rationing of health care services. Attention was diverted away from the previous aim of establishing a desirable level of service provision for all, as new budgetary restraints were imposed by the government.

The Labour Government lost the 1979 general election to a Conservative party which had become firmly committed to the ideology of the private market. Whereas the Labour Government had viewed retrenchment as an unpalatable necessity, the incoming Conservative Government adopted it as a cornerstone of economic policy. Community care was thrust to the fore in an attempt to resolve the political, economic and demographic imperatives.

Summary

- The NHS was the first major attempt to remove all financial and organizational barriers to medical care.
- By the mid-1960s expenditure on health was growing faster than the national income.
- As a consequence of these concerns there were a number of attempts to restructure the organization of the NHS.

The National Health Service: reforms since 1979

The election of Margaret Thatcher and a Conservative Government in 1979 heralded the introduction of market principles into the health and social care arena. Choice, flexibility, competition, charging and contracts became key concepts in the management and running of the National Health Service.

As a result of the Royal Commission's Report on the NHS, the management of the NHS became the focus of government attention. By 1982 a second reorganization of the NHS had begun. District health authorities were introduced (a total of 192 such authorities were created in England), special health authorities were created to deal with the postgraduate teaching hospitals in London, and plans were put in place for Family Practitioner Committees to become employing authorities in their own right.

Further important and substantial changes to the provision of health and welfare services followed, which many commentators believed struck at the heart of the NHS. In 1982, Roy Griffiths, the Deputy Chairman and Managing Director of Sainsbury's, was brought in to give advice on the effective use of management and manpower in the NHS. The major recommendation was the appointment of General Managers at all levels to provide leadership, introduce a continual search for cost improvement and change, motivate staff and develop a dynamic management approach.

Managers who were employed on short-term, renewable contracts quickly became the cutting edge of newly imposed budgets. The threat to managers of not having their contract of employment renewed was sufficient to ensure limited opposition to changes in the funding and delivery of services. Not surprisingly, the major concern of managers at this time was to keep within budget and to balance the books (Harrison *et al.*, 1989). By the end of 1985, General Managers were appointed at all levels of the NHS.

Although tradition and constant public pressure initially forced the Conservatives to retain the overall structure of the health and welfare services, by the end of the 1980s radical changes had taken place. Ideological opposition to public social planning by the New Right placed the traditional practices of health and welfare in jeopardy. Health and social care came to be viewed as commodities that were no different to any other commodity competing in the market-place. Innovation and experimentation, believed to be optimal under conditions which favoured unbridled personal motivation, were said by the New Right to be stifled by the monopolistic hold that the National Health Service had over the provision and practice of health and social care. As well as providing little incentive for advancing medicine, the bureaucratic administration of the NHS was said to foster the conditions under which individuals could not readily be held to account, resources were wasted and personnel acted inefficiently and with relative impunity. In addition, because the state acts as an intermediary, employing a service on behalf of all prospective clients, the traditional relationship between producer and consumer no longer exists. The whole notion of a state-run service implied the imposition of a national standard of care which restricts individuals' ability to make choices about the type of services that they require, and also restricts any comprehensive development of alternatives outside that provided by the state.

The Liberal argument, that 'nobody spends other people's money as carefully as they spend their own', was at this time central to the criticisms of the NHS (Friedman and Friedman, 1980: 146–9). It was argued that services which are provided free at their point of consumption encourage the consumer to overconsume. If people were made to pay for their services more directly, then only affordable services would be consumed. For as long as the health and welfare services remained outside the market-place, they were viewed by the Right as having a destabilizing effect on the social and economic system, draining public expenditure, and creating dependence among those who draw on its benefits. The Welfare State 'rots the individual character with its false promises of security' (anonymous editorial published in *Freedom First Digest* in 1960).

The 1980s were dominated by the debate over the level at which to fund health and social care, how it should be financed and how resources could be used more efficiently through changes to the delivery of services. Cost improvement programmes became a feature of all health authority accounting. Competitive tendering and the rationalization of patient services, which included a reduction in the number of beds and patient facilities, contributed to the substantial savings that were made throughout the Health Service

In 1989, the government announced in the White Paper, *Working for Patients* (Department of Health, 1989a), the separation of responsibility for purchasing services from that of providing services. To this end, health authorities became purchasers, buying services on behalf of their local communities from a range of public, private and voluntary providers. Providers were hospitals and services that opted out of health authority control, as in self-governing NHS trusts. Major changes were made to the way in which resources were allocated, For example, general practitioners were given the opportunity to become fundholders in their own right.

Evidence suggests that the purchaser–provider split created the conditions in which established practices were challenged. NHS trusts were given the freedom to manage their own affairs, health authorities were enabled to use their resources in the way that they thought best suited the needs of their population, and expenditure was made more transparent (Ham, 1996: 26). The evidence on fundholding remains inconclusive and contradictory.

By introducing an internal market in which providers competed to sell their services to health authorities, it was hoped that services would become more responsive to patients and at the same time stimulate a greater efficiency in the use of resources. Under these arrangements the money would follow the patient.

In 1989, the White Paper *Caring for People* was also published. It was based on the Griffiths Community Care Report prepared in 1988 and introduced the key concepts of choice and independence into health and social care provision. In the White Paper, 'choice' is defined as 'giving people a greater individual say in how they live their lives and the services they need to help them' (Department of Health, 1989b: 4). This was to be achieved by giving local authorities the lead responsibility in the planning of community care – they were to become 'enablers' and 'purchasers'. Local authorities were required to prepare community care plans in conjunction with NHS authorities and other agencies and, in addition, to develop the role of case managers working at the local level in the assessment and provision of services. Case managers became responsible for consulting their clients and arranging and buying in care for them from public, private and voluntary suppliers. At the same time, the

Social Security incentives for admission to private and voluntary residential care were removed.

The mixed economy of care portrayed in the White Paper was presented as the solution to the rising social security costs of subsidies to the independent residential care sector. It was also expected to address the level of central government expenditure on health, and the control of quality and exercise of choice.

In 1990, the government White Papers, *Working for Patients* and *Caring for People*, were incorporated into the NHS and Community Care Bill. Although the rhetoric of this Act was appealing and its aims were consistent with what might be considered professional good practice, its implementation proved to be complex, costly and contradictory.

Tensions were quickly exposed between the outlined objectives of self-determination, independence and the need to ration services. The choice of services offered to individuals conflicted with the language of assessment by case managers (Walker, 1995). While choice implies the freedom to select from a range of alternatives, the language of assessment implies a restricted access to services according to implicit or explicit criteria. Eligibility criteria, based on the local availability and pattern of services, became an important factor in the assessment of need and therefore the choice of services available (Means, 1992).

There were also questions about whether the involvement of the independent sector would lead to a greater choice of services, and if it did, whether the diversity of providers would be able to provide quality services or value for money. Nor was it clear what effect competition would have on domiciliary care providers. It is assumed in the NHS and Community Care Act (1990) that the introduction of market elements into the provision of social care would improve efficiency and consumer responsiveness (Hoyes and Means, 1993). What was unclear was whether efficiency and effectiveness would result from competition for finite resources (Leat, 1993).

In order to coax local authorities into the development of a social care market, they were obliged to spend at least 85% of Department of Social Security transfer money in the independent sector. At the time there were widespread concerns that neither the private sector nor the voluntary sector were well enough developed to meet the needs of the local authorities (Waterhouse, 1993: 9), and as Leat (1993) pointed out, planning was made difficult because of the lack of reliable or up-to-date evidence concerning the scale of independent sector domiciliary care. Throughout the mid-1990s, Social Service Departments grappled with the purchaser–provider split, contracting for services, care management, the construction of community care plans, and the development of procedures for quality assurance, complaints and inspection (Wistow *et al.*, 1992; Beyer *et al.*, 1993; Crosby and Vickery, 1993).

Summary

- The 1980s were dominated by the debate about the level at which to fund health and social care, how it should be financed and how resources could be used more efficiently through changes to the delivery of services.

- In 1989, the government announced in the White Paper, *Working for Patients*, the separation of responsibility for purchasing services from that of providing services. Health authorities became purchasers, buying services on behalf of their local communities from a range of public, private and voluntary providers.
- It was hoped that the introduction of an internal market, in which providers competed to sell their services to health authorities, would result in more flexible and cost-effective services.
- In another document published in the same year, local authorities were given the lead responsibility for the planning of community care.

Community care reforms

Community care has been a prominent policy goal since the Second World War.

In order to understand the power of the concept of community care, it is important to understand the connotations attached to the term 'community'. It is the idea of community, enhanced by a reaction against the large institutions in which long-term care was provided, that has proved to be such a powerful influence in the development of community care as a policy.

Philosophically and ideologically, community care appeared to be everything that institutional care was not – that is, individual-oriented and humane. It was what sick and frail people wanted – a service provided to them in familiar surroundings by familiar faces. It even appeared to be cheaper, although in fact it was never costed. Several years later, community care is talked about with less enthusiasm, and those who operate it are stretched taut across the burgeoning demands that are made upon them.

Goffman (1961) and Robb (1967) were responsible for highlighting the dependency which was created through custodial care. In his study on the social situation of mental patients and other inmates, Goffman concluded that 'mental patients can find themselves crushed by the weight of a service ideal that eases life for the rest of us' (Goffman, 1961: 336). Although it was 'easier' for groups of people to be looked after in institutions, increasingly it became regarded as an expensive way of looking after frail, sick and elderly people. The Guillebaud Committee on the costs of the NHS in 1956 suggested that:

> Policy should aim at making adequate provision wherever possible for the care and treatment of old people in their own homes. The development of domiciliary services for this purpose will be a genuine economy measure and also a humanitarian measure enabling old people to lead the sort of life that they much prefer.
>
> (Ministry of Health, 1956)

Not surprisingly perhaps, the precise definition of community care has remained elusive. In a Department of Health and Social Security report of a study on community care in 1981, it was stated that confusion over the term 'community care' arises from 'switches between its use as a description of what services/resources are involved and statements of objectives' (Department of Health and Social Security, 1981c: 7). At different times, three distinctly different types of care in the community have assumed prominence. These are services provided in residential care, services provided through professionals working in the community, and services provided by the community on a voluntary basis (Allsop, 1984: 108).

In 1957, the Royal Commission on the law relating to mental illness and mental deficiency stated that 'community care covers all forms of care (including residential care) which it is appropriate for local health and welfare authorities to provide'. By 1976, the *Priorities for Health and Personal Social Services in England* document stated that 'community care covers a whole range of provision, including community hospitals, hotels, day hospitals, residential homes, day centres and domiciliary support' (Department of Health and Social Security, 1976: 8). It embraces 'primary health care and all the above services whether provided by health authorities, local authorities, independent contractors, voluntary bodies, community self-help or family and friends' (Department of Health and Social Security, 1976: 8).

However, by 1979 it appeared that community care had assumed a much narrower remit. In the Public Expenditure White Paper it was stated that 'Community care is distinguished from expenditure on residential care, day care and other expenditure' (Select Committee on Social Services, 1981). It became clear, as the 1980s progressed, that 'Care in the community must increasingly mean care by the community' (Department of Health and Social Security, 1981a: 3), the general aim of community care policies being to 'maintain a person's link with family, friends and normal life, while offering support to meet particular individual needs' (Department of Health and Social Security, 1981b). Subsequent statements have emphasized the family, as opposed to statutory services, as crucial to care in the community: 'Most people who need long-term care can and should be looked after in the community; this is what most of them want for themselves and what those responsible for their care believe to be best' (Department of Health and Social Security, 1981a).

In line with the prevailing ideology of individualism, in which notions of personal responsibility and individual self-reliance were seen to be paramount, it should not be surprising to find that the family unit was viewed as central to the success of community care. As early as 1977, Patrick Jenkin claimed that 'The family must be the front line of defence when Gran needs help' (Jenkin, 1977, quoted in Cooke and Campbell, 1982).

The family, as the basic unit of self-support, is seen by the 'anti-collectivists' (the modern exponents of nineteenth-century liberalism) to be constantly endangered by the intrusive activities of the state: 'God designed the family to take care of people from the cradle to the grave. The state is no substitute' (quoted in Marshall, 1975: 36).

In the context of Conservative philosophy and our prevailing family structure, community care policies offered a very different alternative to that which was first posited as the alternative to long-term institutional care. Early descriptions of community care, despite theoretical inconsistencies, placed a primacy on the services of which it was comprised.

In the 1990s, the reality was that the commitment to community care had turned out to be little more than a way of reducing public expenditure, using the appealing rhetoric of community. As Means and other authors (Means, 1986: 102; Qureshi and Walker, 1986: 121) point out, the allocation of resources within the personal social services disproportionately favoured residential care throughout the 1960s, 1970s and 1980s compared with expenditure on community care services. In this situation, the public benefits of whole-scale family care are reaped by the state, as public expenditure is reduced and more money becomes available to be spent elsewhere.

> We know the immense sacrifices which people will make for the care of their own near and dear – for elderly relatives, disabled children and so on, and the immense part which voluntary effort even outside the confines of the family has played in these fields. Once you give people the idea that all this can be done by the state and that it is somehow second best, even degrading to leave it to private people (it is sometimes referred to as cold charity), then you will begin to deprive human beings of one of the essential ingredients of humanity – personal moral responsibility.
>
> (Margaret Thatcher, 1978)

By making a virtue of caring within the family, illness, disability and care, all become private matters requiring private solutions. However, family care carries with it major implications for women, who bear the brunt of caring. The personal service that women provide in their caring role is often regarded as just another part of their role in the family (Land and Rose, 1985). By failing to ensure a comprehensive system of community health care services, the Government endorses altruistic actions which isolate women and limit the freedom of carers to fulfil their own potential. Carers are further devalued by the lack of financial remuneration for the specific quasi-professional tasks which they perform and the lack of recognition they receive in the public sphere of work. As Land and Rose (1985) have highlighted, the work of women carers is not distributed through a market nor is it administered by the welfare state. Consequently, they do not receive any wage remuneration. They remain part of the domestic economy moulded by the relationships which govern everyday life in the family and the community.

Summary

- Philosophically and ideologically, community care appeared to be everything that institutional care was not – individual-oriented and humane. It even appeared to be cheaper, although in fact it was never costed.
- In the context of Conservative philosophy and the prevailing family structure, community care policies offered a very different alternative to that which was first posited as the alternative to long-term institutional care. It relied heavily on family care and, in particular, care provided by women.

- Many commentators suggest that community care has been little more than a way of reducing public expenditure using the appealing rhetoric of community.

A primary care led NHS

The term 'community care' has figured less prominently at the close of the twentieth century. An ambitious and far-reaching programme of change has identified primary care as the way forward. The 'third way' of running the NHS outlined in the White Paper *Modernising the NHS* is based on six key principles. Among others, these include:

- the local implementation of national standards;
- the development of partnerships across agencies;
- a focus on efficiency and quality of care.

The model designed to deliver this service involves the devolution of commissioning previously carried out by health authorities to primary care groups (PCGs). Primary care groups consisting of all GPs in a defined area will replace commissioning and fundholding arrangements. Over time these will be superseded by primary care trusts. In conjunction with health authorities, local authorities and NHS trusts, PCGs will develop a Health Improvement Programme. These programmes will form the local strategy for improving health and health care, and will provide the framework within which PCGs will commission services. GPs will need to develop new skills to equip them for this new role, not least of which will be their contribution to the public health agenda (Busby *et al.*, 1999). In recognition of this, PCGs are expected to operate on one of four levels which reflect the amount of responsibility to be assumed for the commissioning of care. The legislative basis for the development of primary care trusts (PCTs) – the point at which PCGs become freestanding bodies responsible for community health services – has yet to be introduced.

In addition to the changes outlined above, there are a number of initiatives to develop the consistent delivery of high-quality health care. These include the following:

- National Service Frameworks – the best evidence of clinical and cost-effectiveness will be drawn together for each of the major care areas and disease groups;
- the National Institute for Clinical Excellence (NICE) – the institute will produce and disseminate clinical guidelines based on relevant evidence of clinical and cost-effectiveness, and will bring together the results of clinical audit and research and development being carried out;
- the Commission for Health Improvement (CHI) – the commission will develop systems for monitoring clinical quality;
- Clinical Governance – this is the process by which clinical standards are ensured.

Thus primary care is the central plank of ambitious and far-reaching reforms of the health service introduced by the Labour Government. These reforms, and their implications, are discussed in more detail in the next chapter.

Health and social care: differences

This section will discuss the many important differences in the ways in which health and social care organizations are organized. However, it is important to bear in mind that neither sector is monolithic – there are also many organizational, managerial, professional and cultural differences *within* each sector.

Box 10.1 Important differences between health and social care

Health care	Social care
Universal access, mostly free at point of delivery	Targeted at those in greatest need; many services charged for (means-tested)
NHS is held in high public esteem	Social Services is unpopular and stigmatizing
Private provision rare; small voluntary sector	Private provision significant; important voluntary sector
Care mostly commissioned for populations	Care mostly commissioned for individuals
Care-providers assess need	Care-commissioners assess need
Professional power is strong	Professional power is weak
Accountable to national government only	Accountable to local and national government
Most interventions offer treatment/cure	Most interventions offer care and some prevention of harm

---

Access

The NHS offers universal access to services which are free at point of delivery. Social Services departments, on the other hand, restrict access to the social care which they arrange to those in greatest need (using explicit criteria for eligibility or prioritization), and may and in some cases (e.g. residential care) must charge clients for some services.

Although the NHS is perceived as universal, there are in fact very few legally enshrined rights of access for individuals. These include the right of every person to be registered with a GP (although not necessarily the GP of their choice), and the requirement that local health services provide services such as genito-urinary clinics which the public can access directly. Many patient contacts with the NHS are with GPs or the primary health care teams attached to general practice, and are initiated by patients. However, most contacts with hospital and community health services (except Accident and Emergency services, where many patients either present themselves or themselves summon an ambulance) are mediated by GPs acting as 'gatekeepers', referring patients on to such services on the basis of their professional assessment of clinical need. Access may then be further mediated by the use of waiting-lists, a different diagnosis by a specialist, etc. Nevertheless, it is generally understood that in principle all those who need a service will receive it. However, in 1996 the introduction of eligibility criteria for continuing health care raised the question of whether 'eligibility' constitutes 'entitlement'. This question has still not been resolved, but is particularly topical because of the debates about rationing, and whether or how services should be targeted at those most in need or most able to benefit, rather than at everyone with any need or who might benefit.

Social care, by contrast, is often perceived as a stigmatizing service. The service is widely associated with undesirable behaviour (e.g. people with mental health problems who are a threat to themselves or others, children who are at risk of harm or neglect) or with need arising from illness, frailty or disability. Social Services are legally required to provide a number of services (e.g. child protection, approved social workers qualified to assist in the compulsory admission of clients to psychiatric hospital, and the assessment of the needs of those caring for relatives at home). However, some of these requirements do not include the provision of services which are valued by clients. The assessed needs of carers do not have to be met. Parents of 'at-risk' children, and those compulsorily admitted to psychiatric hospital, may find the 'services' unwelcome and intrusive. These latter services are provided, at least in part, as a system of social control designed to contain challenging, antisocial or cruel behaviour. (The NHS takes on a similar role in psychiatry, but this forms a much smaller part of the total range of the services which it offers.)

The commissioning and provision of services

During the early 1990s, both health and social care organizations were reorganized in order to create 'internal markets' whereby the functions of commissioning and of providing care were separated. This was done very differently in the two sectors. The basic 'internal-market' structures and processes in each sector remain intact after the passing of the Health Act (1999). First, whereas Social Services departments were intended simply to separate their purchasing and providing functions, the NHS market was more complex. It consisted of health authorities, which provided no services, and GP purchasers (originally fundholders, and now primary care groups), which provided primary care services while also purchasing selected areas of hospital and community health care. NHS purchasers generally had a restricted choice of care providers, because the numbers of locally accessible hospitals and community health services were small. Furthermore, health authorities were expected not to destabilize the local health care system by moving large contracts away from local hospitals. Social Services departments, on the other hand, were expected to contract with a multiplicity of local providers and to deliberately dis-invest from their own in-house provider services. The result was that the development of constructive purchaser–provider partnerships between Social Services departments and large numbers of providers was much more difficult. Furthermore, Social Services departments are expected to use private-sector providers (e.g. residential and home care providers, and private fostering agencies). In the NHS this would be unusual, generally occurring only in service areas of perceived marginality (e.g. physiotherapy, complementary medicine) or as 'quick fixes' (e.g. to reduce waiting-lists for elective surgery). However, it should be added that many doctors work in private practice as well as for the NHS. Social Services departments also use voluntary-sector providers (e.g. Age Concern for home care, the National Society for the Prevention of Cruelty to Children for child protection), whereas such providers are less commonly used by the NHS (cancer and terminal care nursing being examples here).

Most NHS care, and an increasing proportion of social care, is arranged by block contracts and service agreements. These are contracts which specify the quantity and nature of work to be supplied in a set period of time for all patients who require such a service, and which usually detail the scope for flexibility in the case of unexpected fluctuations in demand. In the NHS, it is provider staff who decide the components of care that are required in most cases. However, in social care the components of individual care packages are decided by the commissioners.

Management and accountability

Central government exercises direct control on the 'family' of NHS organizations (trusts and health authorities) via the NHS Executive and its regional offices; while GPs hold personal independent contracts with the Secretary of State, administered through local health authorities. Although health authorities and trusts have boards and chairs, these are limited in the extent to which they are able or willing to challenge central government policy decisions. Chief Executives of trusts and health authorities are expected by central government to be broadly 'on message', and their boards are unlikely to require them to flout central government policy. Moreover, there is a view that such boards lack transparent accountability, particularly since the representatives of local government were removed in the early 1990s.

Directors of Social Services departments, on the other hand, are accountable to the Social Services committees of local authorities. These are the equivalent of trust/health authority boards, but are composed of democratically elected local authority members. Such members may choose to take a position that is explicitly opposed to the policies of central government. For example, some local councillors decided to obstruct negotiations with their health authority about continuing health care because they wished to make a stand against what they saw as years of cost-shunting from the NHS to Social Services (e.g. the closure of long-stay beds, psychiatric hospital wards, etc.).

There are a variety of internal management structures within the health and social care sectors. The chief difference is that whereas doctors, nurses and professions allied to medicine are organized as autonomous professionals with their own powerful organizations for regulation and training, this is not the case with social workers. Most staff in both sectors are salaried and subject to hierarchical line management arrangements, with professional supervision for clinicians. However, doctors tend to work without clinical supervision once they are trained. Hospital doctors do not generally regard themselves as managed by the hierarchy of the trust which employs them, whereas GPs are in any case independent contractors operating small businesses. However, the traditional lack of accountability of GPs is being addressed by the latest NHS reforms, which dictate that they must work together in primary care groups, while not losing independent contractor status unless they wish to do so (Secretary of State for Health, 1997). Another recent policy development is that some GPs have opted for salaried status.

In Social Services departments there are few equivalents of independent contractors, the commonest example being social workers who work as freelances representing children in court proceedings (guardians *ad litem*).

There are particular issues of accountability in social care, where services may be provided by private, for-profit organizations. The evidence suggests that accountability in these may be weak. However, there is growing concern that there is insufficient accountability for the quality of care throughout both sectors, and current government initiatives seek to strengthen accountability arrangements by imposing a duty of clinical governance on NHS trusts and primary care groups (Secretary of State for Health, 1997) and improving inspection arrangements for Social Services departments (Secretary of State for Health, 1998).

Another difference between the two sectors with regard to accountability is the monitoring of outcomes of services. Virtually all social care services are concerned either to provide care and an acceptable quality of life (e.g. residential and home care for older people or for adults or children with disabilities), or to prevent harm (e.g. working with children at risk of harm or neglect, or with people with mental health problems, and if necessary removing them to a place of safety). Many NHS services offer a degree of cure, either by the relief of symptoms or the eradication of disease, although of course there are many NHS services that provide non-curative and preventive care. It is theoretically easier to monitor the success of cure (i.e. restoration of good health) than that of care (i.e. less deterioration, enhanced quality of life). In practice, both health and social care are monitored primarily by the scrutiny not of outcomes, but of outputs – counting the number of episodes of care offered to patients or clients. Such techniques have been much more controversial in health care than in social care. For example, a 30-minute visit to offer personal care by a home carer is less open to divergent interpretations and costings than a 'finished consultant episode', which may include days or even weeks in hospital with a range of diagnostic tests, surgical procedures, administration of drugs and nursing services. The appropriateness of such monitoring is a key issue, given the government's drive for cost-efficiency in the NHS. Similarly, local authorities are required to observe the principles of 'best value' when commissioning and providing all services, including social care.

A further dimension of accountability is that of accountability to the public. Formally, this accountability is to local government for social care and to national government for health care. However, in a wider sense (i.e. the degree to which the public is interested in and concerned about services provided) the two sectors are very different. In the case of Social Services departments, such accountability is weak because the general public takes little interest in their activities except when there is breakdown of mechanisms to care for children at risk of abuse or people with severe mental health problems. In the case of health, there is widespread public interest in and attachment to the NHS. However, it could be argued that the veneration displayed towards doctors and nurses creates a 'halo effect' which is antithetical to a real accountability culture. In any case, recent much-publicized scandals in hospital and primary care are likely to have eroded medical prestige. Community Health Councils do exist in every locality both to deal with complaints from the public and to advise health organizations from a service user's point of view. However, they are not generally regarded as major forces in local health systems. Agencies' own complaints procedures are regarded as inefficient and frustrating for service users. Some user and carer groups can be influential lobbyists, particularly in the case of physical disability, but these represent particular interest groups rather than the public as a whole.

Funding

The budget for the NHS is set nationally by the cabinet, and distributed locally by the NHS Executive. Different mechanisms are used for hospital and community health services on the one hand and primary care services on the other. In the latter case, a standard national contract with GPs sets a multiplicity of criteria for spending portions of the budget for specified activities ('items of service'). By contrast, detailed allocation of funds to specific services is the responsibility of local purchasers and providers in the case of hospital and community health services, as indeed it is in Social Services.

Central government grant-aids local government to a very significant degree, and therefore has a great deal of control over the total income that the local authorities receive. Moreover, central government may veto plans to raise money locally (via council tax) which it regards as excessive. However, decisions about how much of the overall local authority budget is allocated to Social Services departments are taken locally.

Both sectors also benefit from special grants, usually for particular projects, allocated after agencies have bid successfully for money by detailing plans on how it would be spent.

An issue of particular concern to the public is the fact that not all social care services are free at the point of delivery. Residential care, home care, respite care, day care and meal-delivery services are generally charged for, usually after means-testing (although some departments make standard charges for services such as attendance at day centres). Expressions of public concern generally focus on the fact that older people are expected to use their savings to fund long-term residential care, and to sell their houses if necessary (Diba, 1996). This may dash the hopes of themselves and their families that their property would pass on to the next generation.

Although the NHS is regarded as being free at the point of delivery, there are in fact widespread charges, such as prescription charges (although older people, the heaviest users, are exempt from these), charges for dental and eye care, and so on. There are debates about whether some aspects of personal care that are arranged by Social Services departments are in fact health care (e.g. bathing, foot care). Some regard charges for such services as in fact being charges for health care. The frequency of such debates has increased as Social Services departments have withdrawn traditional 'home-help' services (house-work and shopping) in order to provide personal care for people at home.

Professional differences

There are significant differences in the ways in which the variety of profes-sionals understand and maintain their position within the network of care personnel. Doctors work autonomously and have high status, higher incomes than other care professionals and considerable authority. They generally take on the leadership of the care teams with which they work. Nurses, on the other hand, are trained to work efficiently to clear professional hospital guide-lines within a hierarchical framework (Pietroni and Pietroni, 1996). Social workers work more autonomously than nurses but, like them, generally within clear supervisory and management structures.

In health, individual professionals routinely manage their own workload and set their own priorities within those workloads. Social workers' work-loads are usually allocated on a team basis, according to explicit criteria, and social workers generally check frequently with managers about the many legal and financial issues relating to the services that they provide (Mental Health Act, 1983 and Community Care Act, 1991).

Whereas doctors, professions allied to medicine and nurses generally focus on specific medical/clinical problems, social workers, and arguably some community nurses (particularly health visitors), also look for underlying social and emotional problems. They may therefore take time to 'wait and see' (e.g. in supporting parents at risk of neglecting their child, or supporting a frail elderly person living at home but needing ever increasing support). Health professionals, on the other hand, who tend to carry caseloads with greater numbers of patients than social workers typically do, are used to much more rapid decision-making. Such differences in the pace of working may cause friction between professionals.

In both sectors, a significant proportion of care is offered by non-profes-sional staff who lack professional training or membership of professional bodies. Their work is often in reality unsupervised, although in accordance with care plans made by professional staff. They therefore lack status and negotiating power, and are generally low paid.

Summary

- Most NHS care is free at the point of delivery and some (e.g. GPs, Accident and Emergency services) can be accessed directly by the public. Clients may be charged for most social care, and access is restricted to those in greatest need as assessed by professionals. Some free social services are in fact aspects of social control (e.g. child protection, admission to mental hospital).

* Local health systems consist almost entirely of public sector organizations, and most health care is commissioned on behalf of local populations. Social care is generally commissioned on behalf of individuals, and involves a multiplicity of private and voluntary sector service providers as well as those provided by Social Services departments themselves.
* Health services are accountable to central government, whereas Social Services are accountable to local government as well.
* Social Services mostly offer care or seek to prevent harm. Although health services also do this, they predominantly provide treatment and, where possible, cure.
* Social care for those who need help with daily living is not free except to the poorest clients. However, only a minority of health services are charged for.
* The boundary between health and social care is unclear and contested.
* Professional prestige and power are much greater in health care than in social care, particularly in the case of doctors.

Health and social care: joint working

Throughout the 1990s, and indeed before then, successive governments have urged closer and more effective working between health and social care agencies. In part, such exhortations arise from an acknowledgement of the difficulties and differences outlined above. In part, they arise from the recommendations of successive inquiries into incidents when joint working broke down (usually cases of serious child abuse or violence by people with mental health problems). In part, they reflect the fact that health and social care organizations often find themselves serving populations which are not coterminous. Such boundaries change over time due to successive reorganizations in local government and the NHS. In the late 1990s, the establishing of unitary authorities in local government and primary care groups in the NHS suggested that the direction of change was towards smaller groupings in both cases. However, it is expected that some health authorities, NHS trusts and primary care groups will merge during the next few years.

Government advice on better joint working has ranged from simple exhortation to the creation of specific mechanisms designed to encourage (or require) agencies to work in this way. Examples of mechanisms which included financial incentives to better joint working include monies such as the Mental Illness Specific Grant and Mental Health Partnership Fund, designed to encourage the provision of 'seamless services' for people with mental health problems who years ago would have been cared for in hospital, and equivalent monies for people with learning disabilities. Challenge Fund and Winter Pressures monies also encouraged joint commissioning of community services, particularly for older people, to relieve pressure on hospitals.

More recently, The Health Act (1999) has established a new statutory duty of partnership between agencies. The boards of primary care groups must include a representative from the local Social Services department. Joint Investment Programmes are required in each district to improve community services for older people, and will in time also be required for services for younger people. There are new arrangements for joint working, such as pooled budgets, lead commissioning (where one commissioning agency transfers funds to the other, which then commissions both health and social care) and integrated provision (where one organization provides both health and social care). Guidance on national health and social care priorities is now issued jointly to all relevant agencies.

Within this framework of government policy, a wide range of joint commissioning and provision activity can be identified. This range can be schematized as shown in Box 10.2, and examples are discussed below.

Box 10.2   Types of joint health and social care activity

- Local joint strategic planning
- Local joint commissioning/provision of services
- Local joint commissioning/provision of individual care packages
- Mechanisms for improving communication and co-operation between agencies

---

Local joint strategic planning

This may be done on a district-wide basis in order to look at broad strategic issues/tasks (e.g. the setting of joint priorities) or the joint monitoring of processes and outcomes (e.g. the care offered to those discharged from hospital, or the co-ordination of future investment in existing services or in service innovations or developments). Alternatively, agencies may come together to look at how best to meet specific types of need (e.g. mental health, people with physical or learning disabilities) or the needs of particular localities (e.g. reorganizing services so that health and social care teams serve the same geographical areas).

Local joint commissioning/provision of services

Joint commissioning of services may, for example, provide 'seamless care' by ensuring that those with both health and social care needs receive the care they need in a 'joined up' way which both avoids gaps and duplications in services and maximizes continuity of care (Vaughan and Lathlean, 1999). Particular services or projects which can be provided or commissioned jointly include the following:

- transport to enable older and disabled people to access the full range of services and facilities that they need;
- joint stores of mobility aids, and joint teams and facilities to provide adaptations to the home;
- respite care for those whose informal carers (family members and friends) need a break;
- day care for those who need social stimulation, monitoring of health conditions and/or rehabilitation;
- hospital at home and other intermediate care schemes (Vaughan and Lathlean, 1999); rapid response teams, and improved discharge co-ordination.

Local joint commissioning/provision of individual care packages

Two different approaches typify how such joint working has been attempted. Unified assessment seeks to integrate assessment, often by building up a single assessment tool from a number of modules, implemented by different disciplines (e.g. on social needs, nursing needs, carers' needs, mental health needs, etc.). Unified care may be offered by means of a generic care assistant, offering help with feeding, dressing, hygiene, continence, simple dressings, foot care and dental hygiene, or alternatively by means of a multi-disciplinary care team working together to provide services which are integrated and well co-ordinated.

Mechanisms for improving communication and co-operation between agencies

Although simple and unambitious, such mechanisms have been very successful in improving joint working. For example, there may be an agreement between a health centre and a Social Services department with regard to defining tasks, roles and responsibilities, and agreeing procedures for assessment, provision of care, quality assurance and complaints. Many GPs welcome the arrangements whereby a social worker is attached to the practice, thereby facilitating quicker communications and mutual understanding (Rummery and Glendinning, 1997). However, what suits one practice may not suit another, and other models (e.g. social work sessions at the practice, telephone links, etc.) may be more appropriate.

Summary

- Better co-operation between health and social care has long been urged by governments, and new mechanisms have been introduced to make truly joint working between the two sectors more effective and achievable.
- Joint working may take place at different levels, such as strategic planning, the commissioning and provision of services for population groups, districts or individuals, and better arrangements for communication and co-operation.

Discussion

It is apparent from this overview of health and social care in the UK that its delivery cannot be divorced from the political and economic climate in which it is produced. Although there has always been some sort of consensus on the provision of welfare, the level at which it is fixed and the way in which it is administered have always produced a divergence of opinion.

The basis for the separation of health and social care provision preceded the development of the NHS, but has persisted ever since. As this chapter has demonstrated, the services provided by the health service and by local authorities are not always distinguishable in terms of content, although increasingly users of Social Services are expected to make some financial contribution to the service, whereas patients are generally not required to do so.

Throughout the 1990s, and indeed before then, successive governments have urged closer and more effective working between health and social care agencies. Over time the separation of health and social care has become increasingly dysfunctional, resulting in some spectacular failures in the care of sick and vulnerable people. However, attempts at achieving a seamless service have previously been restricted to particular client groups or 'one-off' initiatives. Health Action Zones present the opportunity for much greater integration across a much wider group of public services, including the criminal justice system, the environment, transport and education. There has not yet been enough time to assess how successful this initiative has been. In addition, the 1999 Health Act established for the first time a new statutory duty of partnership between agencies, with primary care group boards appointing a representative from the local Social Services department. Similarly, it will be interesting to see how much progress this will produce towards the provision of a seamless service.

There can be no doubt that many of the problems in delivering an integral health and social care service arise from the separation of responsibility and funding for the service between the Department of Health and local government. It will be interesting to observe whether fundamental progress can be made towards a seamless health and social care service without reviewing this separation.

Discussion points

- How relevant is the history of the development of the NHS to current health and social care delivery?
- What mechanisms have been put in place to ensure the delivery of evidence-based medicine?
- What are the advantages and disadvantages of the separation of health and social care services? Should this separation continue?
- Personal care tasks which are performed by nursing staff in hospital are carried out by social care staff in the community. Is it the responsibility of the individual or the state to fund such personal care?

- Is the accountability of both the NHS and Social Services departments sufficiently democratic? How could democratic accountability be enhanced?

Further reading

Ham C (1999) *Health policy in Britain*, 4th edn. London: Macmillan. This book provides an overview of the development of the NHS and its current structure and function.

Health systems under pressure

Peter Bundred

To achieve a sustainable medical care system we will have to rethink our notions of limitless and continuous progress in medicine. We must be willing to accept illness and death after our normal span of 75 or 80 years has run its course. We should be satisfied with that fate and try to make it available to everyone by targeting the causes of premature death, rather than struggling to survive to an advanced age at all costs and without regard to the quality of life.

(Callahan, 1998)

Models of health systems

There is no doubt that we all aspire to better health, and to achieve this we make more and more demands on the health care system. In the UK the National Health Service (NHS) has for the last 50 years fulfilled the role of the major provider of health care. Like all large organizations (the NHS is the biggest employer in Europe) it has failed to meet the demands being made on it by both patients and employees, and has been in a state of perpetual change. Since its inception there has been a major piece of government legislation almost every year to change the 'system', but despite these Acts of Parliament (or perhaps because of them) the NHS is failing to provide the services that we all perceive we need.

Health systems differ from country to country, but they all have a number of common attributes around which the structure of the system is based. Barr (1990) described the six features required to form a successful health system. These are listed in Box 11.1.

Box 11.1   Barr's criteria for a health system

- *Adequacy and equity of access to care.* There should be basic health care available to all citizens, and treatment should be in accordance with need.
- *Income protection.* Patients should be protected from payments for health care, which threaten their income, and payment for this protection should be related to the individual's ability to pay.
- *Macro-economic efficiency.* The nation's expenditure on health care should consume an appropriate fraction of the country's gross domestic product (GDP).
- *Micro-economic efficiency.* The mix of services provided by the health system should be a balance between those which improve health outcomes and those which satisfy consumer demand.
- *Freedom of choice for consumers.* The freedom to choose should be available in both the private and publicly funded sectors.
- *Appropriate autonomy for the providers of care.* It is important that all health workers should also have some freedom to choose how the other objectives are attained, especially in matters of clinical and organizational innovation.

If all of these criteria were met, a country's health system would supply health care of high quality at a cost that the country could afford. Sadly, most systems fail in at least one area. In the USA, for example, there are large numbers of people who have no access to health care despite the fact that the country spends over 15% of its GDP on the health sector. Over 50 million Americans are unable to afford private medical insurance and earn too much to be covered by the publicly funded system. In Uganda, one of the world's poorest countries, the government can only afford to spend $9 per head per year, which is not even sufficient to pay for a national childhood immunization programme. As a result of this under-investment in health care, medical and nursing staff working in the public sector spend part of each working day earning money outside the public health sector in order to pay for the necessities of life.

The NHS also has its problems. There has been recent debate about the amount invested in the NHS by the government. The current figure of 5.8% of GDP used to fund the NHS is lower than that for any other European country. With the increasing demands being made on health systems, many more countries will fail to meet the criteria for an effective health system.

The way in which health care is delivered is specific for each country. There are four basic 'types' of health delivery system, which can be classified as shown in Box 11.2 (Smith, 1998).

Box 11.2 Basic types of health system

- The 'socialized' system, as found in the UK and Sweden, which covers everyone, and the government acts as the only 'payer' for the care provided. The staff are usually salaried or 'capitated' (paid a fixed fee for the number of patients cared for).
- Socialized insurance, as found in France and Canada. This system also covers everyone and also has a single state 'payer', but staff tend to be paid a fee for each service provided.
- Mandatory insurance, as found in Germany, Japan and Malaysia. This system also covers everyone, but has multiple 'payers' in the form of sickness funds and insurers. Care is provided through a mixture of salaried public servants and private providers who are paid a fee for service.
- Voluntary insurance, as found in the USA and South Africa, which does not cover the entire population, and has many 'payers' and 'providers' and different systems of payment and delivery of health care.

All health systems are under considerable pressure to supply the care which patients demand. The more sophisticated the system, the greater the demands that are placed on it. There are a number of forces which put pressure on the health systems. Hadridge and Hodgson (1994) have described these, and they have shown that the forces acting on a health system are not independent variables but are interdependent on each other.

Using the NHS as an example, there are at least 11 driving forces which can be identified as acting to put pressure on the system to change.

1. *Economic stress.* Despite several years of positive growth in the economy, there is still under-investment in the NHS. The government has to decide into which service it puts more finance – the dilemma faced by all politicians!
2. *Information powershift.* Information has become a powerful commodity, and as patients learn to access information on the Internet so they begin to challenge the dominance of the professional. This puts increasing pressure on the structure of the health care professions, leading to change in the work carried out by each professional within the health team.
3. *Innovation momentum.* More and more high-cost innovations are being introduced into health care. The pharmaceutical industry is continuously introducing new drugs that cost many hundreds of million pounds to develop, and these development costs have to be passed on to the NHS. New surgical techniques are putting up the cost of health care, especially in specialist areas such as cardiology and neurosciences.
4. *System funding.* The financial constraints on the health system are multiplied when we consider that other government departments are also competing for funds to supply care to patients. Social Services supplies a considerable amount of care to vulnerable groups in the community. However, there is often little co-ordination between health and social services in the delivery of such care, leading to inefficiencies.
5. *Changes in the delivery system.* Over the last 10 years the NHS has seen a change in emphasis, with primary care services becoming more

prominent. This has required a change in the funding of the service, leading to financial pressure on hospitals.

6. *International perspectives*. The European Union rules have changed the structure of the care that is supplied by the NHS. The recent legislation specifying the NHS's responsibility to provide free nursing care for the elderly who are being cared for at home has put an additional financial burden on the service.

7. *Social norms*. As society changes, so the demands placed on the NHS also change. Expectations are increasing in a relatively under-funded service. The public's perceptions of health professionals are also changing. Two notable legal cases, namely the Bristol Children's Hospital Case (Smith, 1998) and the Shipman Case (Pringle, 2000) (see Boxes 11.3 and 11.4), have highlighted the vulnerability of the medical profession in an era of rapid change.

8. *Community values*. Linked to these changes in social norms are changes in the values placed on health care by the community. Issues such as genetic engineering, changing ethical standpoints and the role of the media have played a part in changing the views and attitudes of the public towards health care.

9. *Demographic changes*: With an increasing number of elderly patients to care for, the NHS is changing both the intensity and the type of services on offer. Coupled with a decreasing tax base (as the elderly pay less tax), this is putting additional burdens on the service.

10. *Care threshold*. The changes in the public's values and norms have influenced their health-seeking behaviour, affecting the threshold at which they seek care. The public's increased levels of awareness and the availability of complex medical interventions in the NHS have also influenced care thresholds.

11. *Political choices*. Underpinning all of these forces acting on the NHS are pressures from the politicians. Health care in most countries is dominated by political imperatives, and health professionals ignore these at their peril.

Box 11.3 The Bristol Children's Hospital Case

The Bristol Case refers to a report from the General Medical Council into the deaths of a number of children at the Bristol Royal Infirmary after they had undergone heart surgery. They identified several issues that arose during the course of their inquiry that concern the practice of medicine and surgery generally, and that need to be addressed by the medical profession, including the following:

- the need for clearly understood clinical standards;
- how clinical competence and technical expertise are assessed and evaluated;
- who carries the responsibility in team based care;
- the training of doctors in advanced procedures;
- how to approach the so-called learning curve of doctors undertaking established procedures;
- the reliability and validity of the data used to monitor doctors' personal performance;
- the use of medical and clinical audit;

- the appreciation of the importance of factors, other than purely clinical ones, that can affect clinical judgment, performance and outcome;
- the responsibility of a consultant to take appropriate actions in response to concerns about his or her performance;
- the factors which seem to discourage openness and frankness about doctors' personal performance;
- how doctors explain risks to patients;
- the ways in which people who are concerned about patients' safety can make their concerns known;
- the need for doctors to take prompt action at an early stage when a colleague is in difficulty, in order to offer the best chance of avoiding damage to patients and the colleague and of putting things right.

Source: Smith R (1998) All changed, changed utterly: British medicine will be transformed by the Bristol case. *British Medical Journal* **316**, 1917–18.

Box 11.4 The Shipman Case

Dr Harold Shipman was a general practitioner in Manchester who was accused and later convicted of multiple murders. As Pringle has pointed out in an editorial in the *British Journal of General Practice*, the case has caused concern to doctors and patients alike. Shipman broke the trust between himself and his patients, and many doctors now feel that the case may have done irreparable damage to the traditional relationship between a doctor and his or her patients.

Pringle points out that if patients can no longer trust their doctor not to harm them deliberately, how can they possibly trust him or her not to avoid accidental harm? Or covertly to deny the patient access to effective treatment (e.g. on the grounds of cost)?

Pringle also points out that the Shipman Case has highlighted a problem with regard to a basic tenet of professionalism, namely that of self-regulation. The General Medical Council, the body with statutory rights to control the medical profession, has had little success with the introduction of performance procedures for general practitioners. However, the introduction of revalidation on a cyclical basis may help to restore the public's confidence.

The most damaging revelation to emerge from the Shipman Case concerns professional isolation. Pringle points out that single-handed GPs are particularly vulnerable. The solution would seem to lie in the development of professional networks which could include continuous professional development, closer performance monitoring and a formal appraisal system.

Source: Pringle M (2000) The Shipman inquiry: implications for the public's trust in doctors. *British Journal of General Practice* **50**, 355–6.

These forces have led to considerable changes in the ways in which health delivery systems function, especially in those health systems that rely on voluntary health insurance for funding. In the USA, despite the fact that the country's economy is at its strongest for the last 30 years, 25% of adult Americans go without needed medical care. The American system of health delivery requires that individuals who are employed take responsibility for acquiring health insurance. This is usually provided as part of a 'package' from the employer. Budetti *et al.* (1999) have shown that 42% of workers with incomes of less than $20 000 per annum were not offered an insurance plan through their workplace, or were deemed to be ineligible. Moreover, they showed that even those with health cover were finding the cost of health care prohibitive; 24% of insured Americans had failed to get a recommended treatment or test for financial reasons. The report also showed that Americans living in the bottom half of the income distribution, who were least likely to have health insurance, were at high risk for health problems.

Summary

- Health systems can be defined in terms of how they handle access, cost, efficiency, choice and autonomy.
- There are four basic types of health system – socialized, social insurance, mandatory insurance and voluntary insurance.
- Forces that affect the performance of health systems include economic and political issues, social norms and community values, information and innovation, and demographic factors.
- All health systems have flaws and weaknesses.

Inequity

The inability of a health system to provide a comparable level of health care across the entire population is termed *inequity*. When the NHS was set up in 1948, enshrined in its philosophy was the availability of health care for everyone, which was 'free at the point of contact'. Despite 50 years of socialized health care, it is quite surprising that one of the major issues facing the politicians is the continuing problem of 'equity' within the NHS. It is also an important ethical issue, as we saw in Chapter 2, as inequity contravenes the concept of *justice*, one of the four fundamental principles of health care ethics.

There is both economic and epidemiological evidence of differences in the distribution, availability and use of health services in the UK. This difference is not new. In 1977, the then Secretary of State for Health (David Ennells), in a speech to Parliament when he commissioned Sir Douglas Black to examine these differences, is reported in *Hansard* as saying: 'The crude differences in the mortality rates between the various social classes are worrying. To take the extreme example, in 1971 the death rate for adult men in social class V (unskilled workers) was nearly twice that of adult men in social class I (professional workers) . . . when you look at death rates for specific diseases the gap is even wider'. The subsequent Black Report (Townsend and Davidson, 1988) showed alarming differences in mortality rates between those at the top of the economic tree and those at the bottom. Whitehead's *The Health Divide* (1988) confirmed these findings. Epidemiological research conducted in the 1990s has continued to show that the NHS is still failing to provide equitable health cover for the whole population.

There is a view that to improve the health of the population we need merely to improve the health care delivery system. After all, it is easier for politicians to increase spending on the NHS than to address the real causes of health inequity. Could the improved mortality rates and increased life expectancy in the UK over the last century be due to improved health care? It may be so in the middle classes. In men aged 15–45 years in social class I there has been a marked fall in the mortality rate from 88 per 1000 in 1911 to 66 per 1000 in 1981. However, in Social Class V there was an increase from 142 per 1000 to 166 per 1000 over the same time period (Marmot, 1999). It is more likely that these differences in mortality can be explained by traditional determinants of ill health such as poor diet, poor housing, exposure to violence, environmental pollutants, overcrowding and exposure to infectious disease. A longitudinal study on death rates for a number of diseases has shown that the availability of health care has had little effect on the overall mortality. McKeown (1976) pointed out that death rates from tuberculosis in Europe had fallen considerably from the peak in the nineteenth century to the time of the introduction of chemotherapy and BCG vaccination in the mid-twentieth century. This was despite the fact that most adults who were exposed to the bacillus during the course of their lives failed to become 'infected'.

In many countries there is a strong correlation between life expectancy and social status. The more affluent and educated the community, the more likely they are to live longer. In the UK, despite 50 years of the NHS, 'Top people live longer. Moreover, they are generally healthier while doing so'. Marmot and Theorell (1988), in a study of 10 000 British civil servants, showed that the age-adjusted mortality rate over the 10 years of the study was three and a half times higher in the manual and clerical grades than in the senior administrative grades. This difference was more marked when all four civil service grades were compared (see Figure 11.1).

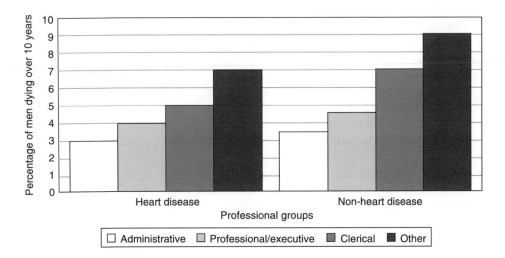

Figure 11.1 Whitehall study of differences in age-adjusted mortality rate between four civil service grades.

None of the individuals in the study could by any stretch of the imagination be described as 'impoverished or deprived', yet there is a significant difference between the groups. The traditional determinants of ill health cannot explain these differences in mortality. In civil servants these differences are more to do with the hierarchy within the civil service than with the simplistic view that they emanate purely from the concept of social inequalities and differentials in the 'wealth' of individuals. The gradients in mortality described by Marmot are seen across most diseases and most causes of death, and are mainly related to smoking behaviour. However, 'top people rarely smoke; bottom people often do' smoking behaviour does not account for all of the risk.

Coronary artery disease – a case study

Coronary artery disease remains the commonest cause of death among middle-aged men in the UK. From a biomedical standpoint it is a disease that can easily be explained. A diet high in cholesterol, in a hypertensive smoker, leads to progressive occlusion of the coronary arteries, which in turn causes angina or, when there is a sudden complete occlusion, a myocardial infarction. Around 25% of patients with myocardial infarction die within the first 24 hours after the event. Those who survive may make a full and complete recovery, usually with the aid of rehabilitation. A substantial number will require further treatment, usually in the form of a revascularization procedure. This in part explains the picture of the aetiology and management of this disease.

Coronary artery disease shows a marked social gradient in both morbidity and mortality. How does the individual's position in this social hierarchy affect their risk of developing this disease? When Marmot and Theorell (1988) examined the death rate for coronary artery disease among civil servants, they were able to show a threefold difference in mortality between the high-ranking and low-ranking groups. Even in non-smokers they found a twofold difference. They also showed that lower-level civil servants were far more likely to have raised blood pressure and raised cholesterol, both of which are major risk factors for heart disease. The overall risk of developing the disease was four times higher in the lower-ranking group. However, the traditional risk factors of smoking, hypertension and raised cholesterol, only accounted for 35% of the total risk. What comprises the other 65% of the risk to the individual?

Possible explanations come from animal models. Sapolsky (1990) showed that in baboons the dominant male in the troop is more physiologically capable of controlling his 'fight and flight' response compared with subordinate males. The latter individuals are subjected to more prolonged levels of stress than the dominant male, and they seem to be in a continuous state of low-level readiness. Could this abnormal response to stress be the cause of increased risk in low-ranking civil servants? Marmot found that the blood pressure response at work (a measure of the response to stress) was similar in all four groups of civil servants. However, in higher-ranking officials it fell more rapidly when they left work. They seemed to have more 'control' over their work environment and were less likely to take their problems home with them. Other primate work in macaques has shown that in an experimental setting, animals of low status who were fed on a diet high in cholesterol were four times more likely to develop atherosclerotic stenosis of the coronary arteries than higher-status animals that were fed the same diet (Kaplan *et al.*, 1982).

A biopsychosocial model for the aetiology of coronary artery disease begins to emerge. Individuals who are 'in control' of their lives, with better job satisfaction, seem to be at much lower risk of developing heart disease, despite the fact that they are exposed to similar biomedical risks in their daily life.

The differences in the responses of patients from different social classes to a disease are not just seen in their risk of developing the disease. There are also quite marked differences in the ways that individuals use the health system. In coronary artery disease this is seen as differences in treatment rates. In a study conducted in a district hospital in London, women were shown to have a poorer prognosis than men, and to receive less vigorous treatment (Wilkinson *et al.*, 1994). Epidemiological data from Wirral, Merseyside, have shown differences in the utilization of revascularization procedures (bypass surgery and angioplasty) between different social classes (Bundred and Todd, 1996). On the Wirral, where the population structure is very similar to that of England as a whole, the standardized mortality rate for those in the lowest socio-economic 10% of the population is 40% above the average for the area. However, the standardized mortality rate for those in the top socio-economic 10% is 40% below the average for the population. Despite similar in-hospital mortality rates, there is a sixfold difference in the hospital discharge rate for the two groups. In terms of 'health need', many more individuals in the lowest 10% require revascularization. However, patients in the top 10% of the population are three times more likely to have a revascularization procedure (720 per million, compared with 230 per million in the lowest 10%). Similar findings were reported in the West of Scotland. This variation in both health-seeking behaviour and access to the service highlights the inequity within the NHS. It is a good example of what Tudor-Hart (1971) has termed the *inverse care law*, whereby more and better health care tends to be provided for those who need it least.

From this case study it is clear that coronary artery disease has both a biomedical and a biopsychosocial aetiology. In general, traditional hospital-based health systems are designed to deal with the biomedical components of the disease. It could be argued that the biopsychosocial elements of the disease fall outside the remit of traditional health services and should be managed in a different way.

Summary

- Health is unequally distributed across the social classes, and so is health care. Unfortunately, the two inequalities do not match.
- Coronary artery disease exemplifies this problem very well.
- The reasons for inequity are complex, and cannot be explained solely by biomedical factors. Psychological and social factors are also important.

Developing primary care teams

The GP should be accessible, attend patients at home or in the surgery, carry out treatment within his competence and obtain specialist help when needed. He would attend childbirth and advise on how to prevent disease and improve the conditions of life among patients. He should play a part in antenatal supervision, child welfare, physical culture, venereal disease and industrial medicine. Nursing should be available, based with the doctor in primary health centres.

(Dawson of Penn, 1920)

So wrote Lord Dawson in 1920, on the establishment of a National Health System for the UK. The NHS was the first of a number of publicly funded comprehensive health systems to be established. At its heart has always been a strong primary care service.

General practitioners and nurses

To examine the role of the general practitioner (GP) in the structure of the NHS and the more recent developments in primary health care, we must look at some of the historical perspectives underpinning the development of the health professions in the UK.

Prior to the establishment of the NHS, GPs had worked exclusively as single-handed doctors. Many of them practised in poor-quality and often cramped accommodation. Others worked from their own homes in what has been described as a cottage industry. It was unusual for the GP to have any professional nursing assistance. Nurses tended to work from local authority clinics or as part of outreach programmes from the local hospital. This dichotomy between the two professional groups has its origins in history. Doctors, who were usually male, had developed from the apothecaries, barber surgeons and physicians. The nursing role (usually female) had developed as a result of a need to care for the destitute sick in the municipal hospitals in the mid-nineteenth century. Florence Nightingale and others had formalized this role, but it was essentially hospital based. With the exception of midwives and district nurses who were employed by local authority clinics, few nurses worked in the community. Primary care and the concept of multiprofessional working in the NHS are a very recent development. First-contact care in the UK has always been structured around the general practitioner. The development of a specific role for nurses in the primary care setting started in the 1970s with the appointment of nurses to work in GP practices.

Over the years, British medicine has experienced a considerable amount of inter-professional rivalry, with each of the professional groups developing along separate lines. A contemporary article from the College of Physicians written in 1669 (cited by Hopkins *et al.*, 1996) described considerable rivalry between physicians and apothecaries in the seventeenth century. Some 20 years later the physicians and surgeons were in dispute as to which professional group should be allowed to prescribe 'internal remedies'. It is at times of change that these professional rivalries tend to be more apparent. This may be due in part to professionalization, but it is also dependent on the rise of consumerism and the demands which patients make on the different professions. Gender also became an important issue in the development of the professional roles. Nightingale wrote:

> of the jargon, namely of the rights of women, which urges women to do all that men do, including medical and other professions, merely because men do it, and without regard to whether this is the best that women can do, merely because they are women.
>
> (Nightingale, 1860)

The setting up of the general practice service at the start of the NHS had not been without difficulties. Only weeks before the NHS was launched on 5 July 1948 the GPs had not agreed to join the new system. The major issue of contention was the status of GPs in the Health Service. They had always practised independently, and financially they had been structured as small businesses. The introduction of capitation (the payment of a fixed fee for each patient cared for) would remove their fee-for-service status, which the GPs saw as a disadvantage. In order to placate them, the Government allowed the GPs to maintain their independence (allowing them considerable tax concessions), but demanded that they follow a contract specifying the standards of care supplied. This 'independent contractor status' still exists and is the way in which the majority of GPs are remunerated.

Within a year of the inception of the NHS, the Collings Report (Collings, 1950) painted general practice in a poor light: 'The overall state of general practice is bad and still deteriorating. . . . The development of other medical services has resulted in wide departure from both the idea and ideal of family doctoring' (Collings, 1950). Collings made two important recommendations. First, he suggested that an attempt should be made to define the function of general practice within the NHS. Secondly, he suggested 'that group practice units should be formed'. As a result of the report, the 1970s saw the gradual formation of group practices. Within these group practices the professional roles tended to remain demarcated along the traditional boundaries. A practice of four GPs might well have a district nurse and a health visitor (public health nurse) attached to the practice by the local authority or hospital, but often they would not be regarded as part of the core practice 'team'. Occasionally the practice may have appointed a nurse to work within the practice on purely nursing duties. The sharing of professional roles and responsibilities was a difficult obstacle to overcome. This was mainly due to the adherence to strict professional codes of conduct laid down by the professional bodies, the General Medical Council and the Central Council for Nursing.

The White Paper, *Primary Health Care – an Agenda for Discussion* (Department of Health and Social Security, 1986), flagged up the need for the development of working teams: 'Primary health care is best provided when family doctors, community nurses and practice nurses work together as members of a primary care team'.

The main issue that prevented the development of primary care teams was the way in which GPs and nurses were paid. The 'independent contractor status' had allowed GPs to continue to run their practices as small businesses, which meant that nurses who worked within general practice were employed by the GPs. From the outset nurses had become salaried employees of the NHS. The difficulty in teamworking arose because of this employer–employee relationship. Some of the more enlightened nurses (and GPs) did not regard this as an issue, and were able to develop strong working relationships in quite complex teams.

In the late 1980s, two further White Papers and the Acts which followed them had a dramatic impact on the structure of primary care in the NHS. *Promoting Better Health* (Department of Health and Social Security, 1987) changed the structure of the contract which GPs had with the NHS, requiring them to concentrate much more on health promotion and the prevention of disease, although they still maintained their 'independent status'. To comply with this Act, GPs began to use nurses in different roles within the practice. It was quite common for nurses to run the long-term management of patients with chronic disease. Asthma, diabetes and hypertension management became the domain of the properly trained practice-based nurse.

The White Paper *Working for Patients* (Department of Health, 1989a) allowed GPs to expand the team further within their practices. The development of the 'fundholder GP' who had control over the budget for the practice allowed for a good deal of innovation. Teams were set up with many different professional groups (Rashid *et al.*, 1996), each of which began to question their role within the team, and it became clear in the early 1990s that nurses had the potential to expand their role within the primary care team. Nurses had already taken over some of the tasks traditionally carried out by GPs (Stilwell *et al.*, 1987). In contrast to North America, where the title of *nurse practitioner* was used from the early 1970s, it was not taken up in the NHS until much later. In many primary care teams nurses now provide a large amount of the care which had been traditionally been supplied by doctors (Venning *et al.*, 2000). Often the nurse is the point of first contact with the health system. New developments in the NHS such as the *NHS Direct* telephone information line are run entirely by nurses, allowing patients rapid access to health advice.

Developing teamwork

Firth-Cozens (1998) points out that all successful organizations are in a state of continuous change. Coupled with the drive for change is the need for individuals within organizations to work as teams. As mentioned earlier, the NHS has been in a state of continuous change since its inception. Primary care has changed beyond all recognition, and if the pace of change is to continue, then the need to ensure the working of primary care teams is paramount.

What is a team? It is most commonly defined as a group of people brought together to work towards a common purpose, so that the individual members are interdependent on each other. They communicate and work with each other to achieve a common purpose, and each has a defined role within the team designed to help to achieve the team's goal.

There is no doubt that effective teams improve the quality of primary care from the perspective of the patient, the organization and the team members. Patients benefit from contact with a wider group of professionals who can achieve much better outcomes for the individual patient. Team members benefit because working with colleagues improves both job satisfaction and the individual team members' mental health (Sonnentag, 1996). Finally, the primary care organization benefits because teams are more cost-effective, there is less staff absenteeism, staff are better motivated and multidisciplinary health care teams allow more efficient use of staff and other resources.

If everyone is a winner, why do some teams fail? Firth-Cozens (1996) found that with the implementation of clinical governance, the main reason why team leaders felt that they had failed was because the team had *failed to work together*. Why don't people want to work together? As Firth-Cozens points out, people may refuse to work in teams because they regard it as politically, economically or socially advantageous to them to stay away. Introverted team members may find the presence of other team members very threatening. However, teamworking presents a fundamental dilemma for all members of the team – that is, the choice of working together in a relationship with others or working alone. In large group practices, minor irritations such as perceptions about the partner with the easiest patients, which partner did not do their fair share of out-of-hours work, or who was landed with the audit work, are all issues which affect the team's functioning. Individual clashes can cause a team to be dysfunctional, as well as clashes between the professional groups that make up the team. Florence Nightingale's perceptions of the roles of doctors and nurses are still as strong today as when they were originally voiced.

The *management structure* of the team can also influence its effectiveness. The more pyramidal the structure, the more stresses are generated. Modern management theory now recommends flat structures with little hierarchy. Differential remuneration between the different groups also leads to poor teamworking, especially when roles traditionally taken on by higher-paid members of a group within the team are delegated to less well-paid members of the team. In the primary care team this can be seen when the nurse has been given responsibility for the running of a specialized service (e.g. the diabetic clinic) with no increase in reward. This situation is made much worse when the nurse is not trained properly to take on the new role.

One of the most important future threats to primary care teamworking concerns the *changing roles* of team members. As existing team members take on the roles of others, and as new members of the team are introduced, so new tensions are introduced into the team. In a rapidly changing health care system, no single professional group within the team has control over a specific set of skills. The whole system is in a state of flux. As hospital-based care is moved into the community, so the work of the GP is changing. The care offered by GPs has expanded to meet the new responsibilities. For example, diabetic patients are rarely admitted to hospital, and are managed almost exclusively in the community, where their care is often superior to the care that they received in the hospital outpatients clinic. As the GP's workload expands with this additional clinical load, so delegation within the team must occur. The rule of professional substitution has been around for years. In principle it states that 'no one should carry out a job which can be done as effectively by someone else who is less qualified'.

The members of the primary care team need to examine their professional roles in the light of professional substitution. Much of the work carried out by each professional group within the team was developed as part of the standards set by professional organizations a considerable time ago. Nurse practitioners with Masters degrees now run satellite practices for GPs and run postoperative intensive-care wards with little or no supervision. They perform surgical procedures such as the collection of the veins from the patient's legs as part of a coronary artery bypass operation, and many other highly skilled tasks that were previously performed by doctors. Yet most nurses may still not prescribe any medication, even simple analgesics such as paracetamol.

Summary

- When the NHS began, general practice was based on the independent contractor model, and was often of low quality.
- There has been a significant move in primary care towards multidisciplinary teamwork, which brings many advantages but also has its own problems.
- The roles of doctors and nurses in primary care are currently in a state of flux.

Continuing changes in primary care

In 1997, the new UK government initiated major changes in the structure of the NHS. In the White Paper *The New NHS: Modern, Dependable* (Department of Health, 1997), the concept of the 'internal market' where hospitals competed for patients was scrapped, to be replaced by an ethos of co-operation between the commissioner of care (the GP) and the provider (the hospital).

The term *commissioning* had been coined during the days of the internal market. It had become clear that purchasing health care was a complex business. First, it is difficult to equate the market-place with the clinical process. Patients do not follow a particular pathway during their illness, and a course of treatment may vary from patient to patient. As Light (1997) has stated, 'in health care there is no clear product, with clear property rights which can define a price in the same way as a price is set for a hotel room or a computer'. Secondly, the internal market soon highlighted the inequities in the NHS. There was a bias towards hospital-based services, with large discrepancies in the provision of those services. The South of England and parts of Scotland were better resourced than areas such as Merseyside and the North East of England. The concept of commissioning began the process of moving towards a more cost-effective approach to health care delivery. It emphasized prevention, health education and patient self-care whilst moving the centre of health care delivery away from the hospital into primary health care, which helped to coin the phrase 'a primary care lead NHS'.

If primary care is the cornerstone of the NHS, how does it address inequity? McNiece and Majeed (1999) have described the difference in the health status of the different social classes attending general practices in the UK. They examined general practice consultation rates among elderly patients taking part in the fourth national survey of morbidity in general practice, conducted over a 1-year period in 1991 and 1992. A total of 60 practices in England and Wales took part in the study. Elderly patients accounted for 71 984 (14%) of the consultations studied. Consultation rates were highest in social classes IV and V (Registrar General's Classification). There was a 23% difference between social classes I and V, patients in social class V having 4.82 consultations in the year compared with 3.93 in social class 1. Of all the individual aspects of the NHS, the general practitioner service seems to be closest to meeting the original concepts of the 1948 Act. However, there are still problems in the provision of an equitable service. Inner-city practices tend to have fewer partners and are less likely to have functional teams. They often deal with the sickest members of society, and only in a few very deprived areas has any attempt been made to provide increased resources.

One of the major problems highlighted in *The New NHS: Modern, Dependable* was the lack of co-ordination between the various authorities providing health care to the population. The service was seen as being very patchy, with some of the ex-fundholding practices providing excellent care whilst there were some practices, particularly in areas of deprivation, where the standard of care was poor.

The development of primary care groups (PCGs) and primary care trusts (PCTs) is seen as the way in which some of these problems can be addressed. PCGs are groups of local health and social care professionals who, together with patients and the local health authority representatives, take devolved responsibility for the health care needs of their local community. They are intended to bring GPs, nurses and other local 'stakeholders' together and give them a lead role in the planning, provision and development of local health services. In particular, they will be responsible for targeting health care at patients who are not receiving the care they need, or whose health status falls below that of the rest of the community.

The three main functions of PCGs are as follows:

- to improve the health of and address health inequalities in their communities;
- to develop primary care and community services across the PCG;
- to advise on, or commission directly, a range of hospital services for patients within their area that meet patient needs appropriately.

Box 11.5 Structure and functions of primary care groups (PCGs)

There will be nearly 500 PCGs in England and Wales, and they will each serve a population of up to 250 000 patients. They will be governed by a Board, which will be constituted as a committee of the health authority. The Board will have between four and seven GPs, up to two nurses, a representative of Social Services, a representative of the health authority, a Chief Executive and a lay member. The Board will appoint a Chair from within its members. The PCGs are seen as being able to operate at four levels, with Levels 3 and 4 being designated primary care trusts.

- *Level 1*: the minimum requirement is that they act in support of the health authority in commissioning care for their population, acting in an advisory capacity to the health authority.
- *Level 2*: the PCG takes devolved responsibility for managing the budget for health care in their area, acting as part of the health authority.
- *Level 3*: the PCG becomes a freestanding body (a trust) accountable to the health authority for the commissioning of care.
- *Level 4*: in addition to the responsibilities in Level 3, the primary care trust will also address the responsibility for providing services for the community.

As well as their statutory responsibilities, the PCGs and PCTs have other important tasks. Each is required to develop a Health Improvement Programme, which targets high-risk groups in their area. Areas covered include specific patient groups (e.g. diabetics) or targeting care towards vulnerable groups in the community (e.g. children or the elderly). They are also responsible for the implementation of *clinical governance* in primary care. Clinical governance is a framework through which NHS organizations are accountable for continuously improving the quality of their services and safeguarding high standards of care. In primary care it is intended to be an open process embracing all members of the primary care team. It is designed to identify poor performance and, where possible, tackle the issues causing poor performance (e.g. lack of resources) and improve skills.

How does clinical governance work? The main principles that underpin the process are as follows:

- the establishment of clear lines of responsibility and accountability for the quality of clinical care within the group;
- the introduction of a comprehensive programme of quality improvement systems, which will include clinical audit, the application of evidence-based

practice, the implementation of clinical standards and guidelines, and the development of staff skills;

- the development of education and training plans to develop a more competent work-force;
- the development of policies for the management of risk;
- the development of procedures for all professional groups to identify and remedy poor performance.

Summary

Recent changes in the organization of primary care in the UK are intended to reduce inequity and improve quality. These include the following:

- the emergence of primary care groups and trusts;
- health improvement programmes;
- clinical governance.

Making health care more efficient

The main problem with most health systems is that they are very inefficient. Attempts have been made over the last decade to reform the delivery of care, and perhaps the most well known of these in the UK is the Thatcher Government's attempt to introduce a 'market-based' system into the NHS in the early 1990s. In the USA, the introduction of 'managed care' has radically changed the way in which patients pay for and receive the care that they need. These system changes have one thing in common – they were designed to remove inefficiencies, and to provide better value for money for the payer. (For a more detailed discussion of the issues surrounding health economics, the reader is referred back to Chapter 8.)

In the UK tight controls over NHS expenditure in the 1980s had produced a financially efficient service. The main area of concern was the variation in availability and outcomes of the health care. Wennberg (1984), writing in the USA, pointed out large geographical variations in the availability of medical services. Similar work carried out in the NHS at about the same time showed similar variations in clinical practice, as well as large differences in the availability of a number of surgical procedures in different parts of the country. What had also emerged were marked discrepancies in the outcomes of surgical procedures. In one example there was a sixfold difference in 5-year survival after surgery for colon cancer between two areas of the country.

Clinical audit

In order to reduce these inequalities, the NHS introduced the concept of *clinical audit*, which is based on two principles. First, the care offered should be compared to a standard set at a national level, and secondly, a mechanism should be in place to improve the quality of care continuously so that it equates with the national standard (closing the audit loop). As a result of the introduction of the clinical audit programme, which was compulsory for all clinical teams in the NHS, a number of important findings emerged. There were variations in the standards of clinical practice, not only between clinical teams in various parts of the country, but also between clinicians in the same team. A good example was the use of low-dose aspirin in the long-term management of patients with ischaemic heart disease. There was strong evidence that aspirin reduced the risk of secondary infarction in these patients (Antiplatelet Trialists' Collaboration, 1994), yet in some areas of the country less than 25% of at-risk patients were receiving this preparation. If this was the case for the use of a simple preparation, were there other variations in the use of more complex interventions? A number of major national audits confirmed that throughout the NHS there was marked variation in practice. Cochrane (1979) had pointed out that many of the interventions used in the NHS had never been shown to be effective when compared with alternative methods of treatment. He emphasized that the better part of efficiency is effectiveness: 'how can a system be efficient if the clinician does not know what works and what does not?' So began a new concept within the NHS, namely the *evidence-based medicine* movement.

Box 11.6 The evidence for the best management of coronary heart disease

The following Internet websites provide an excellent source of information on the primary and secondary prevention of coronary heart disease.

1. The Scottish Intercollegiate Guideline Network: Lipids and the Primary Prevention of Coronary Heart Disease. Report Number 40, published in September 1999: http://www.show.scot.nhs.uk/sign/clinical.htm
2. The Scottish Intercollegiate Guideline Network: Secondary Prevention of Coronary Heart Disease following Myocardial Infarction. Report Number 41, published in January 2000: http://www.show.scot.nhs.uk/sign/clinical.htm
3. Netting the Evidence: A ScHARR Introduction to Evidence-Based Practice on the Internet. http://www.shef.ac.uk/uni/academic/R-Z/scharr/ir/netting.html
4. The Heart of General Practice: http://medicine21.com/heartGP/

Change management

Clinical governance focuses on a comprehensive program of continuous quality improvement. It includes processes for monitoring care and external review, policies for managing risk, and clear lines of responsibility and accountability. It has shifted the emphasis from the cost of health care to the quality of clinical practice. Many clinical teams have experienced considerable problems in translating the concept into routine clinical practice. Changing the way in which professionals work has always been difficult. Ryan and

Gross (1943) first described the 'diffusion principle of change'. They describe five behaviour patterns in any change situation. These include *innovators*, who represent 6% of the population and who need no encouragement to adapt to any changing environment, but who tend not to be trusted by the majority of their peers. The next group, called *early adopters*, represent a further 15%, and they are the key facilitators of change. Early adopters observe and follow the innovators, and are regarded as trusted members of the profession. The *early and late majority* make up the bulk of the group and will only change their behaviour after the early adopters have changed. Finally there is a group which Ryan and Gross refer to as *laggards*. These individuals are set in their ways and are unlikely ever to take on new ideas. Innovators are usually the people who develop the ideas that are taken up by the early adopters and later by the majority of professionals in a changing work environment.

The introduction of new working methods designed to improve the quality of patient care in the NHS is a good example of the diffusion principle of change. One of the best illustrations of this was the introduction of *integrated care pathways* (Kitchiner *et al.*, 1996) (see Box 11.7) into routine hospital practice. Although these pathways were based on scientific principles that had been shown to improve patient care, the innovators who introduced them had the greatest difficulty in convincing the majority of health professionals to use this new approach. Over a period of 6 years, integrated care pathways gradually became established as an effective method of continuously improving care, and they became a vehicle for introducing clinical governance into routine clinical practice.

Box 11.7 Integrated care pathways

Integrated care pathways provide a practical tool for monitoring and improving patient care. They set locally agreed standards for the management of specific groups of patients. These standards or guidelines are based on the best available evidence and are used to develop and implement multidisciplinary clinical plans. The pathway is divided into time intervals during which specific goals and expected progress are indicated, together with guidance on the optimal timing of appropriate investigations and treatment. The care pathway forms part or all of the patient's record, and allows documentation of the care given by members of the multidisciplinary team, together with the progress of the patient. It identifies specific goals or outcomes that should be achieved by the patient and the multidisciplinary team. Variations from these goals are recorded, together with the reasons for those variations. Analysis of aspects of care and outcome allows a continuous evaluation of the effectiveness of clinical practice. The information obtained is used to revise the care pathway in order to improve the quality of patient care.

Source: Kitchiner D, Davidson C and Bundred P (1996) Integrated care pathways: an effective tool for continuously evaluating clinical practice. *Journal of Evaluation in Clinical Practice* **1**, 65–9.

Summary

Health care systems can be made more efficient by the following:

- becoming aware of economic costs;
- clinical audit;

* evidence-based practice (e.g. with heart disease);
* effective management of change (e.g. through integrated care pathways).

Where are health systems going?

> The safety of our patients is more at risk from inappropriate activism than from diagnostic error: more at risk from wishful thinking than from ignorance.
>
> (James McCormick, *The Times Health Supplement*, June 1990)

Donaldson and Muir Gray (1998) suggest that in the management of a rapidly changing health system, 'cultural change needs to be wrought alongside structural reorganisation and systems reform to bring about a culture in which excellence can flourish.' Cultural change has been a central component of all of the changes introduced into the NHS over the past 20 years. There has been a change from a primarily administered service to one in which general management has become a key component. Part of this 'management' revolution involved clinicians because they became much more concerned with the resources that they used in the delivery of health care. This required a major cultural and behavioural change on the part of the medical profession, which took many years to implement. The reforms of the early 1990s took the concept of management further forward, and some would say too far, with the introduction of the 'managed health market' and fundholding. The 1997 change of government saw the introduction of 'quality' as the flagship of the changes introduced by the Labour administration.

All of these reforms have involved substantial shifts in the attitude of the professionals working in the service. The structure of health systems will continue to change, and these changes will increase in magnitude and intensity as the financial resources to fund health care are put under even greater pressure. This will require the professions working in health care to adapt to change more quickly than they have done in the past. Smith (1997), in his article entitled *The Future of Health Systems*, postulates that the four basic types of health system (see Figure 11.2) may in the future expand to become six completely different structures which incorporate much of the existing systems but also take on new concepts such as tools to manage demand (advice lines such as *NHS Direct*, user co-payments and health education) and tools to control professional behaviour (managed care, clinical practice guidelines and evidence-based medicine). More importantly, the role of the consumer becomes much more prominent in the delivery of health care. Smith's most radical model, which he calls the 'informed consumer model', involves consumers using information technology to access information and control their own health care. This inverts the traditional 'industrial age medicine' model of health care into 'information age health care', where the consumer takes control and the large amount of informal self-care is absorbed into the new model, thus 'empowering the consumer'. The observant will also note that 'information age health care' encourages financial expenditure at the low-cost end of the care spectrum, thus reducing the overall cost of the health care provided.

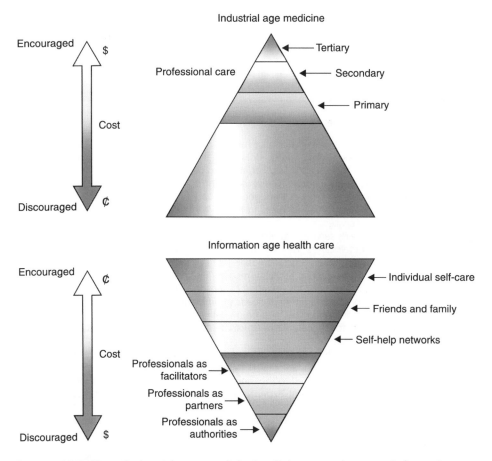

Figure 11.2 How 'industrial age medicine' will invert to become 'information age health care'.

Predicting the future is not easy, and Smith points out in his later article (Smith, 1998) that many of the changes he describes may never come to fruition. However, he concludes that 'Most large sections of developed economies – transport, manufacturing and telecommunications – have been transformed in the past 20 years; health care has not but surely will be'.

The NHS Plan – a plan for investment, a plan for reform

The NHS Plan (Department of Health, 2000) was published in July 2000 and is the blueprint for the future changes in the way that the NHS is both funded and managed. As Dixon and Dewar (2000) have stated, it is impressive in scope and reflects messages coming from both staff and patients about the way in which the service should proceed. It also enshrines many of the concepts discussed by Smith, and its implementation will require enormous cultural change.

Ten core principles underpin the plan (see Box 11.8). They reiterate the underlying principles that were the cornerstone of the original NHS Act in 1946.

Box 11.8 Ten core principles of the NHS Plan

1. *The NHS will provide a universal service for all based on clinical need, not ability to pay.* Health care is a basic human right. Unlike private systems, the NHS will not exclude people because of their health status or ability to pay.
2. *The NHS will provide a comprehensive range of services.* It will provide access to a comprehensive range of services throughout primary and community health care, intermediate care and hospital-based care, and it will continue to provide clinically appropriate cost-effective services.
3. *The NHS will shape its services around the needs and preferences of individual patients, their families and their carers.* The NHS of the twenty-first century must be responsive to the needs of different groups and individuals within society, and challenge discrimination on the grounds of age, gender, ethnicity, religion, disability or sexuality. Patients will have a greater say in the NHS, and the provision of services will be centred on patients' needs.
4. *The NHS will respond to the different needs of different populations.* Health services will continue to be funded nationally, and be available to all citizens of the UK. Efforts will continually be made to reduce unjustified variations and raise standards to achieve a truly National Health Service.
5. *The NHS will work continually to improve quality services and to minimize errors.* The NHS will ensure that services are driven by a cycle of continual quality improvement. Quality will not just be restricted to the clinical aspects of care, but will also include quality of life and the entire patient experience. The NHS will continually improve its efficiency, productivity and performance.
6. *The NHS will support and value its staff.* The strength of the NHS lies in its staff, whose skills, expertise and dedication underpin all that it does. They have the right to be treated with respect and dignity.
7. *Public funds for health care will be devoted solely to NHS patients.* The NHS is funded out of public expenditure, primarily by taxation. Individuals will remain free to spend their own money as they see fit, but public funds will be devoted solely to NHS patients, and will not be used to subsidize privately funded health care.
8. *The NHS will work together with others to ensure a seamless service for patients.* The health and social care system must be shaped around the needs of the patient, not the other way round.
9. *The NHS will help to keep people healthy and work to reduce health inequalities.* The NHS will focus its efforts on preventing as well as treating ill health, recognizing that good health also depends on social, environmental and economic factors. The NHS will work with other public services to intervene not just after but also before ill health occurs. It will work with others to reduce health inequalities.
10. *The NHS will respect the confidentiality of individual patients and provide access to information about services, treatment and performance.* Patient confidentiality will be respected throughout the process of care. The NHS will be open with regard to providing information about health and health care services. It will continue to use information to improve the quality of services for all, and to generate new knowledge about future medical benefits.

The Plan itself is built on four main themes:

1. increasing the capacity of the NHS to treat patients;
2. setting standards for care and developing targets to ensure that the standards are met;
3. improving the delivery of care so that the patient comes first;
4. developing partnerships with other agencies to ensure seamless care for patients.

The Plan is funded by a massive investment in funds which is equivalent to an increase in income of one-third over a 5-year period. These funds will be used to increase the capacity of the NHS and to increase the number of staff as follows:

- 7000 extra beds in hospitals and intermediate care;
- over 100 new hospitals by 2010, and 500 new one-stop primary care centres;
- over 3000 GP premises modernized and 250 new scanners;
- clean wards – overseen by 'modern matrons' – and better hospital food;
- modern IT systems in every hospital and GP surgery;
- 7500 more consultants and 2000 more GPs;
- 20 000 extra nurses and 6500 extra therapists;
- 1000 more medical school places;
- childcare support for NHS staff, with 100 on-site nurseries.

Coupled with these expansions in the infrastructure will be a reform process which will require fundamental changes in both the attitude and behaviour of staff. The Department of Health will set national standards for care, and some of these have already been published in the form of National Service Frameworks for mental health and coronary heart disease. Organizations such as the National Institute for Clinical Excellence will be expanded to ensure that care remains cost-effective, and a Modernization Agency is to be set up to disseminate best practice. Medical staff are to be offered more modern contracts, and coupled with these will be the ability to earn more remuneration through improved efficiency. Nurses are to expand their role, and legislation is being introduced for nurses to prescribe medicines.

The NHS Plan is one of many radical and far-reaching developments in health care delivery systems. As financial pressures increase, the rate of change may also increase, and this will affect the way in which health professionals work. Publically funded health care is a privilege of which the UK is rightly proud. If we are to continue to have such a system we must be prepared to see it change, and to modify our work accordingly.

Discussion points

1. Should the problems exemplified by the Bristol Case and the Shipman Case be seen mainly as the failings of individuals, or should they be regarded as signs that the health care system is not working effectively?

2. How much of the inequity in health, and in access to health care, can be explained simply on the basis of differences in income between members of a society?
3. As nurses take on more of the role of the doctor, what will be the doctor's role in the primary care team?
4. How can we best determine the balance between improving standards of care within health care systems (e.g. through clinical audit and governance) and increasing the amount of resources devoted to health care systems? Should the answer lie in the hands of politicians, ethicists, health care professionals or consumers of health care?

Further reading

Dixon J and Dewar S (2000) The NHS Plan: as good as it gets, make the most of it. *British Medical Journal* **321**, 315–16.

Smith R (1997) The future of health care systems. *British Medical Journal* **314**,1495–6.

References and useful websites

References

Acheson D (1999) *Independent Inquiry into Inequalities. Health Report.* London: The Stationery Office.

Adelstein A, Staszewski J and Muir C (1979) Cancer mortality in 1970–72 among Polish-born immigrants to England and Wales. *British Journal of Cancer* **40**, 464–75.

Ahmad W, Sheldon T and Stuart O (eds) (1996) *Ethnicity and health: reviews of literature and guidance for purchasers in the areas of cardiovascular disease, mental health and haemoglobinopathies.* Centre for Reviews and Dissemination Report No. 5. University of York: NHS Centre for Reviews and Dissemination and Social Policy Research Unit.

Allen I (1991) *Family planning and counselling projects for young people.* London: Policy Studies Institute.

Allen I (1994) *Doctors and their careers: a new generation.* London: Policy Studies Institute.

Allport G (1937) *Personality: a psychological interpretation.* New York: Holt, Rinehart & Winston.

Allsop J (1984) *Health policy and the National Health Service.* London: Longman.

Annandale E (1998) *The sociology of health and medicine: a critical introduction.* Cambridge: Polity Press.

Annandale E and Hunt K (1990) Masculinity, femininity and sex: an exploration of their relative contribution to explaining gender differences in health. *Sociology of Health and Illness* **12**, 24–46.

Anonymous (1974) Stroke and the family (editorial). *British Medical Journal* **iv**, 122.

Antiplatelet Trialists' Collaboration (1994) Collaborative overview of antiplatelet therapy. *British Medical Journal* **308**, 81-106.

Arber S, Gilbert N and Dale A (1985) Paid employment and women's health: a benefit or a source of role strain? *Sociology of Health and Illness* **7**, 375–400.

Aron R (1970) *Main currents in sociological thought 2.* Harmondsworth: Penguin.

Ashton C and Kamali F (1995) Personality, lifestyles, alcohol and drug consumption in a sample of British medical students. *Medical Education* **29**,187–92.

Atkinson P (1988) Discourse, descriptions and diagnoses: reproducing normal medicine. In Lock M and Gordon D (eds), *Biomedicine examined.* London: Tavistock/Routledge.

Atkinson R and Shiffrin R (1971) The control of short-term memory. *Scientific American* **224**, 82–90.

Atkinson RL, Atkinson RC, Smith EE and Bem DJ (1993) *Introduction to psychology,* 11th edn. Fort Worth, TX: Harcourt-Brace Jovanovich.

Bahrick H, Bahrick P and Wittlinger R. (1975) Fifty years of memory for names and faces: a cross-sectional approach. *Journal of Experimental Psychology* **104**, 54–75.

Banks M and Jackson P (1982) Unemployment and risk of minor psychiatric disorder in young people: cross-sectional and longitudinal evidence. *Psychological Medicine* **12**, 789–98.

Banks M, Beresford S, Morrell D, Waller J and Watkins C (1975) Factors influencing demand for primary medical care among women aged 20–44 years. *International Journal of Epidemiology* **4**, 189–95.

Barker D (1997) Intrauterine programming of coronary heart disease and stroke. *Acta Paediatrica* **422 (Supplement)**, 178–82.

Barker D (1999) Fetal origins of cardiovascular disease. *Annals of Medicine* **31 (Supplement 1)**, 3–6.

Barr N (1990) *Economic theory and the welfare state: a survey and reinterpretation.* Welfare State Programme Discussion Paper No. 54. London: London School of Economics and Political Science.

Beattie A (1991) Knowledge and control in health promotion. In Calnan M, Gabe J and Bury M (eds), *The sociology of the health service.* London: Routledge, 162–202.

Beauchamp T and Childress J (1994) *Principles of biomedical ethics.* Oxford: Oxford University Press.

Beck A (1991) Cognitive theory: a 30-year retrospective. *American Psychology* **46**, 368–75.

Belloc N and Breslow L (1972) Relationship of physical health status and family practices. *Preventive Medicine* **1**, 409–42.

Bendix R (1966) *Max Weber: an intellectual portrait.* London: Methuen & Co. Ltd.

Berkman LF and Syme SL (1979) Social networks, host resistance, and mortality: a nine-year follow-up study of Alameda County residents. *American Journal of Epidemiology* **109**, 186–204.

Beyer S, Evans G and Felce D (1993) Service development under the All Wales Mental Handicap Strategy. In Robbins D (ed.), *Community care: findings from Department of Health funded research 1988–1992.* London: HMSO, 64–7.

Binet A and Simon T (1905) New methods for the diagnosis of the intellectual level of subnormals. *Annals of Psychology* **11**, 191.

Blane D (1999) The life course, the social gradient and health. In Marmot M and Wilkinson RG (eds), *Social determinants of health.* Oxford: Oxford University Press, 66–80.

Blaxter M (1990) *Health and lifestyles.* London: Tavistock/Routledge.

Bloor M, Samphier M and Prior L (1987). Artefact explanations of inequalities in health: an assessment of the evidence. *Sociology of Health and Illness* **9**, 231–64.

Botting B (1997) Mortality in childhood. In Drever F and Whitehead M (eds), *Health inequalities. Decennial supplement.* London: The Stationery Office, 83–94.

Bowlby J (1981) *Attachment and loss. Volume III. Sadness and depression.* Harmondsworth: Penguin.

Bowling A (1987) Mortality after bereavement: a review of the literature on survival periods and factors affecting survival. *Social Science and Medicine* **24**, 117–24.

Bowling A (1991) *Measuring health. A review of quality of life measurement scales.* Milton Keynes: Open University Press.

Bowling A (1995). *Measuring disease.* Buckingham: Open University Press.

Breeze E, Sloggett A and Fletcher A (1999) Socioeconomic status and transitions in status in old age in relation to limiting long-term illness measured at the 1991 Census. *European Journal of Public Health* **9**, 265–70.

Brewer R (1986) A note on the changing status of the Registrar General's classification of occupations. *British Journal of Sociology* **37**, 131–40.

British Medical Association (1993) *Medical ethics today: its practice and philosophy.* London: BMJ Publishing Group.

Brown G and Harris T (1978) *Social origins of depression: a study of psychiatric disorder in women.* London: Tavistock.

Brown G and Harris T (eds) (1989) *Life events and illness.* London: Unwin Hyman.

Bruce M (1968) *The coming of the welfare state,* 2nd edn. London: B. T. Batsford Ltd.

Budetti J, Duchon L, Schoen C and Shikles J (1999) *Can't afford to get sick: a reality for millions of working Americans. Report to the Commonwealth Fund.* New York: Commonwealth Fund; http://www.cmwf.org/programs/insurance/budetti_sick_347.asp

Bundred P and Todd P (1996) The economic and equitable distribution of cardiac interventions in the British Health Service: how one health district approached these problems. *Proceedings of the International Health Economics Association Conference, Vancouver, Canada.* Vancouver: International Health Economics Association.

Bunton R (1995) Health off the shelf? *Health Matters 21,* **Spring issue,** 8–9.

Burghes L, Clarke L and Cronin N (1997) *Fathers and fatherhood in Britain.* London: Family Policy Studies Centre.

Bury M (1982) Chronic illness as biographical disruption. *Sociology of Health and Illness* **4,** 167–82.

Busby H, Elliott H, Popay J and Williams G (1999) Public health and primary care: a necessary relationship. *Health and Social Care in the Community* **7,** 239–41.

Callahan D (1998) *False hopes: why America's quest for perfect health is a recipe for failure.* New York: Simon & Schuster.

Calman M (1991) *Preventing coronary heart disease: prospects, policies and politics.* London: Routledge.

Cannon W (1929) *Bodily changes in pain, hunger, fear and rage,* 2nd edn. New York: Appleton-Century-Crofts.

Catalan J, Gath D, Anastasiades P *et al.* (1991) Evaluation of a brief psychological treatment for emotional disorders in primary care. *Psychological Medicine* **21,** 1013–18.

Chomsky N (1975) *Reflections on language.* New York: Parthenon Books.

Clare A (1976) *Psychiatry in dissent.* London: Tavistock.

Cobb S (1976) Social support as a moderator of life stress. *Psychosomatic Medicine* **38,** 300–14.

Cochrane A (1979) 1931–1971: a critical review with particular reference to the medical profession. In *Medicines for the year 2000.* London: Office of Health Economics.

Cohen S and Syme L (1985) *Social support and health.* New York: Academic Press.

Coleman MP, Babba P, Damiecki P *et al.* (eds) (1999) *Cancer survival trends in England and Wales 1971–95.* Deprivation and NHS Region Series No. 61. London: The Stationery Office.

Collings J (1950) General practice in England today. A reconnaissance. *Lancet* **1,** 555–79.

Conger R, Lorenz F, Elder G, Simons R and Ge X (1993) Husband and wife differences in response to undesirable life events. *Journal of Health and Social Behaviour* **34,** 71–88.

Cooke A and Campbell B (1982) *Sweet freedom.* London: Pan Books.

Corbin J and Strauss AM (1988) *Unending work and care. Managing chronic illness at home.* San Francisco, CA: Jossey-Bass.

Cornwell J (1984) *Hard-earned lives: accounts of health and illness from East London.* London: Tavistock.

Costa P and McCrae R (1985) *The NEO personality inventory manual.* Odessa, FL: Psychological Assessment Resources.

Costain Schou K and Hewison J (1999) *Experiencing cancer. Quality of life in treatment.* Buckingham: Open University Press.

Coulter A (1999) Paternalism or partnership? *British Medical Journal* **319,** 719–20.

Crosby D and Vickery A (1993) Development of community care schemes. In Robbins D (ed.), *Community care: findings from Department of Health funded research 1988–1992.* London: HMSO.

Cuff E, Sharrock W and Francis D (1992) *Perspectives in sociology*, 3rd edn. London: Tavistock.

Davey Smith G, Bartley M and Blanc D (1990) The Black Report on socioeconomic inequalities in health 10 years on. *British Medical Journal* **301**, 373–6.

Dawson of Penn (1920) *Interim report on the future provision of medical and allied services. Consultative Council on Medical and Allied Services*. London: HMSO.

Department of Health (1989a) *Working for patients*. London: HMSO.

Department of Health (1989b) *Caring for people. Community care in the next decade and beyond*. London: HMSO.

Department of Health (1992) *The health of the nation: a strategy for health in England*. London: HMSO.

Department of Health (1997) *The new NHS: modern, dependable*. London: The Stationery Office.

Department of Health (1998) *Our healthier nation: a contract for health*. London: The Stationery Office.

Department of Health (1999) *Saving lives: our healthier nation*. London: The Stationery Office.

Department of Health (2000) *The NHS Plan. A plan for investment, a plan for reform*. London: The Stationery Office; www.nhs.uk/nhsplan

Department of Health and Social Security (1976) *Priorities for health and social services in England*. London: HMSO.

Department of Health and Social Security (1981a) *Growing older*. London: HMSO.

Department of Health and Social Security (1981b) *Care in the community*. London: HMSO.

Department of Health and Social Security (1981c) *Report of a study on community care*. London: HMSO.

Department of Health and Social Security (1986) *Primary health care – an agenda for discussion*. London: HMSO.

Department of Health and Social Security (1987) *Promoting better health. The government's programme for improving primary health care*. London: HMSO.

Der G, MacIntyre S, Ford G, Hunt K and West P (1999) The relationship of household income to a range of health measures in three age cohorts from the West of Scotland. *European Journal of Public Health* **9**, 271–7.

d'Houtard A and Field MG (1984) The image of health: variations in perceptions by social class in a French population. *Sociology of Health and Illness* **6**, 30–60.

Diba R (1996) *Meeting the costs of continuing care: public views and perceptions*. York: Joseph Rowntree Foundation.

Digby A (1989) *British welfare policy. Workhouse to workfare*. London: Faber and Faber.

Dixon J and Dewar S (2000) The NHS plan: as good as it gets, make the most of it. *British Medical Journal* **321**, 315–16.

Donaldson L and Muir Gray J (1998) Clinical governance: a quality duty for health organizations. *Quality in Health Care* **7 (Supplement)**, S1-2.

Downton J (1993) *Falls in the elderly*. London: Edward Arnold.

Dowrick C, Dunn G, Ayuso-Mateos J *et al*. (2000) Problem-solving treatment and group psycho-education for people with depressive disorders in urban and rural communities: a multi-centre randomized controlled trial. *British Medical Journal* **321**, 1450–54.

Drever F and Whitehead M (eds) (1997) *Health inequalities. Decennial supplement*. London: The Stationery Office.

Dunnell K (1995) Population review. 2. Are we healthier? *Population Trends* **82**, 12–18.

Eachus J, Williams M, Chan P *et al.* (1996) Deprivation and cause-specific morbidity: evidence from the Somerset and Avon survey of health. *British Medical Journal* **312**, 287–92.

Engels F (1844) *The condition of the English workingclasses in England in 1844* (translated by W Henderson and W Chaloner, 1958 version). Oxford: Blackwell.

Eskenazi B and Bergmann JJ (1995) Passive and active maternal smoking during pregnancy, as measured by serum cotinine and postnatal smoke exposure. 1. Effects on physical growth at age 5 years. *American Journal of Epidemiology* **142**, S8–10.

Eysenck H (1947) *Dimensions of personality*. London: Routledge & Kegan Paul.

Fallowfield L (1990) *The quality of life: the missing measurement in health care*. London: Souvenir Press.

Fenton S, Hughes A and Hine C (1995) Self-assessed health, economic status and ethnic origin. *New Community* **21**, 55–68.

Filakti H and Fox J (1995) Differences in mortality by housing tenure and by car access from the OPCS Longitudinal Study. *Population Trends* **81**.

Firth-Cozens J (1986) Levels and sources of stress in medical students. *British Medical Journal* **292**, 533–6.

Firth-Cozens J (1996) *Clinical effectiveness in health authorities*. Durham: Report to the NHS Executive, 1996.

Firth-Cozens J (1998) Celebrating teamwork. *Quality in Health Care* **7 (Supplement)**, S3–7.

Fisher K and Collins J (eds) (1993) *Homelessness, health care, and welfare provision*. London: Routledge.

Florey C and Taylor D (1994) The relation between antenatal care and birth weight. *Revue d'Epidemiologie et de Sante Publique* **42**, 191–7.

Foot M (1963) *Aneurin Bevan. A biography*. London: Readers Union.

Fox J, Goldblatt P and Jones D (1990) Social class mortality differentials: artifact, selection or life circumstances? In Goldblatt P (ed.), *Longitudinal study: mortality and social organisation, 1971–1981*. London: HMSO.

Friedman M and Friedman R (1980) *Free to choose. A personal statement*. Harmondsworth: Penguin.

Gardner H (1983) *Frames of mind*. New York: Basic Books.

General Medical Council (1993) *Tomorrow's doctors*. London: General Medical Council.

General Medical Council (1995) *Duties of a doctor*. London: General Medical Council.

General Medical Council (1999) *Seeking patients' consent: the ethical considerations*. London: General Medical Council.

Gepkens A and Gunning-Schepers L (1996) Interventions to reduce socio-economic health differences: a review of the international literature. *European Journal of Public Health* **6**, 218–26.

Gillon R (1986) *Philosophical medical ethics*. Chichester: John Wiley & Sons.

Gloaguen V, Cottraux J, Cucherat M and Blackburn I (1998) A meta-analysis of the effects of cognitive therapy in depressed patients. *Journal of Affective Disorders* **49**, 59–72.

Goffman E (1961) *Asylums. Essays on the social situation of mental patients and other inmates*. Harmondsworth: Penguin.

Goldblatt P (1988) Mortality and social classification. Presentation to Economic and Social Research Council Survey Methods Seminar Series, March 1988. *Social and Community Planning Research Survey Methods Newsletter* **Summer issue**, 8–9.

Goldthorpe J (1988) Making 'class' and 'status' operational – concept formation, application and evaluation. *Social and Community Planning Research Survey Methods Newsletter*, **Summer issue**, 5–7.

Gottlieb BH (1978) Development and application of a classification scheme of informal helping behaviour. *Canadian Journal of Behavioral Science* **10**, 105–15.

Graham H (1993) *When life's a drag: women, smoking and disadvantage*. London: HMSO.

Greenberg RS (1983) The impact of prenatal care in different social groups. *American Journal of Obstetrics and Gynecology* **145**, 797–801.

Greenwood (1957) Attributes of a profession. *Social Work* **2**, 45–55.

Hadridge P and Hodgson A (1994). *The Hemingford scenarios: alternative futures for health and health care. Report of a Scenario Planning Workshop*. Cambridge: Cambridge Health Futures.

Ham C (1992) *Health policy in Britain*, 3rd edn. London: Macmillan.

Ham C (1996) *Public, private or community: what next for the NHS?* London: Demos.

Hardey M (1998) *The social context of health*. Buckingham: Open University Press.

Harding S (1995) Social class differences in mortality of men: recent evidence from the OPCS Longitudinal Study. *Population Trends* **80**, 31–7.

Harding S, Balarajan R and Balarajan R (1996) Patterns of mortality in second-generation Irish living in England and Wales: longitudinal study. *British Medical Journal* **312**, 1389–92.

Harris J (1985) *The value of life*. London: Routledge.

Harrison S, Hunter D, Marnoch G and Pollitt C (1989) *The impact of general management in the NHS*. Leeds: University of Leeds and The Open University.

Health Education Authority (1993) *Peers in partnership: HIV/AIDS education with young people in the community*. London: Health Education Authority.

Health Education Council (1994) *Health and lifestyles: black and minority ethnic groups in England*. London: Health Education Council.

Helsing KJ, Moysen S and Comstock GW (1981) Factors associated with mortality after widowhood. *American Journal of Public Health* **71**, 802–9.

Herzlich C (1973) *Health and illness*. London: Academic Press.

Hogan DP and Park JM (2000) Family factors and social support in the development outcomes of very low-birth-weight children. *Clinical Perinatology* **27**, 433–59.

Holmes T and Rahe R (1967) The Social Readjustment Rating Scale. *Journal of Psychosomatic Research* **11**, 213–18.

Hopkins A, Solomon J and Abelson J (1996) Shifting boundaries in professional care. *Journal of the Royal Society of Medicine* **89**, 364–71.

Howlett BC, Ahmad WI and Murray R (1992) An exploration of white, Asian and Afro-Caribbean people's concepts of health and illness causation. *New Community* **18**, 281–92.

Hoyes L and Means R (1993) Quasi-markets and the reform of community care. In Le Grand J and Bartlett W (eds), *Quasi-markets and social policy*. London: Macmillan, 93–124.

Hultsch DF, Hertzog C and Dixon RA (1990) Ability correlates of memory performance in adulthood and aging. *Psychology and Aging* **5**, 356–68.

Jenkinson C, Layte R, Wright L and Coulter A (1996) *The UK SF-36: an analysis and interpretation manual*. Oxford: Oxford Health Services Research Unit, Department of Public Health and Primary Care, University of Oxford.

Kane P (1994) *Women's health: from womb to tomb*, 2nd edn. London: Macmillan.

Kaplan G, Pamuk E, Lynch J, Cohen R and Balfour J (1996) Inequality in income and mortality in the United States: analysis of mortality and potential pathways. *British Medical Journal* **312**, 999–1003.

Kaplan J, Manuck S, Clarkson T, Lusso F and Taub D (1982) Social status, environment and atherosclerosis in cynomologous monkeys. *Atherosclerosis* **2**, 359.

Kehrer B and Wolin V (1979) Impact of income maintenance on low birthweight, evidence from the Gary experiment. *Journal of Human Resources* **14,** 434–62.

Kitchiner D, Davidson C and Bundred P (1996) Integrated care pathways: an effective tool for continuously evaluating clinical practice. *Journal of Evaluation in Clinical Practice* **1,** 65–9.

Klein R (1989) *The politics of the National Health Service.* London: Longman.

Land H and Rose H (1985) Compulsory altruism for some or an altruistic society for all? In Bean P, Ferris J and Wynes D (eds), *In defence of welfare.* London: Tavistock, 74–96.

Lawson R (1996) *Bills of health.* Oxford: Radcliffe Medical Press.

Lazarus RS (1966) *Psychological stress and the coping process.* New York: McGraw-Hill.

Leat D (1993) *The development of community care by the independent sector.* London: Policy Studies Institute.

Leventhal H, Meyer D and Nerenz D (1980) The common-sense representation of illness danger. In Rachman S (ed.), *Medical psychology. Volume 2.* New York: Pergamon, 7–30.

Levine S and Kozloff M (1978) The sick role: assessment and overview. *American Sociological Review* 43, 317–44.

Ley P (1981) Professional non-compliance: a neglected problem. *British Journal of Clinical Psychology* **20,** 151–4.

Ley P and Llewelyn B (1989) Improving patients' understanding, recall, satisfaction and compliance. In Broome A and Llewelyn B (eds), *Health psychology,* 2nd edn. London: Chapman & Hall, 75–98.

Light D (1997) From managed competition to managed co-operation: theory and lessons from the British experience. *Milbank Quarterly* **75,** 297–341.

McClure G (2000) Changes in suicide in England and Wales, 1960–1997. *British Journal of Psychiatry* **176,** 64–7.

McCormick J (1990) The limits of medicine. *The Times Health Supplement* **June issue,** 7–10.

McHale J, Fox M and Murphy J (1997) *Health care law: texts and materials.* London: Sweet & Maxwell.

Macintyre S (1992) The effects of family position and status in health. *Social Science and Medicine* **35,** 453–64.

Macintyre S (1997) The Black Report and beyond: what are the issues? *Social Science and Medicine* **44,** 723–45.

Macintyre S, Hunt K and Sweeting H (1996) Gender differences in health: are things as simple as they seem? *Social Science and Medicine* **42,** 617–24.

McKeown T (1976) The medical contribution. In Davey B, Gray A and Searle C (eds), *Health and disease – a review.* Buckingham: Open University Press.

McNiece R and Majeed A (1999) Socio-economic differences in general practice consultation rates in patients aged 65 and over. Prospective cohort study. *British Medical Journal* **319,** 26–8.

Marmot M (1995) In sickness and in wealth: social causes of illness. *MRC News* **Winter issue,** 8–12.

Marmot M (1999) Introduction. In Marmot M and Wilkinson RG (eds), *Social determinants of health.* Oxford: Oxford University Press, 1–16.

Marmot M and Theorell T (1988) Social class and cardiovascular disease. *International Journal of Health Services* **18,** 659–74.

Marmot M, Shipley M and Rose G (1984a) Inequalities in death – specific explanations of a general pattern. *Lancet* **1,** 1003–6.

Marmot M, Adelstein A and Boluso L (1984b) *Immigrant mortality in England and Wales*

1970–78: causes of death by country of birth. Studies on Medical and Population Subjects No. 47. London: HMSO.

Marmot M, Davey Smith G, Stansfield SA *et al.* (1991) Health inequalities among British civil servants: the Whitehall II Study. *Lancet* **337**, 1387–93.

Marshall T (1975) *Social policy in the twentieth century*, 4th edn. London: Hutchinson.

Mason J and McCall-Smith R (1999) *Law and medical ethics*. London: Butterworth.

Means R (1986) The development of social services for elderly people: historical perspectives. In Phillipson C and Walker A (eds), *Ageing and social policy. A critical assessment*. Aldershot: Gower, 87–106.

Means R (1992) The future of community care and older people in the 1990s. *Local Government Policy-Making* **18**, 11–16.

Mechanic D (1978) *Medical sociology*, 2nd edn. New York: Free Press.

Miller P (1994) The first year at medical school: some findings and student perceptions. *Medical Education* **28**, 5–7.

Ministry of Health (1956) *Report of the Committee Inquiry into the Cost of the National Health Service*. London: HMSO.

Murray C and Lopez A (1996) *The global burden of disease*. Boston, MA: World Health Organization and Harvard University Press.

Nathanson CA (1980) Social roles and health status among women: the significance of employment. *Social Science and Medicine* **14A**, 463–71.

National Service Framework (1999) *National Service Framework for Mental Health*. London: Department of Health.

National Service Framework (2000) *National Service Framework for Coronary Heart Disease*. London: Department of Health.

Nazroo J (1998) The racialisation of ethnic inequalities in health. In Dorling D and Simpson S (eds), *Statistics in society*. London: Edward Arnold.

Newton RW and Hunt LP (1984) Psychosocial stress in pregnancy and its relation to low birth weight. *British Medical Journal* **288**, 1191–4.

Nightingale F (1860) *Notes on nursing – what it is and what it is not*. New York: Appleton & Co.

Nutbeam D (1986) Health promotion glossary. *Health Promotion International* **1**, 113–27.

Nutbeam D (1998) Health promotion glossary. *Health Promotion International* **13**, 340–64.

Oakley A (1992) *Social support and motherhood*. Oxford: Basil Blackwell.

Oakley A (1996) Preventing falls and subsequent injury in older people. *Effective Health Care Bulletin* **2(4)**.

O'Brien M (1994) *Children's dental health in the United Kingdom 1993*. London: HMSO.

Ogden J (1996) *Health psychology: a textbook*. Buckingham: Open University Press.

O'Reilly P (1988) Methodological issues in social support and social network research. *Social Science and Medicine* **26**, 863–73.

Pahl RE (1990) *On work: historical, comparative and theoretical approaches*. London: Basil Blackwell.

Parsons T (1951) *The social system*. New York: Free Press.

Perry I (1997) Fetal growth and development: the role of nutrition and other factors. In Kuh D and Ben Shlomo Y (eds), *A life course approach to chronic disease epidemiology*. Oxford: Oxford University Press, 145-58.

Phares EJ (1984) *Clinical psychology: concepts, methods and professionals*, revised edn. Hoomewood, IL: Dorsey.

Pietroni P and Pietroni C (1996) *Innovation in community care and primary health*. London: Churchill Livingstone.

Pill R and Stott N (1982) Concepts of illness causation and responsibility: some preliminary data from a sample of working-class mothers. *Social Science and Medicine* **16**, 43–52.

Platt S and Kreitman N (1984) Unemployment and parasuicide in Edinburgh 1968–1982. *British Medical Journal* **289**, 1029–32.

Porter M, Alder B and Abraham C (eds) (1999) *Psychology and sociology applied to medicine*. Edinburgh: Churchill Livingstone.

Pound P, Gompertz P and Ebrahim S (1998) Illness in the context of older age: the case of stroke. *Sociology of Health and Illness* **20**, 489–506.

Powell E (1966) *A new look at medicine and politics*. London: Pitman.

Power C, Matthews S and Manor O (1996) Inequalities in self-rated health in the 1958 birth cohort: lifetime social circumstances or social mobility? *British Medical Journal* **313**, 449–53.

Preston G (1986) Dementia in elderly adults: prevalence and institutionalization. *Journal of Gerontology* **41**, 261–7.

Pringle M (2000) The Shipman inquiry: implication for the public's trust. *British Journal of General Practice* **50**, 355–6.

Prior L (1985) Making sense of mortality. *Sociology of Health and Illness* **7**, 167–90.

Pritchard C and Teo P (1994) Preterm birth, low birth weight and the stressfulness of the household role for pregnant women. *Social Science and Medicine* **38**, 89–96.

Prochaska J and DiClemente C (1982) Transtheoretical therapy: towards a more integrative model of change. *Psychotherapy: Theory, Research and Practice* **19**, 276–88.

Pullinger J and Summerfield C (eds) (1998) *Social trends 28*. London: The Stationery Office.

Putnam R (1994) *Making democracy work*. Princeton, NJ: Princeton University Press.

Qureshi H and Walker A (1986) Responses to dependency: reciprocity, affect and power in family relationships. In Phillipson C, Bernard M and Strang R (eds), *Ageing and social policy: a critical assessment*. Aldershot: Gower.

Radley A (1994) *Making sense of illness: the social psychology of health and disease*. London: Sage.

Rashid A, Watts A, Lenehan C and Haslam D (1996) Skill-mix in primary care: sharing clinical workload and understanding professional roles. *British Journal of General Practice* **46**, 639–40.

Reid D (1997) Securing the people's health. *Health Matters* **29**, 8.

Robb B (1967) *Sans everything: a case to answer*. London: Nelson.

Rose D and O'Reilly K (1997) *Constructing classes: towards a new social classification for the UK*. Swindon: Economic and Social Research Council/Office for National Statistics.

Rose G (1992) *The strategy of preventive medicine*. Oxford: Oxford University Press.

Rotter J (1966) Generalised expectancies for internal versus external control of reinforcement. *Psychological Monographs* **80**, 1–28.

Rowlands O and Parker G (1998) *Informal carers*. London: HMSO (with the Office for National Statistics).

Royal College of Physicians (1985) *Research on healthy volunteers: working party report*. London: Royal College of Physicians.

Royal Commission on the NHS (1979) *Report*. London: HMSO.

Rummery K and Glendinning C (1997) *Working together. Primary care involvement in commissioning social care services*. Manchester: National Primary Care Research and Development Centre.

Ryan B and Gross N (1943). The diffusion of hybrid seedcorn in two Iowa rural communities. *Rural Sociology* **8**, 15–24.

Samphier ML, Robertson C and Bloor MJ (1988) A possible artefactual component in specific-cause mortality gradients. *Journal of Epidemiology and Community Health* **42**, 138–43.

Samuelson P (1976) *Economics*. Tokyo: McGraw-Hill.

Sapolsky R (1990) Stress in the wild. *Scientific American* **262**, 116–23.

Scambler G (ed.) (1997) *Sociology as applied to medicine*, 4th edn. London: W.B. Saunders.

Scambler G and Hopkins A (1986) Being epileptic: coming to terms with stigma. *Sociology of Health and Illness* **8**, 26–43.

Schaefer C, Coyne J and Lazarus R (1981) The health-related functions of social support. *Journal of Behavioural Medicine* **4**, 381–405.

Secretary of State for Health (1997) *The new NHS: modern, dependable*. London: The Stationery Office.

Secretary of State for Health (1998) *Modernising social services. Promoting independence, improving protection, raising standards*. London: The Stationery Office.

Secretary of State for Social Services (1972) *National Health Service reorganization: England*. London: HMSO.

Select Committee on Social Services (1981) *The Government's White Papers on public expenditure: the Social Services. Third Report. Session 1979–80*. London: HMSO.

Seligman M (1975) *Helplessness: on depression, development and death*. San Francisco, CA: Freeman.

Selye H (1956) *The stress of life*. New York: McGraw-Hill.

Shaw B (1946) *The doctor's dilemma*. Harmondsworth: Penguin.

Sheldon W (1942) *The variety of temperaments: a psychology of constitutional differences*. New York: Harper.

Siegrist J (2000) The social causation of health and illness. In Albrecht GL, Fitzpatrick R and Scrimshaw SC (eds), *The handbook of social studies in health and medicine*. London: Sage, 100–14.

Simpson R and Armand Smith N (1986) Maternal smoking and low birth weight: implications for antenatal care. *Journal of Epidemiology and Community Health* **40**, 223–7.

Smaje C (1995) *Health, 'race' and ethnicity*. London: King's Fund Institute.

Smith A (1776) Of the nature, accumulation and employment of stock. In Cannan E (ed.), *An inquiry into the nature and causes of the wealth of nations*, 5th edn. London: Methuen, 313–31.

Smith A (1970) Progress in the 1960s and problems for the 1970s. In McLachlan G and Shegog R (eds), *The beginning. Studies of maternity services*. Oxford: Oxford University Press, 7-23.

Smith R (1997) The future of health care systems. *British Medical Journal* **314**, 1495–6.

Smith R (1998) All changed: changed utterly. *British Medical Journal* **316**, 1917–18.

Sonnentag S (1996) Work group factors and individual well-being. In West M (ed.), *Handbook of workgroup psychology*. Chichester. John Wiley & Sons.

Spaulding JA and Simpson G (1951) *Suicide: a study in sociology*. New York: Free Press of Glencoe.

Stanton A (1987) Determinants of adherence to medical regimens by hypertensive patients. *Journal of Behavioural Medicine* **10**, 377–94.

Steptoe A and Wardle J (eds) (1994) *Psychosocial processes and health. A reader*. Cambridge: Cambridge University Press.

Sternberg R (1985) *Beyond IQ*. Cambridge, MA: Cambridge University Press.

Sternberg R (1995) *In search of the human mind*. London: Harcourt-Brace.

Sternberg R and Wagner R (1986) *Practical intelligence*. Cambridge: Cambridge University Press.

Stilwell B, Greenfield S, Drury M and Hull F (1987) A nurse practitioner in general practice: working style and pattern of consultations. *Journal of the Royal College of General Practitioners* **37**, 154–7.

Strauss A and Glaser B (eds) (1975) *Chronic illness and the quality of life*. St Louis, MO: CV Mosby Company.

Strauss A, Corbin J, Fagerhaugh B *et al.* (1984) *Chronic illness and the quality of life*, 2nd edn. St Louis, MO: CV Mosby Company.

Syme S, Marmot M, Kagan H and Rhoads G (1975) Epidemiological studies of CHD and stroke in Japanese men living in Japan, Hawaii and California: introduction. *American Journal of Epidemiology* **102**, 477–80.

Thatcher M (1978) *Community Care* **12 April**, 3.

Todd J (1975) *Children's dental health in England and Wales 1973*. London: HMSO.

Todd J and Dodd T (1985) *Children's dental health in the United Kingdom 1983*. London: HMSO.

Todd J, Walker A and Dodd P (1982) *Adult dental health. Volume 2. United Kingdom 1978*. London: HMSO.

Townsend P and Davidson N (eds) (1988) The Black Report. In Townsend P, Davidson N and Whitehead M (eds), *Inequalities in health: the Black Report and the health divide*. Harmondsworth: Penguin.

Tsuzuki C (1961) *H.M. Hyndman and British socialism*. London: Oxford University Press.

Tudor K (1996) *Mental health promotion: paradigms and practice*. London: Routledge.

Tudor-Hart J (1971) The inverse care law. *Lancet* **i**, 1179–90.

Vaughan B and Lathlean J (1999) *Intermediate care. Models in practice*. London: King's Fund Publishing.

Venning P, Durie A, Roland M *et al.* (2000) Randomised controlled trial comparing cost-effectiveness of general practitioners and nurse practitioners in primary care. *British Medical Journal* **320**, 1048–53.

Wadsworth M (1986) Serious illness in childhood and its association with later-life achievement. In Wilkinson R (ed.), *Class and health*. London: Tavistock, 50–74.

Wadsworth M, Butterfield W and Blaney R (1971) *Health and sickness: the choice of treatment*. London: Tavistock.

Walker A (1995) Integrating the family into a mixed economy of care. In Allen I and Perkins E (eds), *The future of family care for older people*. London: HMSO, 201–20.

Ware J and Sherbourne C (1992) The MOS 36-item short form health survey (SF-36). I. Conceptual framework and item selection. *Medical Care* **30**, 473–83.

Waterhouse R (1993) Community care to receive extra £20m. *Independent* **30 October**, 9.

Webster J (1998) Time to get things rolling. *Health Matters* **34**, 10–11.

Wennberg J (1984) Dealing with medical practice variations: a proposal for action. *Health Affairs* **3**, 6–32

White A, Nicholas G, Foster K, Browne F and Carey S (1993) *Health Survey for England 1991*. London: HMSO.

Whitehead M. (1988) The health divide. In Townsend P, Davidson N and Whitehead M (eds), *Inequalities in health: the Black Report and the health divide*. Harmondsworth: Penguin, 218-356.

Wilkinson P, Laji K, Ranjadayalan K, Parsons I and Timmis A (1994) Acute myocardial infarction in women: survival analysis in the first six months. *British Medical Journal* **309**, 566–9.

Wilkinson R (1992) Income distribution and life expectancy. *British Medical Journal* **304**, 165–8.

Wilkinson R, Kawachi I and Kennedy B (1998) Mortality, the social environment, crime and violence. In Bartley M, Blane D and Smith Davey G (eds), *Sociology of health inequalities*. Oxford: Basil Blackwell.

Williams G (1984) The genesis of chronic illness: narrative reconstruction. *Sociology of Health and Illness* **6**, 175–200.

Wistow G, Knapp M, Hardy B and Allen C (1992) From providing to enabling: local authorities and the mixed economy of social care. *Public Administration* **70**, 25–45.

Wolpert L (1999) *Malignant sadness: the anatomy of depression*. New York: Free Press.

World Health Organization (1958) *The first 10 years. The health organization*. Geneva: World Health Organization.

World Health Organization (1985) *Social justice and equity in health: a report from the Programme on Social Equity and Health Meeting, Leeds, 22–26 July 1985*. Geneva: World Health Organization.

World Health Organization (1986) *Ottawa Charter for health promotion*. Geneva: World Health Organization.

World Health Organization Quality of Life Group (1991) *Assessment of quality of life in health care*. Geneva: World Health Organization.

Wright E (1985) *Classes*. London: Verso.

Zimbardo P, McDermott M, Jansz J and Metaal N (1995) *Psychology: a European text*. London: HarperCollins.

Zola I (1973) Pathways to the doctor – from person to patient. *Social Science and Medicine* **7**, 677–89.

Useful websites

Action on Smoking and Health (ASH); www.ash.org.uk

Agency for Health Care Policy and Research (AHCPR) guidelines clearing house; www.guidelines.gov/index.asp

Altavista (search engine); www.altavista.telia.com

American College of Physicians; www.acponline.org/index.html

Bandolier; www.jr2.ox.ac.uk:80/Bandolier

Bath Interlibrary Data Service (BIDS); www.bids.ac.uk

British Medical Journal (BMJ); www.bmj.com/bmj

Cambridge Public Health; http://fester.his.path.cam.ac.uk/phealth/phweb.html

Centre for Evidence-Based Medicine; http://cebm.jr2.ox.ac.uk

Centre for Social Marketing, Strathclyde; www.csm.strath.ac.uk

Cochrane Collaboration; http://hiru.mcmaster.ca/cochrane/default.htm

Department of Health; www.doh.gov.uk

EU research funding; www.refund.ncl.ac.uk/Sub/Issues/Iss29/contents.html

Faculty of Public Health Medicine; www.his.path.cam.ac.uk/phealth/int-fphm.htm

Health boards; http://rie.cee.hw.ac.uk/sh05001.htm

Health Education Authority Centre for Health Information; www.quick.org.uk

Health Education Board for Scotland (HEBS); www.hebs.scot.nhs.uk/learning-centre

HEBS – Scotland; www.hebs.scot.nhs.uk/research

Health Promotion Information Centre (Health Education Authority); www.hea.org.uk

International Classification of Diseases (ICD) codes; http://dumccss.mc.duke.edu/standards/termcode/icd9/index.html

King's Fund; www.kingsfund.org.uk

Lancet; www.thelancet.com

Netting the Evidence; www.shef.ac.uk/uni/academic/R-Z/scharr/ir/netting

New Zealand Guidelines Catalogue; www.nzgg.org.nz/library.htm
NHS Direct; www.nhsdirect.nhs.uk
NHS R & D; www.epi.bris.ac.uk/rd/publicat/ebpurch/index.htm
Office for National Statistics (ONS); www.ons.gov.uk
Organizing Medical Network Information (OMNI); www.OMNI.ac.uk
Public health; www.public-health.com
Public health links; www.trigon.demon.co.uk/part1.htm
Public Health Knowledge; www.ukph.org
Public Health Mailbase; www.public-health@mailbase.ac.uk
Royal College of Nursing; www.man.ac.uk.rcn
Scottish Guidelines Network; http://pc47cee.hw.ac.uk/sign/home.htm
Scottish Health on the Web; http://pc47cee.hw.ac.uk/show
Scottish Office; www.show.scot.nhs.uk/cso
St George's Health Care Evaluation Unit; www.sghms.ac.uk/phs/jceu/guide.htm
Stationery Office; www.the-stationery-office.co.uk
Super search engine; http://meltingpot.fortunecity.com/pakistan/360/page1.htm
Users' guide to literature; http://hirunet.mcmaster.ca/ebm/userguid/1_intro.htm
World Health Organization (WHO); www.who.ch
WHO publications; www.who.dk/tec/hcp/index.htm

Index